HOLD TIGHT GENTLY

ALSO BY MARTIN DUBERMAN

HOLD
TIGHT
GENTLY

Michael Callen, Essex Hemphill,
and the Battlefield of AIDS

Martin Duberman

THE NEW PRESS

NEW YORK
LONDON

Requests for permission to reproduce selections from this book should be mailed to:
Permissions Department, The New Press, 120 Wall Street, 31st floor, New York, NY 10005.

Published in the United States by The New Press, New York, 2014
Distributed by Perseus Distribution

CIP data available
ISBN 978-1-59558-945-3 (hc.)
ISBN 978-1-59558-965-1 (e-book)

The New Press publishes books that promote and enrich public discussion and understanding
of the issues vital to our democracy and to a more equitable world. These books are made
possible by the enthusiasm of our readers; the support of a committed group of donors,
large and small; the collaboration of our many partners in the independent media and the
not-for-profit sector; booksellers, who often hand-sell New Press books; librarians;
and above all by our authors.

www.thenewpress.com

Composition by Westchester Book Composition
This book was set in Janson Text

Printed in the United States of America

2   4   6   8   10   9   7   5   3   1

———

There's a certain slant of light,
On winter afternoons,
That oppresses, like the weight
Of cathedral tunes.

Heavenly hurt it gives us;
We can find no scar,
But internal difference
Where the meanings are....
—Emily Dickinson

Contents

CONTENTS

Introduction

Since the midnineties, public concern in the United States about the AIDS pandemic has continued to decline, even as the disease continues to spread. The number of Americans who consider AIDS the most urgent health problem facing the nation dropped from 44 percent in 1995 to 6 percent in 2009. One reason, surely, is that AIDS has become less and less a white disease and more and more a disease associated with people of color. Globally, fewer than half the people afflicted with AIDS are receiving treatment, and in light of recent budget cuts reducing AIDS expenditures, that number is likely to decline further. Even in the most "developed" countries, suppression of HIV through antiretroviral medication remains incompletely effective.

In its most recent (May 2012) report, with data through 2009, the Centers for Disease Control (CDC) shows a vast disparity of new infections among racial-ethnic groups in the United States. Though African Americans make up only 12 percent of the population, black men who sleep with men account for 45 percent of new AIDS diagnoses. This is despite the fact that young gay black men have fewer partners, less unprotected sex, and lower rates of recreational drug use than other gay men. Some Latino men who sleep with men—who made up 20 percent of new AIDS diagnoses in 2009—like some African American men do not primarily self-identify as gay (not least because many consider "gay" a white term). Those who sleep with women as well as men help to account—especially in hot-spot cities such as Washington, D.C.—for the recent realization that new HIV and AIDs cases among African American women are now comparable to rates for women in sub-Saharan Africa. Infection rates continue to rise among white gay men as well, but the mortality rates aren't comparable: the proportion of deaths among whites (and especially among those with high levels of education—and the income and access that follow) has declined, but HIV and AIDS among men and women of color in the United States of all sexual preferences continues to skyrocket, especially among lower-income populations. African American women are now dying at fifteen times the rate white women do. Self-identified gay men of all colors, however, are still fifty times more likely to contract AIDS than any other demographic group.

One would expect to find mainstream LGBT organizations and spokespeople still vociferously active in pressuring pharmaceutical companies and researchers to come up with better treatments and preventative strategies, and governmental agencies—the CDC, the National Institutes of Health—offering greater services to those already ill. But that isn't the case. The sense of urgency *among gay people themselves* is seemingly gone; a portion of the new generation dislikes using condoms for safer sex and tells itself that with the advent of protease inhibitors, AIDS is now a "manageable" disease. It is, for those who can afford and who can tolerate the medications, though no one knows how long they'll remain effective and what secondary damage they're doing along the way; for some people the drugs don't work at all, for others only briefly.

The older generations of white gay men who have physically survived the epidemic have buried their dead—and to a regrettable degree, their heads in the sand. As the longtime AIDS journalist John-Manuel Andriote has put it, the "traditional donors—middle-class and affluent white gay men—have 'moved on' since they can now get their HIV-related medical care from their private physicians. . . . The old ACT UP slogan of 'Silence = Death' still holds, if by 'silence' we mean withholding of support." Since the midnineties the mainstream gay agenda has demoted AIDS from its top priority and replaced it with what those of us on the left call the assimilationist items of legal matrimony and the "patriotic" right to serve openly in the armed forces.

In Africa, AIDS is primarily a heterosexual phenomenon, but in the United States it remains a profoundly gay one, with poor, young, nonwhite men disproportionately impacted—though children, intravenous drug users, and heterosexual women are hardly immune. But self-identified gay men in the United States do still make up 48 percent of the 1 million people currently living with AIDS. We haven't even reached the point where the annual increase in gay male patients being treated exceeds the number of gay men being newly infected.

My hope is that this book will shed additional light on our current approach to AIDS by scrutinizing more closely the earlier years (1981–95) of the epidemic, and in particular the pre–ACT UP (1987) period. I've chosen to tell this story through the lives of two gay men, the singer and activist Michael (Mike) Callen and the poet and cultural worker Essex Hemphill. The two never met and had little in common. Mike was a white midwesterner who came to New York City after college to pursue a singing career. Essex was an African American gay man who grew up in Washington, D.C., and knew early that he wanted to become a writer, and specifically a poet.

Both men were diagnosed with AIDS early in the epidemic. Mike became a leading maverick in the organized efforts to fight the disease as one of the earliest originators of "safe sex" and the People with AIDS Self-Empowerment Movement. Essex largely avoided the white-dominated public protest campaign, primarily devoting himself to participating in and fostering the black gay male and lesbian cultural flowering in the 1980s now widely referred to as the "second Harlem Renaissance." The experience of the AIDS epidemic was in critical ways dissimilar for the white gay community and the black gay one, and that distinction is one of the major themes of this book.

I knew both Mike and Essex, though only slightly. What I did know, I admired greatly—and I wanted to know more. I viewed Mike as an undersung hero of the AIDS protest movement and Essex as an undersung poet of major importance in black cultural circles. In Mike Callen's case, the search for previously unknown material proved comparatively easy: not only did he have a temperament frank to the point of transparency—or, in the eyes of his detractors, to a fault—but he left behind a very large archive of letters, speeches, diary notes, organizational materials, and—as a performer and songwriter—lots of music.

Telling Essex Hemphill's story proved more difficult. He left behind one published collection of poems; an anthology that he edited of writings by black gay men; appearances in Marlon Riggs' and Isaac Julien's films; and a smattering of correspondence, much of which remains in private hands. At the end of his life, Essex told a number of close friends that he wanted his papers to go to the Schomburg Center, the branch of the New York Public Library devoted to black culture. But they never arrived. My own polite letters of inquiry to Essex's mother, Mantalene, went unanswered. However, she did, some fifteen years ago, send a batch of his letters and manuscripts to his literary agent, Frances Goldin. Luckily, I know Frances well; she generously gave me full access to the material, which it turns out includes the manuscript of Essex's unpublished and presumed lost novel in progress, "Standing in the Gap." I've quoted from portions of this treasure trove throughout the book. To further fill out Essex's story, I've conducted lengthy interviews with many of his close friends and have also been given access to letters and other materials in private hands.

Essex's temperament was considerably more guarded and enigmatic than Mike's. A person of charismatic charm and mischievous guile, Essex could often be enchanting, but he keenly guarded his privacy and—while not at all prudish—persistently warded off those who probed for details about his personal attachments or the state of his health. He was so intent on protecting his inner life from unwanted scrutiny and so quick to react to any threat to his principles that some mistook this integrity for hauteur. His poetry, often autobiographical, makes it possible to map certain aspects of his inner life, yet I suspect that even if Essex had left behind a massive archive, it would most likely contain little about his intimate feelings and struggles.

For all these reasons, this book contains more personal information about Mike than about Essex; that reflects both the nature of their respective personalities and the kinds of material each left behind. Though they were very different from each other, I hold these two exceptional men in equal regard and have made an equal effort to bring their remarkable stories to life.

1

Before the Storm

Soon after Mike Callen completed college at Boston University in 1977, he moved to New York City, and soon after that, he became ill with shigella—intestinal parasites. At first, he thought he'd gotten food poisoning from the Kentucky Fried Chicken stand on Forty-Second Street that he frequented. Trying to shrug off and explain persistent, exhausting bouts of diarrhea, he told himself that he'd always been more or less sickly, which was true: as a sensitive, scrawny youngster in Hamilton, Ohio, he'd gotten an ulcer in the fifth grade, a second one in the eighth grade, and yet a third in the eleventh. Then, during high school, he'd been hospitalized twice, once with mononucleosis and once with hepatitis.[1]

A tender, hyperactive child, Mike was playing canasta with some older family friends one day—cheating and winning, "screeching" (his description) with delight—when one of the women put down her cards, gave him a stern look, and said, "If you don't watch out, Michael, you're going to become one of those homosexuals." He had no idea what that meant, but he caught the overtones of imminent doom and realized that the prediction was meant to frighten him. Did that explain, he asked himself, why he often felt nervous and was repeatedly cautioned about being too "animated"? At age eight, for instance, he twirled a baton at the head of a neighborhood parade with such giddy glee that eyebrows were raised; and he remembered running into the house at a young age, "flapping his arms like a little sissy," and his father slapping him hard across the face and yelling, "Don't you *ever* do that again!"

The neighborhood lady's use of the word "homosexual" piqued Mike's curiosity and he decided to ask around. It turned out that everyone in the town of Hamilton knew that "homosexual" meant Delmore Knight, that "dirty old man" who hung around the Greyhound bus station and enticed young boys to do "nasty" things. Although Knight was said to have a doctorate from Oxford University and was even rumored to have won some academic prize, no one in Hamilton seemed to doubt that he deserved the regular beatings that a cadre of high school jocks dished out to him. Republican and evangelical, Hamilton was a Dixie border town known as well for its strict adherence to racial segregation. According to Jennifer Jackson, who went to high school with Mike, Hamilton was "a town with secrets, with a polite midwestern refusal to acknowledge how many were hurt and excluded," exemplified by the crumbling Victorian Poor House Hill, which sat on a visible precipice, initially serving as a debtors' prison, then an orphanage, then a home for the mentally ill—"a perfect storm of misery and entrapment."[2]

When Mike and his brother, Barry, a year older, were in their early teens, their parents decided the time had come to tell them about "the facts of life" (their younger sister, Linda, was exempted from the talk). The boys' mother, Barbara Ann, was a part-time elementary school teacher and their father, Clifford, a factory worker at General Motors. Both were deeply religious Baptists and the topic of sex was at least as embarrassing to them as to their two young sons. During her part of the "birds and the bees" session, Barbara fell back on traditional church teachings. Mike remembered her saying that sex was "dirty and disgusting, messy and a bother, but beautiful if it resulted in a child." After the three children had been born, she and Cliff still had sex once a week to prevent him from getting headaches and hemorrhoids, or turning grumpy.

Mike's father uncomfortably expanded on the theme: "The man puts his penis inside the woman and they make a baby," he told the two boys. "Do you understand?" Cliff asked. Barry, who'd broken out in a cold sweat, nodded yes. Mike, bright and stubbornly outspoken, said he was confused; why, he asked, should he concern himself with putting his penis "inside some stupid girl and peeing inside her just to make a baby; what if the baby turned out to be dumb like my sister?"

Cliff's response was a non sequitur: "Never be afraid to ask us anything." Fine, except that Mike's main fear was his father himself. He always "smelled of grease"—Cliff worked at GM's Fisher Body, welding doors—and was remote and unemotional. Mike became convinced that his father "hated" him and often dreamed that Cliff was stabbing him "with one of those cheap steak knives they kept giving us free for a fill-up at Shell." His closed-down, evasive father was, in fact, a decent, if embittered, man, liberal (considering his time and place) in his political views and struggling to understand his children—though as a devout Baptist he would always find homosexuality repulsive, even immoral.

Life hadn't been easy for Cliff. After his own father's early death, he'd had to forgo college to support his mother and sister. After he married Barbara Ann and had children of his own, he worked ten hours a day, seven days a week, at GM—enduring a ninety-mile daily commute round-trip. According to Barbara Ann, he refused every chance to climb the corporate ladder since he felt that would entail the "sacrifice of his beliefs and his morals," would force him, if he became a foreman or superintendent, to treat employees below him in a "degrading and demeaning" manner that would make them "feel like just so many cattle."

Cliff dreamed of leaving GM altogether, but every idea he had of another way to make a living—starting a restaurant, moving to Arizona to open a small store—somehow broke down. He struggled to avoid seeing himself as a failure, but the effort further closed him off emotionally, made him a hard-shell Baptist in all but name. Trapped himself, he "forced" (as Mike saw it) his wife, Barbara Ann, to go to college and get a teaching certificate, though she preferred being a stay-at-home mom. They'd had "terrific fights" about it and Barbara Ann finally yielded, but in her unhappiness she put on a great deal of weight and according to Mike "had a nervous breakdown."

During his senior year in high school Mike took over the running of the house and did all the shopping, cooking, and cleaning, with little assistance from his siblings. (Cooking would become a lifelong pleasure for him; he deeply associated it with "sensuality and hedonism," and he reveled in "cooking for his man.") In retrospect, he felt the "house-wife" role had been thrust on him, or perhaps he assumed it, because he was frequently mocked in high school as a "sissy," a sort of substitute woman. He had his admirers: Jennifer Jackson, two years behind Mike, was one of them. She recalls his sensitive response to her one day when he spotted her standing in line to audition for a school play, "twisting and turning behind the curtain, ready to run." Mike went over to her, asked her if she'd ever acted before (she hadn't), and drew her out about her difficult background and family life. "He listened," Jackson recalls, "and he wouldn't let you stand there feeling alone and irrelevant. He sensed despair somehow and didn't turn away. . . . There he was, with those hands waving around, perfectly articulate, telling me things *wouldn't be okay, but eventually I'd get out of Hamilton somehow.*" She never forgot his kindness.

But Mike's detractors in high school far outnumbered his admirers. He was frequently bullied, baited as a "faggot," and at least once pissed on in the locker room after gym class by a circle of male classmates. All of which made Mike feel self-conscious and insecure about his appearance. He avoided all mirrors, refusing to look at his own image. As a result of the constant harassment, he attempted suicide twice before the age of twenty-one. Remarkably, he somehow managed, despite excessive chores and excessive ridicule, to maintain a straight-A average throughout high school.

He was not only bright, but exuberantly articulate and musically gifted. From an early age, he idolized Barbra Streisand as "the most brilliant artist of the time" and especially appreciated her "willingness to be awkward and gawky if needed to get the sound out." Bette Midler was another favorite, and Julie Andrews—he sang in her register. He dismissed both Neil Diamond and Elton John as "fake" when expressing pain. A friend told Mike that he sang in "the same sweet vein as Barry Manilow—but was better." As early as high school, Mike started to dream about becoming a cabaret singer, a dream that his married music teacher did his best to sabotage: when Mike was a junior, the teacher tried to rape him, and when Mike successfully fought him off, the man retaliated by writing denunciatory letters about him to try to thwart his efforts to get a music scholarship.

Mike's first choice for college was Boston University. Though he'd never before traveled out of the sixty-mile radius around Hamilton,

Ohio, he flew to Boston for a voice audition. Sitting nervously on the hard bench outside the fourth-floor audition room, he suddenly had to go to the bathroom. To his astonishment, all the stalls were occupied and several men were waiting in line. It suddenly dawned on him that they were there to relieve themselves in several senses. Later, a jubilant Mike would claim an epiphany: "I knew. I knew I was where my destiny was bringing me." When his turn came to enter a stall, his heart was pounding.

The walls of the stall were covered with gay graffiti—"meet me here 7-8-73." Two large holes had been drilled between the stalls and Mike became aware that through the holes "two eyeballs on either side" were looking at him. Then a mouth appeared where an eyeball had been. Mike immediately got an erection and started to sweat. A note on toilet paper arrived from underneath the stall: "STICK IT THROUGH." He did—and instantly ejaculated. As he later wrote, "My body was at peace for the first time ever." He sang his heart out at the audition and won a full vocal scholarship to BU. If he was fated to be Boston's Delmore Knight, he told himself, that was just fine.

Despite its auspicious start, Mike's first year in Boston was the most difficult of his life to date—at one point he told his parents he was going to give up school and return home ("I can't take it"). He stayed, but his triple adjustment—to college, to the Northeast, and to being gay—brought him close to despair. He wrestled with thoughts that "the Bible would damn me if I admitted my [homosexual] feelings to myself." But he decided—bravely, given the limited support systems in those years for a young person coming to terms with a tainted sexual orientation—that no sin was "more deadly than battling the self." By his last year in college, he'd become conscious of "how wrong society was" about homosexuality, a discovery that made him "question *everything*." It was, he later said, "a very painful period; I didn't know what to believe or who I was." By the time he graduated, he'd declared himself an atheist and written to friends and family back home that society, not him, "had a long way to go" toward accepting gay people. In this—as would prove the case with much else—Mike had rapidly jumped to an "avant-garde" position.

Whatever Mike did, he did with zest and intensity—including the pursuit of sex. He would later say that his "shamed-based" sexual fantasies—"quick and dirty"—had been formed "pre-Stonewall." From freshman year on at BU he haunted the fourth-floor men's room in the music building, then broadened out into the gay baths and gay bars (never his favorite—he disliked alcohol, felt that contact took too long, and he was too horny). Initially, he let others suck him off. The first time he reversed roles, he put Saran Wrap—he'd grown up in a germaphobic home—around the other man's cock, but he never took to sucking and professed to being somewhat puzzled and repulsed by oral sex. It didn't help that he early on got gonorrhea of the throat and ever after had a recurring fear of contracting a syphilis chancre on his vocal chords—a terrifying prospect for someone planning a singing career.

He discovered the orgiastic gay male bathhouses while still in college; one of his first partners there told him that he was "built to get fucked," positioned Mike to sit on his erect cock—and voilà! Mike had a moment of "sheer revelation." That same night he got fucked five times and decided that he'd unquestionably found his sexual destiny. From then on, he made a habit of announcing to a potential trick, within the first few moments of their encounter, that he was a "stone bottom." But unlike some other bottoms, Mike never became interested in fist fucking; he heard too many stories of anal fissures and serious injuries. In New York City a few years later, for the first and last time he fisted somebody at their insistence—and promptly threw up; "it was so gross to me."

As an undergraduate Mike started to read gay-themed novels, especially Edmund White and Andrew Holleran, and plays, in particular, Tennessee Williams. In his spare time he was practical enough to pick up some secretarial skills and several part-time jobs, realizing that he had to prepare for the hard-knock life of trying to make it post-college as a singer. He stayed shy, though, of gay politics, then in its infancy—the Stonewall riots had occurred only in 1969 and the modern gay rights movement still had few troops.

One day Mike picked up a copy of the alternative weekly the *Boston Phoenix* and was astonished to read about an organized gay and lesbian group on the BU campus that was planning a picnic by the Charles River. On the given day, he circled warily near the picnic site and was spotted by a member of the gay group, who called over, "I think you're looking for us." (Mike fit the "loose-wristed" stereotypical view of what a gay man was supposed to look like.) Three months later, Mike, verbal, smart, and archly, campily funny, was elected president of the group. But that first foray into gay politics proved disillusioning. As is often the case with political groups, especially college ones, people would sign up to help out on a committee or at an event and then not show up at all or fail to follow through. This ran directly counter to Mike's highly organized temperament. He'd drive himself, even under difficult circumstances, to complete whatever he'd promised to do; he had little patience for sunshine soldiers. Yet his overall experience with the BU group convinced him that politics was antithetical to his personality. He'd dutifully march in the gay pride parade once a year, but as an individual, not as a member of any group.

Looking back on his college years later in life, Mike would describe himself as "paralyzed by regret." He'd had to hold down a job nearly full-time while going to school and could "barely remember classes. A time that should have been joyous was not." Part of the problem was that it felt "DEVASTATING . . . to plop down into completely unfamiliar territory." He felt like a "social cripple. I discovered that the way I did things—dressed, ate, talked, etc.—was NOT the way others did them and I got very embarrassed and shy and insecure." Mike perhaps overstated his devastation—as any drama queen would. He excelled at school and, thanks to a few of his professors, became a lifelong, voracious reader.

In his senior year, Mike came out to his family. His brother, Barry, took the news in stride and they remained close and supportive. The news was received badly by the rest of his family—Mike and his father didn't speak for two years. It hadn't helped that Mike had also declared that he was a nonbeliever, an atheist. His deeply religious mother, despite having thoroughly internalized the Baptist view of homosexuality as sickness and sin, nonetheless reiterated her love for Michael ("You can expect that to remain steady, regardless") and even wrote him that she would "respect your right to believe what you choose to believe." Younger sister Linda maintained a cool distance, cowed perhaps by the vehemence of the family dynamics.

Michael had dated girls in high school and had several close female friends; they told him that his gentleness and respect attracted them (he would soon in fact become a pronounced, outspoken feminist, later on somewhat campily branding himself a "lesbian feminist"). But he'd never "done anything" with a woman, unless kissing Maria Lingley inside the abandoned A&W Root Beer warehouse counted. The girl he dated longest was Lisa Gaylord, and she later explained to Mike "the agony" she went through because he never made any sexual moves on her: she blamed herself for not being pretty or smart or talented enough; later in life Mike apologized to her and to another young woman he'd dated for "fanning such flames of self-doubt." When his parents suggested that "before locking himself into a dead-end life-style" he seek counseling, he dutifully presented himself for the eight free sessions the university provided, but no spark of sexual desire for women resulted. He was a confirmed Kinsey "6," exclusively attracted to his own gender—a status he'd proudly embrace throughout his life.

Following graduation, Mike moved to New York with the goal of becoming a singer, a cabaret performer, but he arrived with minimal financial reserves. After paying his first month's rent on a dingy apartment, he had a mere $20 to his name. He haunted the employment agencies, but it was the late 1970s: New York had been hit by the national economic downturn and Mike's hard-earned secretarial skills failed to land him a job. When the twenty dollars went, he made the practical decision to head up to Times Square—then a hustling mecca—where he gave some guy a blow job for $4 (he didn't feel in a position to haggle).

That enabled him to eat, but he began to feel "really helpless, like ready to cry," fearful of "a nervous breakdown." He'd initially seen the move to New York as a gutsy risk, but relocating to a very tough city to break into a very tough profession—during a recession, no less—now seemed like a mistake. In his early twenties, broke and jobless, he was also without friends, let alone contacts in the entertainment field. While still in college, he'd done a few auditions and had been told that he "had the stuff to make it"; he'd even had a nibble from a manager that didn't pan out.

But Mike had a tenacious streak and an internal strength that be-lied his scrawny looks, histrionic ways, and a less than validating up-bringing. He refused to throw in the towel and crawl back to the Midwest—not even when he was awakened by a rat crawling over him in bed one night, or when a fire broke out in his apartment. Develop-ing insomnia, he turned to sleeping pills. But then the symptoms that he'd initially ascribed to "food poisoning" began to proliferate—mysterious fevers, weight loss, night sweats, fatigue, and relentless diarrhea. Ever since his arrival in New York, Mike—enchanted with the multiple opportunities for sex—had freely indulged. He made no connection, initially, between his superactive sex life and his burgeoning list of physical ills. Finally, after he'd begun to hyperventilate, he got scared and crawled over to a gay men's health clinic in the West Village.

The doctor on duty happened to be Joseph Sonnabend, a South African–born specialist in infectious diseases who'd trained at Edinburgh's prestigious Royal College of Physicians, done his medical fieldwork in South Africa's shantytowns and impoverished villages, and then gone to work as a laboratory virologist under Alick Isaacs, one of the discoverers of interferon, the antiviral agent, at London's famed National Institute for Medical Research. The field of molecular biology was just coming into its own, and Sonnabend shared in the discovery that cellular protein synthesis was needed for interferon to work. He'd moved to New York City in the early 1970s to work with the noted virologist Rostom Bablanian at Downstate Medical Center, and became an associate professor and associate attending physician at medical centers in Brooklyn.

In 1977 Sonnabend began working for the Bureau of Venereal Disease Control, part of New York City's Department of Health, and then, in 1978, he opened a private practice in Greenwich Village specializing in infectious and sexually transmitted diseases, with a mostly gay male clientele. With the arrival of a perplexing cluster of symptoms in a growing number of his patients, Sonnabend's background as a microbiologist, virologist, and infectious disease specialist, as well as his experience in the South African townships, proved ideal for coping with this mysterious and mounting phenomenon. As early as 1982, he created a network of experts, independent of government agencies, to run tests on the samples he'd regularly send them from his patients. He also continued to do basic research on the properties of interferon both at Jan Vilcek's lab at New York University and at St. Luke's–Roosevelt Hospital Center.[3]

When Mike Callen arrived in his office on West Twelfth street in the Village, Sonnabend took one look at him and said, "You're very, very sick. Who is your doctor?" "You are," Mike croaked in response. That was the beginning of a relationship that would have profound consequences in the years ahead, not only for the two men but for the gay community and what would become the AIDS movement. Sonnabend, at age forty-eight, was already well along in his career, having been an assistant professor of microbiology at Mount Sinai School of Medicine before opening his private practice. Though he'd fathered three children (with three women) and been briefly married, Sonnabend openly self-identified as a gay man.

At this point in time, the gay liberation movement was still in swaddling clothes, though following the Stonewall riots, its initial thrust had been radical. In the early seventies, the Gay Liberation Front (GLF), the most visible and active organization, had called for substantive social change, had denounced oppression of all kinds (not merely of the antigay variety), and had tried to form alliances with the Black Panthers and the Latino Young Lords. But as is typically the case in this country with protest movements, GLF had run into the centrist roadblock of American ideology and had given way in short order to the less radical Gay Activists Alliance. That group, in turn, had been superseded by the National Gay Task Force, which confined its agenda solely to what it defined as "gay rights" and adopted the traditional tactics of electoral politics and lobbying as its chosen means. These organizational transformations involved only a small fraction of the gay community. Most gay people remained closeted and apolitical.

What did attract hordes of adherents were the slogans and practices of *sexual* liberation. A segment—according to most estimates, about 20 percent—of the gay male population redefined "promiscuity" as "adventuring," and the baths, the "trucks," and the back rooms of bars and bookstores became jammed with the tangle of eagerly experimenting bodies. Many of those bodies came down with hepatitis, herpes, syphilis, gonorrhea, shigella, amoebiasis, and an assortment of other sexually transmitted diseases. The stricken multitude kept Sonnabend's waiting room packed.

A caring and compassionate man, Sonnabend was widely admired for his brilliance as a diagnostician but was no less notorious for his disorganized, eccentric ways. He was devoted to his patients but not to keeping a tidy or time-efficient office. When Mike would refer friends to Sonnabend, he'd tell them to "take *War and Peace* because you might finish it in the waiting room before you get seen." Mike himself had to wait four hours on one day and was then subjected to watching Sonnabend eat his lunch in front of him during their consultation—some of the food dripping into his beard, while the loud, ancient air conditioner drowned out part of what he was saying. Mike decided it was time to look for a different doctor. But one visit to another well-known gay physician, "Phil Williams," sent him fleeing back to Sonnabend. Williams proved not only "imperious" but moneygrubbing. When Mike called him back into the examining room to ask a belated question, the good doctor added $25 to his bill. Sonnabend, by contrast, saw his patients as part of an unfairly ostracized community—"the health and well-being of gay men were of little concern to society at large"—not customers to be bilked for maximum profit, and he would often forget to bill them—to the admiration and irritation of his beleaguered staff (according to Abby Tallmer, who worked there for several years).

By then Mike had finally landed a job doing office work for the Bradford National Corporation, and he'd switched to a more livable apartment as well. He kept reminding himself that he had to make contacts, find an agent, get his singing career going. But he *loved* sex and spent much of his spare time hunting for and having it. During his first two years in New York he took to heart the popular gay lament "so many men, so little time" and cheerfully referred to himself as a "slut"—a label he would proudly proclaim all his life. Disliking alcohol and disdaining the chitchat of the bars, he opted for the gay baths (St. Mark's was his favorite) and the stalls at the Hudson Street Bookstore in Greenwich Village.

At all times—who can predict a street encounter?—Mike carried with him a jar of lube, 25-cent packets of K-Y to ease entry, a bottle of poppers (amyl nitrate, which produced a disinhibiting rush), two (before and after) five-hundred-milligram pills of tetracycline as anti-STD prophylaxis, and Handi Wipes for the cleanup. Though Mike hardly resembled the muscled gym-built physique then coming into fashion, he had no trouble attracting partners. He was delicately, willowly, handsome: six feet tall, olive skinned, green eyed, and thin (around 135 pounds), with naturally curly dark brown hair—through the right kind of spectacles, something on the order of a Renaissance cherub (minus the wings). Mike wasn't interested in most of the "extreme" sexual practices then in vogue (fist fucking, water sports, scat, or S/M). His single-minded focus was on getting fucked. When he totted up his sexual scorecard in 1982, at age twenty-seven, he figured that since coming out, he'd been "penetrated by an average of 3 men once every 3 days." Deducting for sick days, that put him in gold medal contention with a total of 2,496 partners, of whom he professed to know the first names of no more than a hundred.

He was outspoken and unashamed about his "sluthood." Not every fuck had been magical, but the vast majority, he insisted, had given him pleasure. And what, he wanted to know, was wrong with that? No coercion had been involved, no pederasty, no exchange of cash, no pretense at faithfulness or romance. Like other gay male sex radicals of the day, Mike denounced the puritanical fuzziness that sanctioned multiple monogamous orgasms in order to produce children but frowned on a comparable number with multiple partners to produce pleasure. He did "not accept the concept of sexual addiction at all." A bit later, after he'd become a spokesperson for a segment of the People with AIDS (PWAs) movement, he'd read his sexual history somewhat differently, referring to his generation of sexual liberationists as "predatory, shame-based, dark, use-once-and-throw-away, no contact sex— [all of which went] deep into our wiring." Later still—in part as a result of reading books by "sex-positive" feminists—he'd reclaim and celebrate his "slut" years.

There was one hitch: the escalating number of STDs. Mike was in and out of Sonnabend's office so often that they eventually shifted to a first-name basis. Mike was fond of saying that "if it isn't fatal, it's no big deal," but Joe was less nonchalant about his multiple, incessant infections. When Mike contracted hepatitis for the third time and developed fevers, night sweats, and bloody diarrhea, Joe hospitalized him. Consommé and a battery of tests were his diet for a week. His acne and hemorrhoids improved but a firm diagnosis remained elusive. Sonnabend called in a tropical disease specialist, but the best he could come up with was "atypical malaria." Mike had never been to the tropics, and the paracytology tests failed to confirm that diagnosis or any other. The doctors were back to where they began—scratching their heads.

And not just those in New York. The appearance of other, seemingly anomalous symptoms among young gay men was beginning to puzzle physicians elsewhere. The most perplexing were Pneumocystis carinii pneumonia (PCP), typically associated with the suppression of the immune system; and the appearance of purplish spots on the skin. Sonnabend was among the first to recognize that the spots were indicative of lymphatic tumors, a rare cancer known as Kaposi's sarcoma

(KS) that was traditionally associated with elderly men of Mediterranean origin. Mystified, doctors began to compare notes with colleagues around the country.

Mike wasn't Joe Sonnabend's only patient to experience night sweats and weight loss. As the numbers mounted, he decided to send blood samples to the University of Nebraska, the only place at the time with up-to-date T cell testing technology. Joe drew blind samples from three groups of patients whose histories he knew well: ten were in monogamous relationships; ten were in sexually open-ended relationships, both partners "dabbling" with third parties; and ten were, like Mike, "sluts." Sonnabend's theory was that the degree of immune deficiency would correlate differently for each group—a theory confirmed by the test results: the monogamous group had on average the highest count of protective CD4 cells, the sluts the lowest.

Knowing that Mike was "highly suggestible," Joe refused at first to provide his individual results. He gave Mike assorted excuses: the technology was new and its reliability not fully tested; yes, the three groups did have distinctive patterns, but no one knew why; and so on. "Well, you must think it means *something*," an impatient Mike persisted, "so you might as well tell me. I promise to keep my blabby mouth quiet." And so Joe finally did: "Your immune system is shot—your crucial CD4 cell count is lower than I'd hoped." "How low?" Mike persisted. Joe retreated to generalities: "I can't tell you for certain. Obviously it's better to have more CD4 cells than less, since they indicate the health of your immune system. But the CD4 count is known to fluctuate considerably for a given individual—so don't start getting crazy on me." Within days, Mike fell into a clinical depression that lasted some six months. The year was 1980.

In June 1981, the CDC reported in its prestigious journal *Morbidity and Mortality Weekly Report* (*MMWR*) that between October 1980 and May 1981, five young men in Los Angeles, "all active homosexuals," had come down with PCP and two of them had already died. A few weeks later the *MMWR* added twenty cases of KS among gay men in New York and six in California to the puzzling count. That led the *New York Times*' medical reporter Dr. Lawrence Altman to write a short article in July 1981, reporting that a fatal "gay cancer" had been found among homosexual men who'd had "multiple and frequent sexual encounters with different partners." Thus was the equation drawn early on between gay male promiscuity and terrifying disease.

It was a familiar pairing. The view that equated homosexuality with "sickness" had long held sway both in the general population and among the medical "experts." Thanks to pressure from the post-Stonewall political movement that arose in the early 1970s, some progress had been made in disassociating the two phenomena; the American Psychiatric Association dropped homosexuality from the category of disease as early as 1973. But the new gay political movement had drawn only a small number of adherents; many gay men (lesbians much less so) associated gay liberation during the 1970s with sexual freedom, not with attempting to shift public opinion through educational efforts or pressure politics.

In the historically significant election year of 1980, the fledgling gay movement played little role, its issues ignored by the major political parties. Ronald Reagan's ascension to the presidency marked the onset of a conservative retrenchment that would have horrific ramifications for the mounting epidemic and—in tandem with economic distress—heighten the plight of the disadvantaged in general, bringing the era of civil rights to a screeching halt. Within a year of his election, Reagan's Omnibus Budget Reconciliation Act inaugurated massive cuts in social welfare, soon followed by several-billion-dollar reductions in food stamp and child nutrition programs. Funding for the construction of subsidized housing fell from nearly 145,000 starts in 1981 to a mere 17,000 in 1986, disproportionately affecting low-income African Americans and Hispanics. By 1982, much of the limited progress that had been made in this country, starting with Lyndon Johnson's Great Society initiatives against poverty, would be wiped away.

The Reagan agenda had a different set of priorities: increased spending for combating "communism" (especially in Central America), an emphasis on traditional family values ("Just Say No"), and a "trickle-down" theory of supply-side economics that envisioned a future harkening back to Herbert Hoover. The key spokesmen for the administration, Gary Bauer and William Bennett, held traditional values about gender and sexuality that reached back beyond Hoover to the late nineteenth century. Reagan did appoint a few African Americans to high judicial office, but they were uniformly tried-and-true conservatives opposed to affirmative action and to extending federal action on school desegregation: to chair the Equal Employment Opportunity Commission, for example, he chose Clarence Thomas, that exemplar of deafness to human suffering, who would later be elevated to the Supreme Court.

To further ensure that the underclass would fail to improve its lot, Reagan embraced states' rights—that traditional weapon of white supremacists—and mocked "welfare queens." In a speech he gave in Philadelphia, Mississippi—the town where three activists against segregation had been brutally murdered in 1964—Reagan made it clear that "states' rights" would indeed retain its long-coded meaning of "white supremacy." Those other undesirables, homosexuals, sex workers, and intravenous drug users, would be treated dismissively as well. As Congress gradually increased funding over the years for AIDS education and research, it would always be *more* than the Reagan administration had requested or would spend.

During the 1980s as well as today, Washington, D.C., itself was something of an anomaly. It simultaneously has a high median income level and a nearly 20 percent poverty rate (exceeded only by Mississippi). During the economic restructuring in the country as a whole during the 1960s and 1970s, technological advances had led to the loss of many manufacturing jobs; they were replaced by low-paying service jobs and a high level of unemployment—which disproportionately affected black workers. In the public sector, ironically, blacks with college degrees were able to find professional jobs in the federal government, leading to a significantly larger black middle class whose comparative prosperity contrasted sharply with the decline in economic security for the majority of blacks.

D.C. has always had a large African American population—in 1970 it reached a peak of 70 percent of the whole, since declining to about 50 percent. After the assassination of Martin Luther King Jr. in 1968, rioting that raged for three days had broken out in black neighborhoods and been quelled only by some fifteen thousand federal troops. It wasn't until 1973 that Congress had given the District home rule, providing for an elected mayor and a thirteen-member council. In 1975 Walter Washington became D.C.'s first elected mayor and first African American to hold the office. He was succeeded in 1979 by Marion Barry, another African American leader, but one—he'd been chair of the radical Student Nonviolent Coordinating Committee (SNCC)—of a quite different stripe.

Not surprisingly, few blacks—fewer than one in ten—had voted for Reagan in 1980 or supported his draconian measures, but that shouldn't be taken as the measure or proof of a unified local black community. Many members of the churchgoing black middle class in D.C. feared Barry as a dangerous extremist, a threat to whatever "betterment" they'd managed to attain, and in the Democratic primary for mayor they'd supported his opponent, Sterling Tucker, former director of the cautious Washington Urban League. Neither Barry nor his antagonists, moreover, had as yet shown any awareness or concern for the all but invisible black gay men and lesbians living in their midst, often in isolation from each other.[4]

In 1980, the largely hidden, unorganized world of black gay people stood in stark contrast to the visibility and assertiveness of the white gay community, as spearheaded by the newly radicalized D.C. chapter of the pre-Stonewall Mattachine Society. Though its membership never exceeded a hundred people, with a mere dozen serving as the activist core, D.C. Mattachine had successfully challenged the discriminatory policies of the Civil Service Commission and had gone on to pressure the federal government for concessions on additional issues.

To its credit, D.C. Mattachine had attempted to recruit members from the African American gay bar Nob Hill, though with scant success. Mattachine, like many white-dominated gay organizations, then and now, never understood that the issue of sexual orientation was merely one, and not necessarily the most important, issue that afflicted black gay people on a daily and ongoing basis. Washington, D.C., was segregated in all but name—meaning not just the bars, but schools, housing, medical facilities, and employment opportunities as well.

A black gay presence was just beginning to emerge openly in D.C. and in the nation at large. As early as 1975, a group calling itself the Baltimore Gay Alliance had appeared, and by 1978 the D.C. Coalition had emerged as well. Then in August 1979, just two months before the first national gay march took place in Washington, the initial issue of *Blacklight* magazine appeared under the editorship of Sidney Brinkley (it would continue publishing until 1986).

Simultaneously, a somewhat select core group of openly black gay men and lesbians—from writers to filmmakers to service organizers—

emerged into prominence, among them Billy Jones, Delores Berry, Gil Gerald, Essex Hemphill, Michelle Parkerson, and Renee McCoy. The D.C. black gay community realized fairly quickly that it had the potential to form a national organization, and among their first actions was to ensure that the 1979 March on Washington included their voices. They formally incorporated in October 1980 as the National Coalition of Black Lesbians and Gays (NCBLG). By 1984, it had chapters in half a dozen cities and, unlike some other African American organizations, actively committed resources to fighting AIDS. Though some well-known figures would be involved over the next decade— including Audre Lorde, Barbara Smith, and Joseph Beam—NCBLG had to wage an ongoing struggle, which it ultimately lost, to raise money and build its membership rolls. Marginalized communities, even when comparatively well educated and gifted, usually lack an abundance of all resources except suffering.[5]

The reasons are many. It's probably safe to say that, despite individual variations, for many black gays, race—a shared history and marker of oppression—was and is the primary source of identity, with gender and sexual orientation often secondary (particularly since the latter can be usually hidden if necessary). That was certainly true for the poet Essex Hemphill. "My race," he once wrote, "even at the point of birth, was more important than my sexuality. That's going to always be the case. . . . I love my race enough to know that I'm a Black man first and foremost and that my sexuality falls in line after that."[6]

It's often been argued that homophobia in African American communities is more deeply entrenched than in white ones, but that assertion, I'd suggest, mistakenly equates the black church with the black community—and even the church, it can be further argued, has in recent years come around somewhat on the issue. When *Blacklight* began to publish in 1979, the comment of Bishop William A. Hilliard that "the Church is diametrically opposed to homosexuality" or the publicly stated view of Bishop Jasper Roby to the effect that unless homosexuality ceased, it would "destroy us all," probably typified the view of most traditional black church leaders and goers. After all, heterosexual blacks had themselves been caricatured for so long as (among other things) "lustful sexual beasts" that upholding middle-class white norms of monogamous pair-bonding and excluding noncomplying members of their own community had become an instrument of self-defense.

Since then, as attitudes toward homosexuality have grown more progressive in general, so have those within the black church.[7]

Even back in 1979, black families, arguably, didn't disown or "throw away" their nonconforming children to the same extent that white families did (and still do). When the poet Essex Hemphill, for one, spoke of "home," as he often did, he quite literally meant his own family—not the white-dominated gay "community." The implicit agreement between black parents and their gay offspring often hinged on keeping the news tightly confined within the family circle. This was not the case with Essex. "I exercise the same candor with my parents," he once wrote, "that I exercise with most people." And candor was among his most marked characteristics.[8]

Essex had been born prematurely and with a heart murmur in 1957—he was two years younger than Mike Callen. The second oldest of five children (three sisters and one brother), he was born in Chicago but raised mostly in Washington, D.C. His parents, Mantalene and Warren, had a stormy relationship that ended in divorce. Essex had a deep love/anger bond with his mother, Mantalene, a strong, dignified woman who would later hold an administrative job in the copyright division of the Library of Congress. But he rarely had a positive word for his alcoholic and abusive father (only once did he refer to *both* of his parents as having been "inspiring" to him). In his poem "Vital Signs," Essex recalled witnessing his father's violence: "I . . . always see him punching and pushing, slapping and yelling." One of Essex's close friends in adulthood recalls him saying that once he was even witness to his father stabbing his mother. In the poem "Fixin' Things," Essex describes the family's dynamics:

> In retrospect, it wasn't the sound
> Of my mother crying that hurt most,
> It was the sound of my father leaving
> His marriage, his house, his familiars.
>
> In the debris of ruptured bloodlines,
> In the domestic violence of our families,
> In the turbulence we call love was bred
> The possibility of my dysfunction, and yours.

I tell you of the hatred
That seized the boyhoods
Of my brother and me,
How we fought violently in public,

Drawing blood as if it would
Allow us to see
What was wrong with it,
With him, with me . . .

As a youngster, Essex spent summers with his maternal grand-mother, "Miss Emily"—for whom he felt "pure love"—at her home in Columbia, South Carolina. Her late husband had owned a small res-taurant in town, but because it attracted a "risqué" crowd it had been declared off-limits to Mantalene and her siblings—except to deliver the peach cobblers Miss Emily made at home (though the kids would sneak by after school for lemonade or soda pop). Among other things, Miss Emily taught Essex to cook and praised him for turning out food that reminded her of her husband's.

As a growing boy, Essex wasn't inclined toward athletics: "In the black neighborhood I came from, there was an emphasis on being able to play basketball or football. I, instead, was attracted to gymnastics because of the way the body looked. But I knew instinctively that if I had said, 'I want to be a gymnast,' among the fellas I ran with I would have been labeled a sissy." Essex's tight, slender frame never grew much beyond five feet six inches. As he later put it, "I was the smallest of the fellas that I ran with when I was growing up. When you're the smallest, you absorb the blows of other people trying to be 'manly.' I guess it's an awful fact of adolescence. That drove me to writing, I think."

But though small, Essex was a handsome boy, with a symmetrical face marked by intense, searching eyes and an engulfing smile when he chose to bestow it. His soft, caressing voice could also, especially when speaking on serious matters, ring with passionate conviction. He began writing poetry at age fourteen, while still in high school: "After dinner I would wind up going back to my room and writing in my notebook. I didn't realize I was writing poetry. I was just writing about the events and thoughts of my day." But poetry was from the beginning his most congenial medium, though he would later try his hand at a novel, and some of his adult essays would profoundly influence his generation of black writers.

I was fortunate enough when researching this book to discover a batch of some fifty of Essex's unpublished early poems (mostly from 1974–75, during his seventeenth and eighteenth years), which he bundled together under the rubric "Talking with a Friend . . ." The disarmingly casual title was aptly chosen, for though these first efforts have autobiographical value, Essex made scant claim for their literary merit and never included any of them in the chapbooks he began to publish in 1982 at age twenty-five. He even entitled the first poem in the batch "Act I":

> like a baby realizing it has legs to walk with
> like a bird realizing its need to spread its wings and fly
> so in act I I have filled a need
> which in the beginning was only the need to
> let thoughts, ideas, and my feelings
> come forth, and speak
> the language of 17 years of living

In another poem in the series, he spelled out why he'd felt the need this early to turn to verse:

> The essence of these poems
> is the me
> locked inside of me
> trying to express
> the turmoil
> sometimes felt within
> sometimes hard to express
> but always holding
> meaning

In one of these poems, dated May 25, 1974, Essex begins to convey the "differentness" he felt from most other young men, and the value he placed on it:

> I cry sometimes
> knowing it won't take nothing away from my blossoming
> manhood

You cry don't you
or
are you just another
one of those
uptight and totally in control
of my emotions type of people
who wouldn't be able to cope
with themselves
if any emotion was shown . . .

and sometimes
I cry
for you, too . . .

As a teenager, Essex continued to make other cherished self-discoveries:

Walk alone
little boy
never move with
the maddening crowds

Never forget
where you came from
because no one else
ever will . . .

Walk alone little boy
tomorrow
you'll be a man

In some of the later poems in the series, the maturing Essex reflects back with tender regret on certain aspects of his childhood:

when I was a child, I walked in the woods
on hot July afternoons,
that were cool and dark,
holding secrets,

which sent slight chills up my spine,
when I knew that I would never know
of them completely.
taking mother nature's children,
like the birds that never sang for me,
and the turtles that always stayed in their shells,
and frogs that croaked in disgust at my probing
fingers,
. . . and soft brown baby rabbits I had found
died,
because my hands and my love was not gentle enough.
. . . crying I ran home to my mother
whose hands were gentle enough love warm
enough to calm my broken heart.
I didn't know they needed more then I could
give them so that they could live.

In a piece Essex entitled "A Woman Our Mother We Love You . . ." he expressed the lifelong devotion he felt for his mother, the family peacemaker, in lines amply, if awkwardly, expressive:

And you know that whenever we've found the
heat in the kitchen too hot, to handle
we've come back into the living room
where you are, so that you could help us
sort out, the experience, feeling, or whatever
it was that we confronted on life's battlefield
and with all of that,
you also give us the encouragement to go back
and try again

Yet Essex's deeply religious mother, Mantalene, would hardly have been pleased with the January 12, 1975, poem he wrote about churchgoing:

and the preacher asks the smartly dressed
HOLY ladies
to pass the basket

and give/pleas [*sic*] give
if only a dime/but a dollar
let your SOUL be cleansed
for   a   dime???????????????????
Its for the church
he takes ¾ of what they give
and puts it in a saving account, in his name
the name of the Lord
who likes those who give
so that others may receive . . .

The hurt and disappointment that Essex experienced at the hands of his father is the likely subject of the poignant poem he dated February 23, 1974:

You built my hopes up high
knowing that you wouldn't
be at the bottom to catch them
when they fell

You promised you would be there
whenever I needed you
but you never came

You promised me I wouldn't be hurt by you
but the pain is still here
because
you and your promises are gone

The simmering anger that Essex felt for anyone—perhaps including his father—who dared to mock his dreams comes out strongly in the poem he entitled "Revenge," dated January 21, 1975:

Step on my dreams, and I'll break your legs
and feet into pieces which will never, ever
fit together again,
You will be crippled.
call me names, and I will still your mind,

23

Busting it in half with a brick,
which has your name signed on it,
it is there that the names were thought . . .

By age twenty, encouraged by the prominent African American children's writer Sharon Bell Mathis, Essex would start trying to get some of his poems published. Though little literary merit can be claimed for most of them, an occasional fragment provides some foretaste of the powerful poet he'd later become:

The radio plays syncopated rhythms
To soothe and relax
Black bodies in the quiet of night
that have met
and come/together/apart
from one another
saying something to each other
that words weren't made for
and these same
syncopated rhythms
raise the hand
that will slap a face
and crack, what could've been
but now isn't
while she walks the streets
syncopated rhythmically
to do her thing
with whoever is willing to/for a couple of sheets
of green stuff
moving her body to a beat
that will feed the baby
and pay the rent
for an apartment
which creaks too/to
syncopated/sad rhythms
and a baby breathes
to the rhythms
and cries syncope tears

of want/inquiet

during a very Black night . . .

If Essex began writing seriously at seventeen, his sexual explora-
tions had begun some years earlier. By age fourteen, he'd had his
first sexual encounter that went beyond the usual "messing around"
among neighborhood youngsters. At a convenience store near his
home, a white male clerk in his midforties named George had been
whispering in his ear for weeks about how much he wanted to suck his
dick, how good he was at it, how many others in the neighborhood had
let him, and so on. Essex later recalled that he knew from the start
that his answer would be yes, and finally he said it. Then the sucking
led to fucking and soon Essex would regularly mount George early in
the morning before the store opened or at George's house after it
closed—George's mongrel dog watching the action nonchalantly. The
sex between them went on for nearly two years, with Essex finally
ending it out of fear that it was only a matter of time before they'd be
caught.[9]

In D.C., Essex attended Ballou Senior High School, just a few blocks
from his home, and had a part-time job downtown as a file clerk. He
was by then well aware of his sexual attraction to men but realized, "as
a way of protecting myself from being identified as a faggot around
the school," that he needed always to have a girlfriend. "It would be
my luck," he'd later write, "to date girls who were 'good,' girls who were
not going to experiment with sex beyond kissing and fondling, and
even that was often only tolerated at a minimum if tolerated at all."

During his senior year in Ballou High School in 1975, a more resonant encounter took place when his journalism instructor assigned him
to interview the local Episcopal minister of a church known for providing daily meals for the down-and-out. Essex called the church for
an appointment, but the man who answered the phone told him that
the minister was out. He then chatted pleasantly with Essex, asking
him why he wanted to see the minister. Essex found the man's voice, a
cadenced, leathery baritone, enticing, and when he boldly suggested
that Essex "come on up here and meet *me*," a startled—and turned-on—
Essex required little coaxing.[10]

The voice on the phone turned out to be attached to a tall, broad-
shouldered man in his late forties with salt-and-pepper hair. He'd once

been a promising professional boxer, but an automobile accident had cut short his career. His jacket, Essex later wrote, "constrained obvious arm muscles and an expansive chest," and "his hands were thick and strong." The man, as it turned out, was a volunteer at the church in one of its community programs, and he gave Essex a courtly, unhurried tour.

Perhaps too unhurried; like most seventeen-year-old boys, Essex had (in his words), "raging hormones and an embarrassing erection." When the older man finally closed and locked a heavy wooden door in one of the unoccupied rooms and suddenly said, "Take down your pants . . . I want to suck your dick," Essex eagerly complied. "Orgasm and high-spirited ecstasy" followed, and the two continued to see each other for nearly two years. Essex would borrow his mother's royal blue Dodge sedan "to study at the library" and the two would rendezvous. And more than sex was involved, though that continued to be passionate.

The older man turned out to be "the most well-read adult black male" Essex had known, other than for some of his teachers, and he had a "beautiful, stimulating" mind. In adulthood Essex credited his older friend's counsel with diverting him from making some "foolish choices"—he would never, for example, feel the need "to strike cool poses on the corner and father numerous children to prove my manhood." His older friend pointed him toward the only acceptance that matters: "acceptance of myself." It was an uncommonly lucky coming-out for any day and age, but especially for that one.

Following high school, Essex in 1975 enrolled at the University of Maryland. He was assigned to room with another black gay man, Wayson Jones—probably a deliberate racial slight since they were the only blacks on the entire floor of the dormitory and the room was designed for one person. Wayson came from a military family and, having grown up in a more integrated environment than Essex, recalls no noticeable friction with white students in the dorm—one of his good friends was in fact "a real hippie type." In any case, Essex decided to leave the University of Maryland after one year—not because of endemic racism or because he was in any sort of academic trouble, but rather, as Wayson has put it, because he "needed to 'reinvent' himself." Essex spent some time in Los Angeles in 1976 and then returned to D.C. and completed his degree at the University of the District of Columbia.

During the year that they roomed together, Essex and Wayson "clicked," bonding particularly around music—and smoking pot. Essex favored female jazz vocalists but was also into progressive jazz performers like Bennie Maupin and George Duke. Wayson leaned more toward rock—they both loved the groupies—and more dissonant jazz like that of John Coltrane. In general they (in Wayson's words) had "a great time" together as roommates. Essex had a hot plate and after getting the munchies from smoking pot, they'd devour batch after batch of pancakes. They also shared a small TV set, their special favorites being *Monty Python* and *Saturday Night Live*. Essex showed Wayson some of his early writing, and though not a fan of poetry, Wayson to this day remembers the telling image in one of Essex's poems: returning home in the evening to "count the brown pennies of this day." Wayson, in turn, invited Essex to hear him play saxophone in a jam session and took to heart his opinion that Wayson held back too much when improvising. They were, as Wayson puts it, "very much in tune emotionally and spiritually."

Wayson was already "out" as a gay man, both sexually and politically, had already told his parents—and told Essex, too, the very first time they met. According to Wayson, Essex wasn't at that point really open yet about being gay; he still dated girls and rarely talked about his private life. (Essex's first public declaration of his homosexuality would come during a poetry reading at the library of Howard University in 1980.) Though Essex and Wayson tended to have separate friends, they did some occasional gay socializing together. Wayson took him to Pier 9, D.C.'s first "superdisco," and at another time to a party—at which Essex was "visibly uncomfortable"—at the home of his former high school band director, Doug Hinkle, who'd been really helpful to Wayson when he was coming out during senior year in high school, and who went on to become a photographer for D.C.'s gay paper, the *Washington Blade*. Wayson belonged to the Maryland chapter of the Gay Student Alliance, and unlike Essex at that point was already "very much a gay activist," even giving talks and holding Q and A sessions in front of university classes—a rare act of bravery at this relatively early stage of the gay rights movement. When Essex left the University of Maryland after his freshman year, he and Wayson stayed in touch and within a few years, after Essex's return to D.C., reconnected as part of the city's black artistic circle.

By then Essex was fully out of the closet and eager to explore black gay life. The District's gay history went back at least to the nineteenth-century annual drag balls and up to the ongoing cruising area in La-fayette Square across from the White House. But it wasn't until the cultural revolution of the 1960s that segregated gay life slowly began to give way to interracial contact—a process still far from complete. Even when white gays and their bars didn't adopt exclusionary policies—and many did—their frequent condescension, or worse, made black gays uncomfortable and angry.

By the mid-1970s, an independent parallel movement by and for black gays was starting to form and coalesce in D.C. Concerned about the fact that "black gays were not getting a fair share of the political, social and economic advances of the gay community," in the fall of 1976 a group called the Association of Black Gays formed and for a brief time published the newsletter *Rafiki.* Then, in 1978, the D.C. Coalition of Black Gays emerged—one of the first black gay organiza-tions in the country—which subsequently became the still-active D.C. Coalition. It was determined to take legal action against bars that "carded"—the polite euphemism for denying admission to blacks—and it also intended to expose the racism that characterized white-dominated gay organizations.

The feminist movement in D.C. had also done little to encourage the participation of women of color, heterosexual or homosexual. As a result—expecting neither white women nor black men to address their specific issues—a Washington, D.C., chapter of the National Black Feminist Organization came into being at Howard University in 1974. That same year, Salsa Soul Sisters emerged, and then in 1980 a group of black lesbians formed Sapphire Sapphos; their primary sym-pathies lay not with the feminist movement but with their black gay brothers and with the struggle in general for black liberation. Some D.C. black lesbians may have read the white feminist journal *Quest* (founded in 1974 and including Charlotte Bunch and Rita Mae Brown among its guiding spirits) for its strong positions against oppression of any kind, and of apartheid in particular. As well, many African Amer-ican lesbians embraced feminist issues of reproductive rights, day care, ERA, and equal opportunities in the workplace, while rejecting male definitions of what it meant to be a woman. Nonetheless, many black lesbians also believed—as did many black gay men—that racial solidarity took clear and necessary priority over gender oppression.

Essex would later frame the issue this way: "I always tell people I can be gay in only a few cities in this country, but I'm Black everywhere I go. . . . That's going to always be the case, at least within my lifetime. I don't see any major changes happening in the consciousness of this country around issues of race." In saying this, Essex wasn't prescribing for others; it was up to each individual, he felt, to establish his or her priorities among the multiple strands that make up one's "identity." Even for himself, he acknowledged that varied strands made up his personhood—"it's all hand-in-hand, it comes as one package. I can't just be Black and then just be gay. I'm all of these things." Further, he acknowledged that it would take him "a very long time to arrive at a love of myself that allows the integration to work. Each thing plays off of the other. Each part of me empowers me. So I can't say, well my left hand is gay and my right hand is Black."[11]

Washington, D.C., in 1973 became the first large U.S. city officially to outlaw discrimination based on sexual orientation in housing, employment, and public accommodations. The catch, of course, was that black and Latino/a gay men and lesbians still remained subject to the prevailing racist mind-set among whites—and the prevailing homophobia among heterosexual people of color. It's possible to argue—though the argument is far from conclusive—that within gay circles discrimination against blacks and Latinos was less pronounced in D.C. than within straight ones. During a three-day conference at the University of Houston to plan for the 1979 National March on Washington for Lesbian and Gay Rights, for example, the organizers set aside 25 percent of all leadership and policy positions for Third World delegates, and the black D.C. Coalition, led by Billy Jones, actively participated. The day before the march, the conference agenda included three panels on racial issues, and both Marion Barry and the well-known writer Audre Lorde spoke at the event itself. Judging by numbers alone—estimates vary but are generally upwards of 150,000 attendees—the march was counted a great success.

Yet as Essex and other black gay people well knew, social and cultural circles in D.C. were mostly divided along racial grounds. One of the best-known hangouts for black gay artists was (Valerie) Papaya Mann's brownstone in Northeast D.C.—a salon-like setting reminiscent of 1920s Harlem Renaissance gathering spots in New York City, of which A'Lelia Walker's and Carl Van Vechten's were probably the most famous. Papaya herself had come out in the midseventies and immediately gotten involved in D.C. lesbian and gay life, organizing a variety of social events and becoming a central figure in Sapphire Sapphos, Washington's first organization for African American lesbians. It was at Papaya's that Essex first met his future good friends Chris Prince and Garth Tate and then, through them, any number of other black gay singers, writers, painters, and filmmakers.

One of the early (1979–80) products of these gatherings was the publication of the short-lived but handsomely produced bimonthly *Nethula Journal of Contemporary Literature* (the name "Nethula" had come to Essex in a dream). He co-founded *Nethula* with two young women, Kathy Anderson, whom he'd known at the University of Maryland, and Cynthia Lou Williams. Essex served not only as the journal's publisher, but also as its graphic designer—he'd learned offset printing and typesetting at one of his part-time jobs, and showed a striking gift for it. With wonderful paper stock, stunning cover design, and challenging content, both poetry and prose, *Nethula* was a state-of-the-art publication devoted largely to the work of the newest generation of black artists. Both Sterling Brown and E. Ethelbert Miller of the older group of black writers were among the journal's five contributing editors. Miller especially—a poet on staff at the Howard University library—served as an important bridge between the generations.

In 1980, Miller arranged for Essex and the black lesbian poet and filmmaker Michelle Parkerson to share a bill together at the citywide Ascension Poetry Reading Series at Howard University's Founders Library, which Miller coordinated. Michelle had graduated from Temple University, was then working at the local NBC television affiliate, and had just completed her first film, *But Then, She's Betty Carter.* The two had never met before and the connection proved immediate and consequential for both. As Michelle recalls the evening of their joint reading, "I was just struck by this young brother, whose poems were incredible . . . beautifully sensual and homoerotically brave, which was right where I was at with my own work." After the event concluded, Michelle approached Essex: "Hey, where you been all my life?" she laughingly asked, and told him how much she loved his work. Essex felt the same about hers and the two became fast friends. In the mid-1980s Michelle wrote a poem, "Highwire," that celebrated the friendship:

> We poise above teetering earth
> Defying limitation
> Mere lines suspend us
> We do not know fear
> A precision for danger
> Instructs our hand
> Chaperones the passions
> Propelling us:
> Partners
> Skin to skin
> Flung vast beyond gender
> The sweaty grip of Spirit
> is all that joins us
> Sequined
> Caped
> We test precarious
> air.

The two had much in common. Both came from the Anacostia section of Southeast Washington, both were living in the "gayborhood" of Adams Morgan, and both were gay writers who (in Michelle's words) "loved to push edges." Anacostia sat beyond the army/marine barracks at the southern edge of Capitol Hill and was mostly black and poor. As Essex would later put it, "the city doesn't think kindly of Anacostia. . . . [It's] viewed as a jungle of sorts, breeding crime, poverty and other social ails and traumas no-one really wants to discuss." But Southeast D.C. had been the home of Frederick Douglass, and a number of black artists had lived there. Essex felt a strong attachment to the area, which he made clear in a later poem, "My Funny Valentine/for Southeast":

> Green Dolphin Street is Kind of Blue.
> Cool cats lean on the Avenue.

They keep swing and bop alive.
They brew rhythms, cook blues
In mumbo sauce . . .

Some people can't see Southeast
For the Harlem it is.
They hear go go and call it noise,
Fear its criminal,
But it's the best of our blood
Dignified without violins.

In addition to Michelle, Essex began to work with other writers he was meeting at Papaya's and elsewhere, including Gideon Ferebee Jr. and Larry Duckett (Larry would for a time become a close friend and performance partner). What followed within a few years in the early eighties was a proliferation of contacts, multitasking (Essex, for one, became poet, graphic artist, organizer, set designer, and actor), artist collectives, publications (the first, *MOJA*, would last for only a few issues but led to a host of others, including *ARISE, BGM, Women in the Life*, and the *Au Courant* group in Philly), performance sites, and personnel—all of which helped spawn the widely shared sense that an outburst of creative energy was in play strong enough to warrant being called a second Harlem Renaissance, "second" in relation to time, not quality, and this time around, moreover, centrally, *overtly* gay. "Every week," as photographer and writer Ron Simmons tells it, "there would be an opening, or a reading, or an exhibition—it was incredible." The multiplicity of events from roughly 1980 to 1985 made for animated high spirits, a heady, intoxicating buzz—and a hectic, hazy chronology:

—in 1980 Essex became a founding member of the performance poetry group Station to Station. Its first performance, at D.C.'s Gala Hispanic Theatre, was also the first time Wayson heard Essex read publicly. The poem he chose was "Balloons," his intense take on the serial killer John Wayne Gacy. It left Wayson feeling "awed by the audacity and freakishness of the subject matter":

In black plastic bags
tied at the top

they were buried.
Their faces
swollen with death
rise in my dreams.
I was seventeen
when I read of them:
young boys, young men
lured to a house in Texas.
Their penises were filled
with excited blood:
first hard then soft they became
as Death with its blistered lips
kissed them one by one . . .

—in late December 1981, Essex made his first appearance on the late Grace Cavalieri's WPFW radio show *The Poet and the Poem* (he would appear again in 1985 and for a third time, with Wayson, in 1986).

—*Nethula* continued to publish for a while longer, with Essex assuring the poet (and future biographer of Audre Lorde) Alexis de Veaux that it would no longer be as "thematic" as the initial number. He told her, too, that he was "pleasantly stunned" to read her piece on "Sister Love" in *Essence*: "I could feel the courage it took to name and say what is real on this human journey we are all making. . . . You made me proud. . . . I seem to be realizing how important coalescing is going to be among our variousness [*sic*] in order to make change and survive. This is no place to rest. There must be 'freedom . . . for all of us.' The synthesizing of politics and culture, and who we are . . ."[12]

—Essex now began to self-publish his poetry chapbooks. After a number of commercial publishers told him that they liked his work but "you're a poet and a young one and come back some time later," Essex decided, "with no concern about accusations of vanity and the like . . . to get my words out . . . to take a chance on myself. Trust my own judgment a little more. Become self-sufficient." He felt that the first step "in self-empowerment and control of your image is to do it yourself; from that point of view there is less of a chance of your message being distorted or diluted." He decided to call his venture Be Bop Books—"because there is so much music in my life now." In 1982 he published *Diamonds Was in the Kitty* and *Some of the People We Love Are Terrorists*; the following year he issued four hundred copies of *Plums*. In 1985 would come the more ambitious *Earth Life*, which the *Washington Post* would favorably review, Essex telling its reporter that he drew most of his subjects "from personal experience," and citing Langston Hughes, Gwendolyn Brooks, and Billie Holiday as his "influences." In 1986 he'd publish *Conditions*, his most substantial work to date; the critic Donald Hutera would praise it as "rarely didactic . . . not experimental . . . more of a tender-tough confessee . . . he pares down his words and phrases carefully, for maximum rhythmic impact."

—starting in 1982, Essex and Larry Duckett found a group they called Cinque (named after the West African Joseph Cinqué, the legendary hero who led a successful mutiny on the slave ship *Amistad* in 1839). The following year Essex invited Wayson to join them, adding music to their poetry performances. The trio started to perform publicly, including at the black gay bar Bachelor's Mill. Cinque's performances blended jazz, pop, and words, which Essex named "choral poetry—a kind of melodic and intelligent rap music." As Wayson describes it, the three "would recite in unison or would weave their voices together, dividing the lines or stanzas between voices, the pattern varied to suit the particular poem." All the words were memorized in advance of a performance, the three men meeting at least twice a week for two to three hours and then, as a performance date approached, increasing rehearsal time to three to four times a week. They recorded all rehearsals and listened intently to the recordings in order to critique their own process. This strenuous schedule was eased by smoking a joint or two before each rehearsal.

In "Brass Rail" (named after a black gay bar)—which Essex called his "breakthrough piece" (and which would later appear in Marlon Riggs' film *Tongues Untied*)—"one voice starts at the end of the poem and another at the beginning, so that they cross, repeating a line in the middle." They were using the speaking voice as an instrument of musicality, employing the "ecstatic call-and-response of the Baptist church to convey the erotic urgency of a night in the black gay bar":

> I saw you last night.
> Many occupants are never found

in the basement.
Many canoes overturn
of the Brass Rail.
Your dark, diva's face.
a leg
lushing and laughing.
I hear the sea,
your voice
screaming,
falling from the air,
dancing with the boys on the edge of funk,
twilight.

Another main feature of the performance style that began with Cinqué and continued throughout their work during this period was (in Wayson's words) "the idea of considering the natural spoken inflection as musical pitches and trying to match between the voices, so it sounded like one person speaking." This gave the sound richness and resonance; in some pieces they actually sang, providing a continuum between normal speech and music.

—Cinqué developed a loyal following. Wayson was quoted in the *Washington Post* saying "there is a big tradition of jazz poetry, which we are a part of but not limited to. We're trying to overlap between some already established traditions [to develop something] that, if not brand new, is creative and fresh." Wyatt O'Brian Evans, a friend of Essex's, attended one performance on a sweltering night in 1985 and found it "absolutely mesmerizing." The writer Jim Marks, of the gay bookstore Lambda Rising, was so enthralled with Cinque that he attended not once, but three times. Wayson recalls that the stillness of their audiences during a performance was so profound that "the cliché 'you could hear a pin drop' was literally true."

—Wayson briefly left Cinqué for about a year to work in a band and was replaced by Chi Hughes, both a poet and a performer. In 1984 Essex, too, left to form a duo with Wayson, billing themselves simply as "Essex Hemphill and Wayson Jones." They performed at D.C.'s Blues Alley and at the ENIKAlley coffeehouse. Larry and Chi carry on Cinqué together.

—The Coffeehouse became the most prominent nurturing ground

and outlet for gay black artists in D.C., and Ray Melrose its chief figure. Located between I and K Streets in Northeast Washington in an old two-story carriage house owned by Ray's partner, in what some Washingtonians viewed as an "unsafe" part of town—meaning that to reach the Coffeehouse you had to come off the street and walk down an alley. Ray was (according to Wayson) "irreverent and in your face . . . charismatic, extremely intelligent, arrogant, creative, connective." He would bring people together, was (as the photographer Sharon Farmer describes him), "a great unifier, a hero who tied all the threads together." Ray was also one of the founders of the D.C. Coalition of Black Lesbians and Gays, and an activist in other regards as well. A few years later he would share a house with Wayson for a time. Later still, in 1994, he would be one of many from the black D.C. artistic community who would die of AIDS. But in the early 1980s, according to Wayson, AIDS wasn't "a real issue. . . . It was around then, but we didn't know about it." When the *Washington Blade* ran a brief story in July 1981 that a few cases of some rare "gay cancer" had occurred in New York City and California, the news hardly registered. Such weird, isolated incidents—like Legionnaires' disease or toxic shock syndrome—were always surfacing, and would, it was assumed, just as suddenly disappear.

The Coffeehouse had a fireplace, a welcoming atmosphere, and an open loft with a rail around it that overlooked the main floor. Chris Prince remembers it as a "very special" place, "vibrant artistically," a cutting-edge outpost for mostly (but not entirely) African American gay and lesbian artists. They chipped in a few dollars each to keep logs in the fire (the place was unheated) and to pay for minimal snacks. The Coffeehouse when crowded held at most thirty or forty people. Performances were predominantly by local African American artists, but not solely—the black lesbian vocal duo Casselberry and DuPree and the New York poetry collective Other Countries were among the many well-known figures who performed there early on. Later, in 1985, the Coffeehouse would play host for three days of performances to the Blackheart collective, which included Joe Beam, Craig G. Harris, Donald Woods, and Assotto Saint—by then all well-known figures in the black gay artistic world. For Essex, the Coffeehouse proved an artistic awakening ground. He met a large number of other black artists there and watched them "work out the butterflies." He and Wayson not only performed there together, but Essex did some of his first solo readings.

—Michelle Parkerson, who'd been friendly with Essex since 1980, became part of a circle of friends that also included Sharon Farmer (the well-known community photographer) and her lover Joyce Wellman, the painter. Michelle joined Alexis de Veaux in a joint reading sponsored by *Nethula* at the Market Five Gallery, which the African American journalist Dorothy Gilliam praised in the *Washington Post* as another important marker of the growth of a creative community among black gays and lesbians in D.C. Another marker came in 1983 when Michelle and Essex received a collaborative performance grant from the Washington Project for the Arts (WPA) to co-produce *Murder on Glass*, an experimental dramatization of their poetry, for which Wayson mixed sound and provided music. The WPA was a nonprofit visual and performing arts space in operation since 1975 that had become the premier venue in D.C. for postmodern work; it was particularly devoted to showcasing new artists who lived in the D.C. area. *Murder on Glass* was staged in 1983 at the WPA's Monday Night Performance Series in its black box theater, which accommodated two hundred people.

Murder on Glass was conceived by Essex and Michelle in the context of a crack epidemic, accompanied by drug wars, that by the early 1980s had become rampant, especially in their own Southeast neighborhood in D.C. Serial murders occurred along the freeway, chopped-up bodies of young men and women showing up randomly in garbage bags on the strip of Interstate 295, the borderline between Southeast and the rest of Washington. The duo described *Murder on Glass* as "contemporary urban poetry" visually underscored through a "stark and minimalist" backdrop. On entering the performance space, the audience was confronted by DayGlo body outlines and black plastic bags that moved and rustled on the stage floor, eighties club music with an avant-garde edge sounding in the background. Suddenly the lights came on, a target-practice figure unscrolled onstage, and the live torsos of young men crept from the garbage bags as Essex, standing in the foreground, started to read from his powerful ode "Homocide (for Ronald Gibson)," a young transvestite hustler whose

chopped-up body had been one of those found in a trash bag on Interstate 295:

> Grief is not apparel.
> Not like a dress, a wig
> Or my sister's high-heeled shoes . . .
> While I wait,
> I'm the only man who loves me.
> They call me "Star"
> because I listen
> to their dreams and wishes.
> But grief is darker.
> it is a wig
> that does not rest gently
> on my head.

Essex, Wayson, and Michelle continued to work collaboratively, but
one theater piece, due to be performed in Brooklyn, produced conflict
between the two men. Apparently at some point Essex insisted ("adamantly," according to Wayson) that Wayson quit his day job, move in
with him to save money, and that the two devote themselves full-time
to becoming artists. The idea was "way too much" for Wayson; he
"couldn't imagine not having a regular paycheck—I had absolutely no
talent for frugality," he humorously admits. With hindsight, he acknowledges that he was also afraid of being "totally subsumed" in Essex's vision. Wayson felt that Essex was "the most ambitious person
I've ever known, and had a backbone of steel." His response to Wayson's hesitation was to tell him that he "needed to grow a spine." If he
had, Wayson later wryly commented, that would have produced still
more conflict in their relationship.

Though the two men continued to care deeply for each other, the
rift led Essex to announce that he wouldn't do the planned performance in Brooklyn—wouldn't even call the theater to tell them so.
Wayson placed the call instead, canceling the gig. But it made him feel
humiliated and put out. It reminded him of the time he got busted
when, at Essex's request, he tried to score some pot for him in Merid-
ian Hill (now Malcolm X) Park; Essex had never even offered sympathy to Wayson for the scrape he'd gotten him in—which led Wayson

to tell Essex that he was "very full of himself" and "an arrogant bastard." Cancellation of the Brooklyn gig led to "a major falling-out" between the two men that lasted for about a year: "We kind of had a little alienation thing going on there for a while," is how Wayson later put it—"in fact, we had bookings for the two of us that we couldn't stand to be around each other enough to fulfill. One of which, I think, was at the Kitchen in New York. So he did those with other people. . . . We were sort of walking on eggshells with each other at that point."

But the two men did finally have what Essex called "a very positive airing out, a refueling of our focus." Essex ended up feeling certain that Wayson "is truly a 'brother' to me and I only hope to be as much for him." Reflecting today on their temporary estrangement, Wayson is honorably frank in acknowledging that it hadn't helped their relationship that as Essex's reputation as a poet continued to grow over time, "the instrumental music aspect of our collaboration became less significant." It helped even less when Essex at one point suggested that Wayson tone down the volume of the music so that the poems could be more clearly heard.

The assertive, feisty side of Essex's personality dated as far back as childhood. On one occasion, after being badly teased by some neighborhood kids, he went to the second floor of the Hemphill house, pulled down his pants, and through the window mooned the boys below, shouting that they could kiss his ass. He got a whipping but felt it was worth it. Essex was especially likely to flare up in anger when he perceived an assault on his dignity or on the integrity of his work. Meticulous and exacting about all aspects of how and where he presented his poetry, he did (as one acquaintance puts it) "butt heads" if details for a presentation were overlooked or sloppily organized.

Far more dangerously—for his own safety—Essex would fiercely react to any suggestion of racism on the part of authority figures. In D.C.'s Union Station, he was once stopped by a police officer while traveling to fulfill a public engagement—stopped simply because he was dressed in jeans, a down jacket, and a Raiders baseball cap—in other words, as Essex put it, "in the standard attire of what we will call the 'butch queen' look, the home-boy look, the look of the ghetto." He boldly, adamantly refused to cooperate with the officer or to allow himself to be searched for drugs or weapons. He told the officer to search the white women and men in the station first, and loudly accused him of harassment. When a white man in a suit handed Essex his business card, suggesting he would testify for him in court, the officer nervously relented and let Essex go. It was a narrow, and highly atypical, escape for a black gay man. "You don't mess with Essex," became a byword.

Despite his deserved reputation for feistiness, Essex, as Wayson has put it, "had a very warm, gentle, and nurturing side." As an example, he offers Essex's treatment of his younger brother, Warren (called "Dimp"— for his dimples). Though they'd had considerable conflict with each other while growing up, Essex did all he could to encourage Dimp's ambition to become a singer, and asked Wayson to work with him. Wayson tried but found Dimp's ambition greater than his talent—and somehow found a diplomatic way of conveying that to both brothers. Wayson was touched at Essex's effort to help his brother. To him it was emblematic of his friend's "boyish, sweet side," the side he felt "that many people probably never saw."

Their relationship restored, the two men continued to work together for several more years, often joined by Michelle. Probably the most impressive of their collaborative efforts would come in 1987, when Gerry Givnish, head of the prestigious Painted Bride Art Center in Philadelphia, invited the three to present a collage of performed poems and stories, which they called *Voicescapes*. Together they created their own lighting and stage design, with (in Wayson's words) a minimalist "postapocalyptic feel" (days were spent painting huge chunks of Styrofoam orange, leading Michelle to swear off the color forever). The piece opened with a slide montage of people telling their own stories in 30-second slide/poems put together by Sharon Farmer, Leigh Mosley, and Ron Simmons. Other poems with different themes followed, many of them performed "in a ripple-style syncopation or in unison as a recitation . . . with music providing an effective poetic transition." *Voicescapes* drew considerable praise, the reviewer in *High Performance* describing the evening as "highly engrossing . . . dramatic performances par excellence and a rhythmic choreography of movement, sight and sound." In 1989 *Voicescapes* would be successfully repeated, once again at the Painted Bride.

During this same period, and sparked by poet and playwright Garth Tate, six black male poets formed the group Station to Station. It became a wonderful incubator for Essex and others to try out differ-

ent styles for reading poetry aloud. Among other efforts, Essex utilized Wayson's music to add live synthesized sound to some of the
poems he performed in public. Yet after a time, a certain amount of
friction developed and Essex dropped out of Station to Station. Chris
Prince, another member and one of Essex's friends, ascribes the friction to Essex's demand that the group recite more gay-themed poetry.
Several members weren't gay and several others weren't "out." Chris
ascribes Essex's insistence to his "thick-headed, fierce" side; he could,
like his mother, Mantalene, become stubbornly uncompromising when
convinced, rightly or wrongly, that some important principle was at
stake. As Ron Simmons, another close friend of his, has put it, "sometimes Essex was difficult to get along with."

Absorbed though they were in honing their artistic abilities, Essex
and his friends did manage to spare time and energy for political work.
The D.C. Coalition of Black Gays and Lesbians had transformed itself
into the National Coalition of Black Lesbians and Gays, and according to Renee McCoy, herself active in the Coalition, Essex "provided
significant support and guidance when we were building" the group.
Though he wasn't temperamentally well suited to the give-and-take of
organizational work, he and Michelle as early as 1983 did show up for
an ad hoc meeting to plan for a black arts component to D.C.'s annual
gay pride celebration. On that occasion, a variety of artists and writers
each performed a kind of "audition," and Jim Marks (who thinks he
"may have been covering the meeting for the *Blade*"), remembers listening "to the first few poets thinking that their work consisted primarily of hackneyed 'he done me wrong' self-involved efforts." Then
it was Essex's turn. He began by reading a brief obituary from the
Washington Blade for a murdered street transvestite/prostitute, and
then performed the dramatic monologue he'd written in her voice.
Recalling the event, Jim says, "it still raises the hair on my neck."
Michelle read as well, and Jim felt that the two "were clearly head and
shoulders above the other poets there." Unfortunately, there was
no follow-up meeting—and apparently no arts component to the gay
pride march.

In regard to both the National Coalition of Black Gays and Lesbians and the meeting about the gay pride celebration, Michelle has
made the important point that "there wasn't so much of that social separation, that hard-core, entrenched kind of division between lesbians

and gay men" in D.C.'s black community as was found among white gay activists during this period. Additionally, during the 1980s there was a kind of cooperative New York–D.C. connection among artists, performers, and writers. Isaac Jackson, for instance, the New York City experimental videographer—who was also managing editor of the *Blackheart* collective that included writers David Frechette, Assotto Saint, and Colin Robinson—helped Michelle out with the research for her film *Stormé* (about Stormé DeLarverie, the only female member of Harlem's legendary drag "Jewel Box Review"). "Not that women didn't have their own spaces and the brothers didn't have theirs," Michelle says, "but we were more or less together." Occasionally, allied white people also became involved—like Mary Farmer, who ran Lammas Books, or Deacon Maccubbin, who would offer his Lambda Rising bookstore as a place to have book signings.

Michelle sums up the mounting fervor and excitement in black gay circles: "We were beginning to put flesh on the bones of our gay identities . . . our black gay identities . . . and seeing those as primary voices from which we wrote, spoke, and were politicized."

2

Reading the Signs

Having made some friends and begun psychotherapy, and in general feeling far more settled in New York than earlier, Mike decided to take the initiative and try to set things right with his parents. He wrote them at length and with the kind of blind candor that he characteristically admired in others and aimed for in his own close relationships: "My primary purpose is to *communicate*. To clean up our relationship." He made it clear at the top that he had no intention of "trying to prove worthy" of their love. He already had his mother's—that much he knew—and it was to his father that he mostly addressed his complaints. Clifford, his son felt, was by nature a loner, reluctant to express affection. Mike wanted more from him. He wanted his father to talk openly—"talk to me about your joys; your terrors; your plans for a happy future" (Clifford was in the throes of thinking about retirement). Above all, he wanted a more extended dialogue with both his parents about the pivotal fact of his being gay.[1]

Mike did his best to approach the subject with a straightforward sharing of his own feelings. He'd been hurt, he made clear, that when his parents recently visited him in New York and Mike had tried to broach the topic, his father had pointedly said that he did not want to discuss it, nor—when Mike suggested a book or two on the subject—did he wish to read about it. But Mike, ever persistent, wanted to share with his parents the exhilarating joy he'd felt during the National Gay March on Washington, the sense that change was happening "at a mind-boggling pace. The eighties," Mike presciently predicted, "would be the out decade"—it would, but for reasons Mike could never have imagined.

He wanted his parents to know, too, that he was about to quit his job at Bradford "and risk all to try to make a go of it as a singer." He'd saved up enough money to buy a piano and some sound equipment for his new apartment on Jones Street in the West Village, had made a few tapes that had impressed people, and had already hooked up with a musical director who believed in him.

In response, Clifford made an effort to meet Mike's entreaty that he be more expressive and honest about his feelings. He admitted flat out that he'd felt "anxiety, anger, hurt, and disappointment" when Mike revealed his "choice of lifestyle." And Clifford used the word "choice" deliberately: "You consciously and freely chose your lifestyle with the full realization and knowledge that the relationship of family and most friends would be adversely affected" and, moreover, that "conventional religious practices" would be "precluded" and "any service toward your nation would be severely limited."

And that was for starters. Clifford felt that no conflict need arise when the family gathered, since he felt it "unlikely we will spend large blocks of time together." When they did see each other, furthermore, he didn't feel that it was "asking for the moon" to expect Mike to "play it straight." If Mike felt the effort would be too "draining," then the solution Clifford suggested was to "minimize contact. . . . I shall continue to try to prove 'worthy' of *your* love; if you do not wish to reciprocate, then do not." He ended with his version of an upbeat note: he thought Mike talented and intelligent but he, Clifford, wasn't "comfortable with the public, physical expression of love."

Mike responded with a generosity bordering on sainthood. "I was overcome with emotion," he wrote back. He felt that his father had given him exactly what he'd asked for: "honesty and directness"—two qualities that Mike held most dear. "For the first time," he went on, you "articulated your feelings for me." That, Mike felt, was grounds for hope about their future relationship. However—Mike was about to demonstrate just as much steel as Clifford—there could be no question about trying to act "straight." To do so would be to deny who he was and, further, to corroborate the common view that there was something wrong with being gay—"as if there is something to admit—something hidden and dark and secretive and dirty."

He asked his father to imagine "a society where [his own] love was viewed as a 'strange and unnatural act,' or a 'crime against nature.' . . . Since you don't know what 'caused' your sexual direction, I suggest you stop flailing about trying to figure out what 'caused' mine. . . . Quite frankly, I just like to think I was lucky. . . . gay people are clued in at an early age to the duplicity in all things . . . [and] have a unique perspective that make us particularly adept at art." Mike wasn't merely defending his gayness as normal, he was suggesting that it might well be superior—politically, intuitively, and aesthetically. Overstatement was a common ingredient in the early rhetoric of gay liberation, a trope Mike indulged in with glee, viewing it as necessary compensation for the disparagement of gay lives that had long been common currency. After the extended reign and deep internalization of homophobic self-hatred, affirmation for Mike and others surfaced in the form of strenuous counterclaims. Hyperbole was a strategy for liberation, not itself liberation.

Joe Sonnabend wasn't the only doctor in the early 1980s puzzling over some of his patients' unusual symptoms. Alvin Friedman-Kien, a virologist at New York University Medical Center, was so surprised when the biopsies from two of his gay male patients' "bruises" came back from the lab with the diagnosis of Kaposi's sarcoma (KS) that he asked some of his colleagues if they'd seen anything comparable. Within a few weeks he learned of twenty such cases. A call to a San Francisco colleague, Marcus Conant, brought the total to twenty-six. In Los Angeles several doctors reported a slew of puzzling symptoms: diarrhea and "wasting," chronic fevers, thrush, swollen lymph nodes, and a decline in CD4 cells. Something was clearly in the wind, something awful. But not everyone was alarmed. One member of the gay doctors' organization Bay Area Physicians for Human Rights asserted that peculiar symptomatologies appeared more often than people realized—and just as quickly disappeared. Jim Curran of the CDC also sounded an optimistic note, and New York City's most widely read gay newspaper, *New York Native*, initially published a piece largely dismissive of the earlier alarmist *Morbidity and Mortality* reports.[2]

45

One San Francisco physician suspected the culprit was cytomega-lovirus (CMV), a herpes virus that can produce disease in those with impaired immune function. Joe Sonnabend, on his own, had also suspected CMV and theorized that those of his patients—like Mike— with a repetitive history of STDs had overloaded and compromised their immune systems, thereby allowing the virus to take hold. Sonna-bend saw a certain consistency in the personal histories of all his patients who came in with symptoms of anal gonorrhea, herpes, CMV, fissures, and warts—all were self-described "bottoms" (their primary sexual pleasure was getting fucked), and all showed signs of immune deficiency. One out of three gay men were shedding CMV in their sperm and urine—as opposed to one out of twenty heterosexual men— and CMV was known to be immunosuppressive. So said not merely Sonnabend, but in the early years of the epidemic, the most respected scientific journals, including the *Lancet*, the *New England Journal of Medicine*, and the *Annals of Internal Medicine*.

Sonnabend felt certain that it was going to take years to sort out the complex symptomologies and causative factors. He also felt early on that some people might have a certain degree of genetic protection against immunological assaults. One early finding that suggested ge-netic variables was that those gay men with tissue type HLA-DR3 were more prone to get Pneumocystis carinii pneumonia (PCP), and those with tissue type HLA-DR5 were more likely to develop KS. Given all the variables, it seemed to follow that there would never be one formula, one explanation, for charting the progression of the mys-terious new disease. Sonnabend also insisted early on—and this gave Mike a great deal of hope—that a decline in the immune system's T4 cells was *not* tantamount to an inexorable death sentence (though it would be a number of years before the importance of a high level of T8 suppressor cells would be recognized as essential to warding off infections).

One day when Mike was in Sonnabend's office, legs in the stirrups so Joe could check for anal warts, his assistant came in to tell him that he had a call from a scientist in Japan. Mike was impressed and dutifully waited for Joe to come back. And waited. He was used to Joe's delays but not when his legs were up in the air. Finally pulling on his pants, Mike started to wander around the office. When he bent over the typewriter, he saw the final page of an article in progress that Joe had been working on—a "multifactorial model" to explain the bizarre and mounting number of gay men who were falling ill. At least two other infectious disease researchers were tentatively suggesting that a bombardment of sexually transmitted infections might be responsible for the drastic weakening of the body's immunodefensive capabilities.[3]

Mike sat down and read the entire article. As he later wrote, with characteristic hyperbole, "it changed my life." When Joe finally returned, outspoken Mike told him straight out that he had to publish the article in the gay press, had to get it out quickly so that people could be warned; it was "a moral imperative." Joe halfheartedly protested that it was a highly technical piece, and besides, he had no journalistic contacts. Mike volunteered to write up the material in everyday language and also to get it into the *New York Native*. Ethically, he insisted, it was essential to reach people with the double message: if you stop having multiple sexual encounters and change your behavior, you'll stop getting STDs—and you'll save your life. Joe thought for a second, then said, "I have another patient who feels the same way you do. Maybe if the two of you meet, you can do something." It was August 1982.

The "other patient" was Richard ("Rich") Berkowitz. Born the same year as Callen, he'd grown up in a working-class Jewish family in New Jersey and had come out sexually in his early teens. Hard up for money, and blessed with Italianate good looks that fueled his self-confidence, Rich had started to hustle while still in college at Rutgers. Though he came on as "know-it-all arrogant," he was well aware that his strutting, "I'm in charge" machismo covered over the fear of being called a "faggot" even as it served as a magnet for the increasing numbers of paying customers who came to him for S/M sex.[4]

Berkowitz's bank account was growing nicely and his apartment was filling up with the harnesses, cock rings, studded belts, and boots that his adoring customers lavished on him. He was good at what he did, and he understood "why it was difficult for men to reveal the human desire to relinquish control in sex because it transgressed our culture's definition of what it meant to be a man in much the same way that homosexuality did." Rich was rarely bored, rarely broke, and rarely at a loss to come up with an erotic fantasy that would satisfy his multiplying list of loyal, repeat clients. He loved the easy money and the flexible hours.

Better still, his customers rarely asked Rich himself to reach climax, which freed him up after work to enjoy his own sexual revolution, to cruise the bars, prowl the abandoned piers off West Street in the Village for outdoor sex, and, when the famed Saint disco opened in 1980, to dance with several thousand other muscled, shirtless, drugged young men under the laser lights of the "planetarium-like" ceiling and then to fuck until dawn in the balcony overhanging the dance floor. But Rich was smart as well as hot; he did his best to come only at the baths—where at least you could shower between partners, thus reducing the risk of catching STDs and passing them on to his partners or his regular clients.

He did sometimes wonder what had ever happened to his belief in the early gay liberation ideal of androgyny—men and women sharing the traits that society arbitrarily parceled out to one gender or the other—or to the little kid who'd been frightened of any suggestion of violence, or to the initial movement slogan he'd joined in chanting about "men *loving* men." He felt certain that S/M and love could co-exist and were not mutually exclusive, but he did wonder what the consequences would be of having let the hunt for sexual pleasure eclipse the activism he and many of his friends had been involved in before they let themselves become demoralized and cynical about politics following Reagan's election in 1980.

He worried, too, that despite his efforts at risk reduction, he was paying more frequent visits to Dr. Sonnabend's office to get treated for this or that STD. Rich knew, after all, that he was basically "a germophobic, hygiene-obsessed Jewish boy." After he finally came down with a severe case of hepatitis, Sonnabend quietly read him the riot act about further changing his behavior and gave him a pile of medical papers and journals to take home and read. "I need to get the message out," Joe told him. "I have another patient interested in helping. Perhaps you should meet him." As it would later turn out, Rich had a sky-high T8 cell count that—despite a nasty spell with crack cocaine in the mideighties, from which he eventually recovered—kept him free of opportunistic infections until 1995; he remains very much alive today and in 2003 published a memoir, *Stayin' Alive*.

Rich jumped at Joe's suggestion, eager to lend a hand in getting Joe's findings published. A significant number of medical articles had been appearing since the initial CDC and *New York Times* accounts, including a series of detailed reports in the *New England Journal of Medicine*. It seemed increasingly clear that the most important marker in these strange cases of immune suppression in gay men was a decline in "helper" (or CD4) cells, though the reason for the deficiency remained unknown. The picture became additionally confused when a few cases were discovered among heterosexuals, including one woman. They were mostly intravenous drug users and their partners. As far back as 1979, moreover, a Bronx pediatrician had reported a number of "inexplicable infections among the children of drug users." Nonetheless, clinicians and researchers continued to speak of the spreading *gay* disease—to the point where, by early 1982, the label GRID (Gay-Related Immune Deficiency) had become affixed.[5]

This was tantamount to declaring that homosexual behavior was the key risk factor; the more one engaged in it, the greater one's chances of contracting the disease. There was no disputing the fact that it was mostly gay men who were falling ill. But the *equation* of homosexuality with disease ignored the diversity of current gay male "lifestyles"—to say nothing of the near total absence of the "gay" plague among lesbians. Yes, some gay men had hundreds or even thousands of sexual contacts, but many others were either monogamous or, for varying periods, celibate. The comparatively small subset of gay men who came down with STDs or with GRID were not inherently "immoral"—was it the number of orgasms or the number of partners that critics objected to?—nor was this statistically small group synonymous with *the* gay lifestyle. (In fact only one of the first four cases seen in L.A. had a sexual history that might accurately be called "promiscuous.") Besides, promiscuity among heterosexuals, ever since the pill had become available, was hardly unknown.[6]

What did become clear early on was that the country in general, and the federal government in particular, was simultaneously bent on ignoring or condemning GRID and those who had it. The pious Jerry Falwells of the land were quick to raise their gleeful voices in praise of God's judgment against the "wicked practice" of homosexuality, while the Reagan administration bent its energies not to expanding health and social services to the afflicted but to cutting them. Diseases relating to sex have long been viewed in Western culture as the result of divine retribution. As Peter Lewis Allen has demonstrated in his splendid comparative study, *The Wages of Sin: Sex and Disease, Past and Present*, the link between "debauchery" (variously defined) and punishment has a long history in the West, with "unbridled lust" widely cited by physicians and clerics alike as attributable to everything from leprosy to syphilis to bubonic plague.[7]

Allen makes the additional and crucial point that the latest plague would be marked—as none had been previously—by the afflicted banding together and beginning to see themselves as "a group of people defined by their illness and entitled to rights because of it." In the same way that Mike Callen, Joe Sonnabend, and Rich Berkowitz were on the verge of combining their resources, others, too, were beginning to realize that they need not sit passively by while their country abandoned them. They could unify and become proactive in their own behalf.

In San Francisco, a group of activists formed the Kaposi's Sarcoma Research and Education Foundation (which later became the San Francisco AIDS Foundation). In August 1981, following President Reagan's proposal to make sharp cuts in the budgets of both the CDC and the National Institutes of Health (NIH)—even in the face of the growing likelihood that a significant epidemic was in the wings—eighty men gathered in the New York City apartment of the gay writer Larry Kramer to hear Dr. Alvin Friedman-Kien describe the crisis and to try to raise funds for researching the new disease and possible treatments for it. That night they raised a little over $6,500; the Gay Men's Health Crisis (GMHC) had been born.

Rich read through the materials Joe Sonnabend had given him and promptly contacted Mike Callen. His initial impression was that Mike was "queeny," but after they talked, he found in him "a calming thread of sanity." They agreed with Sonnabend's emphasis on a multifactorial model for explaining what would soon be called AIDS, though none of the three ruled out the possibility—which other researchers, including the CDC, were beginning to lean toward—that a single new killer virus, as yet unidentified, was the culprit. Even if that view was confirmed, Mike and Berkowitz felt that Sonnabend's ideas should be circulated widely in the community and debated. And the best way to do that was to write an article for *New York Native*, one that would eschew the technical language of the medical journals and be understandable to the average gay man.[8]

That was the task Rich and Mike set for themselves. Every gay man they met who'd come down with the syndrome turned out to have a sexual history similar to their own: namely, multiple partners followed by multiple STDs. Both agreed with Sonnabend's view that sexually transmitted diseases had a cumulative and weakening effect on the immune system, and both were determined to become active in their own behalf. Mike, while in college, had begun to read and be influenced by feminist literature, including early critiques of the health system ("just because somebody says they're looking out for your best interest doesn't mean that they are").

And both, finally, were determined to change their own behavior. When drawing the connection between repetitive sexually transmitted infections and the weakening of the immune system, Joe Sonnabend insisted that he was drawing a *factual* connection that he'd found among those of his patients who came down with the disease. But, he also insisted, "it's got nothing to do with judgment" of the behavior involved. Sonnabend explicitly separated himself from the disapproving view Larry Kramer had taken in his notorious 1978 novel, *Faggots*, in which he'd deplored and deprecated the promiscuous sexual behavior of the fast-track gay male lifestyle. Sonnabend was widely and wrongfully accused of sharing Kramer's moral disapproval of multiple, anonymous partners.

Mike, nonetheless, decided on temporary celibacy for himself, and Rich decided to kick out his S/M clientele. Mike also vowed to get on with his career—or with his hopes for one. He became a soloist with the New York City Gay Men's Chorus and told himself that "however much time I have left to live, what I really want to do is be openly gay and sing gay music." He managed to get a few solo cabaret dates, but then decided to try to form a rock band.

To that end, he placed an ad in *New York Native* looking for musicians. Pam Brandt, a lesbian musician who'd been in a somewhat successful all-women's trio called The Deadly Nightshade, and a drummer named Richard Dworkin, formerly with the San Francisco–based band Buena Vista, responded. They met in Mike's studio apartment at Jones and Bleecker Streets, which had a small kitchen, wall-to-wall carpeting, an upright piano, a small Yamaha sound system—and no furniture, except for two fold-up director's chairs and a typing table. Mike made sherbet, then they ordered Chinese food, chatted pleasantly for a while, tried out a little music, and soon agreed to work together. They subsequently named themselves—after considering

The Amoeba Farts, The Scandells, and Take Back the Nitrites—Lowlife. Mike insisted on gender parity for the group and guitarist Janet Cleary soon joined them. Lowlife, for some two years, would play various clubs, blending an infectious variety of styles with between-the-songs banter that, as one critic put it, "never loses sight of the group's gay roots."

That first night, Pam went home after their initial discussion. Richard knew he was interested in something more, and stayed.

Mike sensed it too. Never reticent, always direct, he told Richard that same night that he had "it." Richard shrugged. Years later, Richard thought that he'd never have become involved with Mike if his own father hadn't committed suicide when he was ten years old—it had given him the double sense that all deep relationships were transient and that the death of a loved one was familiar and could be survived. Besides, he found Mike charming, warm and funny, big-hearted, genuinely interested in people, and gifted with a remarkable capacity for drawing out almost anyone within half an hour into a sort of "conspiratorial intimacy."

Richard had an unorthodox background. His parents—so different from Mike's—were confirmed atheists, and when he was barely out of his teens, Richard had helped run a failed city council campaign in Minneapolis. He'd then lived on a commune in rural Minnesota and spent most of the 1970s in San Francisco, where he attended the Conservatory of Music and played free jazz with various gay musicians, including Blackberri, Steven Grossman, the Angels of Light, and the gay male rock/soul band Buena Vista, which was featured in the pioneering documentary *Word Is Out*. He also met Jim Fouratt—well known in the 1980s as the co-founder of Danceteria, which became one of the most popular downtown nightclubs in New York City—who encouraged Richard to move east and for a few months gave him a place to stay. Richard felt that his whole time in San Francisco somehow contributed to his willingness to get involved with Mike—some sense about the wildness and spontaneity of life, about following unexpected impulses, about valuing the inconclusive, the impermanent.

A week after the two met—in late June 1982—Mike was hospitalized with cryptosporidium, formally diagnosed with GRID, and told that he had six months to live. From the time Mike's T-helper cells had first been tested in 1981, he never had a count of more than 200, and he had consistently high levels of CMV, which was known to be immunosuppressive. Sonnabend immediately put him on two double-strength Bactrim tablets daily to prevent Pneumocystis pneumonia (PCP). It was a crucial decision: Mike would never develop the often-fatal pneumonia. Yet more than thirty thousand would die of the preventable disease in the years to come, simply because the CDC and the medical community failed to prescribe Bactrim as a prophylaxis. Many could have been saved had federal agencies formally announced—as the CDC finally did in 1989—that a daily dose of Bactrim should be the standard of care for patients at risk.

There was no excuse for the seven-year delay: Bactrim was hardly an unknown, recondite, or expensive drug. It was readily available as a cheap generic product in 1981–82 and had been frequently used to prevent PCP in other kinds of immunocompromised hosts—for example, in kidney transplant patients. (Sonnabend, when part of the infectious diseases service at Downstate Medical Center in the 1970s, had had experience in its renal unit.) The CDC and the NIH's failure to recommend it for GRID/AIDS patients seemed to both Joe and Mike, in Joe's words, "a glaring example of a discriminatory response—that is, its selective denial to gay people . . . of the brutal indifference of federal health officials." Many years later, he would express "bewilderment" at "the trust placed in authorities representing institutions that had such an abysmal record regarding concerns for the health of minorities."

Many AIDS patients, out of understandable panic to do *something*, would increasingly grasp at a variety of rumored cures. As underground networks and buyers clubs began to spring up to get hold of any drug thought to be effective, the list would grow long: ribavirin (which had been used in Europe and Mexico against various viral diseases); suramin (which produced no rise in CD4 cells but led to unintended and dangerous adrenal insufficiency); HPA-23, acyclovir, imuthiol, and dextran sulfate in various combinations. All were equally ineffective. Other patients underwent chemotherapy and full-body radiation, submitted to bone-marrow transplants and high-dose regimens of interferon, attached themselves to spiritual guides, or swallowed vast quantities of herbal compounds. Mike stuck to Sonnabend's advice: except for taking Bactrim, which was known to work against PCP, avoid all the touted drugs du jour.[9]

53

During his June 1982 hospitalization, Mike was surprised to get a visit from the undemonstrative, reserved Richard Dworkin, the new drummer in his rock group. The visit meant a great deal to Mike and cemented the two men's initial attraction to each other. After Mike's release from the hospital, they began to date and soon became lovers. It was one of those miraculous cases of "hooked atoms." Richard was as dependable and principled as Mike, but far less histrionic and verbal. Taciturn and forceful, he was Mike's ideal version of a "top." As he once put it, "Richard never had the history of self-torture for feeling different that I, early a sissy, always felt." He would bring a solid strength to Mike's life, much-needed ballast for the storms that lay ahead.

By this point in his life, Mike had had lots of sex, but never a lover. For brief periods, he'd had a boyfriend—the psychologist Richard Pillard in Boston, and in New York City a cop named George. With Richard, sex became something of an issue. Labeled terminally ill due to sexually transmitted infection, Mike now began to associate sex with disease and death, not love. He also had very specific health issues, like anal fissures, which in these early days of AIDS and the widespread fear of contagion, doctors were reluctant to treat surgically. The result, as Richard put it, was that "our sex life was not everything I wished it could be." Mike said the same and more to close friends like Abby Tallmer, a young lesbian and recent graduate of Vassar who began working full-time in Sonnabend's office in May 1983. She became especially close to Mike, with whom she shared a campy wit, a relish for sexual candor and gossip, and a deep concern for social justice. According to Abby, Mike expressed sadness and regret that he and Richard couldn't indulge fully in the anal sex both preferred.

Adding to the problem was Mike's image of himself as essentially nonmonogamous. "I'm really a whore," he told Abby. "I am built to be a whore—or fate and circumstance made me a whore. Once a whore—always a whore." Richard seemed to be exactly the sort of man he thought he'd been looking for: "He's really nice, he likes to fuck, and he's a musician, and there are all these reasons why I should stay with him. But I also was on the lookout for reasons to *not* stay with him." Mike decided that the problem was his, and he had "a couple of intense weeks—almost psychotic—of 'I don't really love him.'" But the feeling passed.

Besides, Mike was dumbfounded that Richard, who was in good health, would choose to get sexually involved with someone possibly contagious and probably fatally ill. With typical directness, Mike simply asked him—and was amazed at Richard's matter-of-fact response: "I'm a gay man living in New York City. I'm going to have to deal with this disease sooner or later. I may as well begin now." Richard, too, had had numerous partners in the past—though he couldn't match Mike's high numbers—yet he'd had few sexually transmitted diseases and didn't have a compromised immune system.

It was at just this critical juncture—July 1982—that the CDC released new findings that further muddied the waters. Within a two-week period the CDC announced three cases of PCP among hemophiliacs and thirty-four cases of Kaposi's sarcoma among Haitians living in the United States. The CDC offered no commentary to accompany the figures, but obviously the "gay disease" had now been found in several other populations and wasn't strictly confined to gay people. Reactions ranged from excitement to rage. The excitement was mostly felt by gay men relieved of the singular onus for the plague (the term "GRID" quickly gave way to acquired immune deficiency syndrome, or AIDS) and hopeful that a substantial rise in federal funding and research would follow. The rage was felt among hemophiliacs who had previously assumed that the blood supply was uncontaminated, and among Haitians for being unfairly singled out for discrimination. AIDS had also been found in Denmark in 1981, but that was all but unmentioned, as Haiti—in a clear case of racism—was highlighted. Within a few months, the Haitian Coalition on AIDS was founded to challenge, successfully, the designation of Haitians as a risk group.[10]

With Mike's health improved, he and Rich Berkowitz set to work on the Sonnabend-inspired article. It took three months to complete and Mike, ever the perfectionist, was ready for yet another rewrite until Rich called a halt by pointing out that the number of diagnosed cases in New York City had doubled from three hundred to six hundred during the time they'd been at work. They entitled the piece "We Know Who We Are," and it appeared in the November 8–21, 1982, issue of *New York Native* with a byline that added "with Richard Dworkin" to Callen and Berkowitz. It minced no words: "Few have been willing to say it so clearly, but the single greatest risk factor for contracting AIDS is a history of multiple sexual contacts with partners who are having multiple sexual contacts."

"Other factors may contribute," they acknowledged later in the piece, but went on to insist that to date "no evidence supports" speculation about a new or mutant virus. It was true that the CDC had found a cluster of nine gay men who'd had sexual contact only with one another over a five-year period, and yet each man had developed Kaposi's— thus suggesting that a virus, not promiscuity, was centrally involved. Yet in a footnote, the CDC had acknowledged that the nine "tended to report having more sexual partners in the year before onset of symptoms (median: 50)." As for hemophiliacs, the U.S. blood supply comes of course from many different donors with many different viruses, and "continual re-exposure and re-infection" over the years may have weakened the recipients' immune systems. In regard to the infected Haitians, CDC scientists reasoned that in the course of frequent visits to and from the island, with its poor sanitary conditions, they may have picked up "a variety of tropical viruses."

Mike and Rich argued in their article that "whichever theory you accept, promiscuity is the way AIDS is being spread among gay men"; they specifically cited, as did a number of specialists in the early years, the known fact that repeated re-infection with a common herpes virus—cytomegalovirus (CMV)—"produced a mild sperm-induced immunosuppression." Both were forthright about acknowledging in the piece their own sexually active histories and went to great lengths to avoid being misunderstood as saying that there was something inherently wrong with having a large number of sexual contacts. Not only did they still believe in sexual liberation, they argued, but they were *not* suggesting *legislating* an end to promiscuity—like passing laws to close the baths or back-room bars. *The* underlying cause of AIDS, they insisted, was homophobia: "Hatred has forced too many of us into the ghetto of the bathhouse circuit . . . disease settings equivalent to those of poor Third World nations, and junkies."

Instead, Rich and Mike called for "sexual alternatives"—like " 'fuck buddies' . . . circles of healthy individuals who can be trusted to limit their sexual contacts to members of that closed group"—until greater understanding of AIDS and treatments for it had developed: "The epidemic of AIDS need not result in abstinence or even monogamy

for everyone. Not everyone who wishes to discuss alternatives to promiscuity," they insisted, "is sex-negative or a sexual fascist."

Their article caused an immediate uproar. It should be remembered
that in November 1982—just one year into the U.S. epidemic—a significant number of gay men were still in denial about both how extensive and how lethal the plague could become. Thanks to assorted CDC
reports, there was also a fairly widespread conviction, bordering in
some quarters on hope, that heterosexuals would become infected in
mounting numbers. It was a message that the new organization the
Gay Men's Health Crisis (GMHC) eagerly promoted in the expectation that it would prompt the federal government and the medical establishment to respond with a massive research effort and a quick
cure—since heterosexual lives *mattered*.

At the time, GMHC, under the conservative leadership of Paul
Popham, a Republican gay man and ex-marine, had in an "educational"
brochure only gone so far as to say that the disease *might* be sexually
transmitted. David Goodstein, the even more conservative owner of the
national gay magazine *The Advocate*, expressed far more concern about
the rise of the Religious Right than about "the gay cancer." At the end
of 1982 he listed AIDS as ninth among the top ten stories affecting
homosexuals that year. As for most of the national media—the *Boston
Globe* and National Public Radio were among the few exceptions—they
either entirely ignored or profoundly downplayed the mounting health
threat. It wasn't until May 31, 1982, that an American newspaper, the
Los Angeles Times, ran a front-page story about the disease now known as
AIDS. And during all of that year, the three major television networks
devoted a combined total of thirteen minutes to the epidemic, though
853 people had already died from it.

Not even the countercultural *Village Voice* had opened up its pages.
Dr. Lawrence Mass had been consistently providing reliably sober
articles for *New York Native* about the epidemic, but the *Native* had
only fourteen thousand regular readers in a city with an estimated gay
population of six hundred thousand to a million. Since the *Native*'s
circulation was only about 10 percent of the *Village Voice*'s, Mass submitted an article there in an effort to reach a larger audience. He was
turned down on the grounds that "it isn't a *Voice* piece."

Given the general climate of dismissiveness and denial, Mike and
Rich could have logically expected little or no reaction to their own

article. But they'd been so deeply engaged with the epidemic and knew so many young men who'd been afflicted (both were members of the first AIDS support group, which met weekly) that they felt and hoped that the piece might have real impact. It did—but not in the way they intended. The response was almost entirely negative, the prime objection being that they'd turned their backs on the sexual revolution and joined forces with Larry Kramer, who in his 1978 novel *Faggots* had famously and controversially excoriated gay male "promiscuity."[11]

Charles Jurrist, a dance critic for the *New York Daily News*, published a retaliatory article, "In Defense of Promiscuity," in the *Native* accusing Mike and Rich of "the unleashing of hysteria." Only 716 cases of AIDS had been reliably documented, he argued, and many more people than that "were injured or killed last year in automobile accidents." After all, he wrote, "life can't be made risk-free. . . . You can't very well ask every man you meet to go for $400 worth of laboratory tests and give you a notarized copy of the results before you'll go to bed with him." He intended, Jurrist went on, to lead his life pretty much as he had been: "I will continue to be 'promiscuous.' I won't be scared out of seeking fulfillment. Nor will I consider my behavior in any way as self-destructive." Jurrist died from AIDS in 1991.

In the *Native*, Dr. Peter Seitzman, president of the New York Physicians for Human Rights, agreed with Mike and Rich that "it is the number of *different partners* that increases risk, not the amount of sex itself," but he objected to the "vehement" tone they'd employed and accused them of "shout[ing] guilt . . . from the rooftops." In the *Advocate*, Nathan Fain, a GMHC board member, similarly claimed that Rich and Mike were urging gay men to "follow along in self-flagellation." And even Dr. Lawrence Mass joined the chorus of contempt, inaccurately accusing them of linking hands with the Religious Right in demanding that the baths be closed down.

Nor was the negative reaction confined to New York. A number of the early male leaders of gay rights activism, including Marty Robinson and Jim Owles in New York, Morris Kight in L.A., and Frank Kameny in D.C., actively and publicly resisted any suggestion that recreational sex could be linked with disease. In Toronto, the radical paper *Body Politic* published a piece by Michael Lynch and Dr. Bill Lewis denouncing the efforts of some gay men to "rip apart the very promiscuous fabric that knits the gay male community together. . . . Gays are once again allowing the medical profession to define, restrict, pathologize us." Such a response was perhaps understandable, given the fact that the medical community had for generations pathologized gay people, but it was also a misunderstanding of Mike and Rich's basic argument. In a sharp reply to the *Body Politic*, Mike fought back:

> Lewis and Lynch are at a loss to understand all the "fear and para-noia" which the AIDS epidemic has caused. It astounds me that I have to point out that all this "panic" is because *gay men are dying.* . . . However much gay people have suffered at the hands of medicine, we cannot allow our knee-jerk defensiveness to delay urgently needed, rational discussion about the medical hazards of promiscuity. Promiscuity may indeed be the warp that "knits together the social fabric of the gay male community," but this lifestyle is clearly killing us. . . . By refusing to see that our lifestyle is potentially fatal, we may permit the ultimate triumph of the Moral Majority: we will kill *ourselves.*

In a 1983 interview on the TV show *Freeman Reports,* Berkowitz went still further, likening promiscuity to "alcoholic addiction," agreeing with his fellow panelist Larry Kramer that "homophobia"—not pleasure—was "at the heart of promiscuity"; the denial of civil rights, the two men claimed, forced people "into the ghetto" and a life of promiscuity. Thus began an ugly schism within the community of gay male activists, one that would at times take on a fiercely acerbic edge.

In a further attempt to rebut the angry critiques, Mike and Rich submitted a fourteen-page reply to critics of "We Know Who We Are," in which they justly claimed that their views had been misread, misunderstood, and misrepresented: "Neither of us has experienced a moment of guilt about our own promiscuous behavior. . . . Neither of us has problems with our gayness or with sexuality; we have problems with disease." They wrote understandingly of a community "dazed by tragedy" but insisted that the best defense was to "educate ourselves about how our bodies work." The *Native* refused to print their response and turned down as well another piece that specifically replied to Jurrist's critique.

As the debate raged on, New York City hospitals were reacting to the mounting number of AIDS patients with a harshness reminiscent of the medieval treatment of lepers: as contagious sinners kept in de facto isolation from "innocent" human beings. It wasn't yet clear whether AIDS was most efficiently transmitted through blood or semen, and tales abounded of nurses, gowned and masked from head to toe, ignoring patients or approaching them only with the utmost wariness, frequently sliding meals somewhere in their vicinity—like outside in the hall—rather than risk actual contact. Some AIDS patients, refused a room, ignored by orderlies, died on hospital gurneys in the corridors.

Nor was funding for research on AIDS remotely keeping pace with the exponential rise in case numbers. During the 1982 Tylenol scare, in which seven people died after taking cyanide-laced pills, the federal government allocated—within two weeks—$10 million to investigate the contamination. In New York City, it was the theater community, not city or state officials, that led the way with fund-raising efforts. As early as 1982, cabarets like Don't Tell Mama, the Saint disco, and the restaurant Claire did small-scale benefits for AIDS research, and the pace quickened in 1983 when Mike Callen, along with Tammy Grimes, Rex Reed, and others, performed *Pal Joey* as a benefit for GMHC at Town Hall.[12]

During the first year and a half of the AIDS crisis, Washington did little—other than indulge in repetitive, homophobic speeches from congressmen like Jesse Helms and William Dannemeyer in which they applauded the Lord's righteous punishment of homosexual immorality and recommended a large-scale quarantine program. In these early years of the epidemic, Representative Henry Waxman was nearly alone among congressmen in declaring himself "very disappointed with the government's response."

On the state and city levels the record varied somewhat. New York had more than one-third of all AIDS cases in 1982 but reacted more lethargically in the early years than San Francisco or Los Angeles during the same period. Mike and the GMHC leadership had their differences, but they thought and acted on parallel lines when it came to trying to activate city officials. Mayor Ed Koch, though widely rumored to be gay, had essentially disassociated himself from the epidemic. He assigned Herb Rickman as his "liaison" to *both* the gay and the Hasidic Jewish communities—an action akin to sending the same ambassador to Iran and Israel.

Earlier in his career, Koch had positioned himself as an ally of the

LGBT movement; on his very first day in office as mayor, January 1, 1978, he'd issued an executive order banning sexual orientation discrimination in municipal employment. But when he moved in 1985 to extend the order to cover city contractors, his good friend and ardent homophobe New York's Catholic Archbishop John O'Connor threatened to go to court to block gay people from working with children. Koch agreed to let the courts decide—and they overturned the order.

Koch did testify yearly on behalf of New York City's gay civil rights bill—introduced annually until finally passed in 1986—but he failed to use his position to exert pressure for passage from behind the scenes. And nearly two years passed after the onset of the AIDS crisis before GMHC or any AIDS group succeeded in getting a meeting with the mayor. Koch did subsequently establish an Office of Gay and Lesbian Health Concerns, under which AIDS was subsumed—but it lacked the funding needed to develop a coordinated citywide response. He also seemed oblivious to the ravages AIDS was inflicting on minority communities. It would be the Manhattan Borough president David Dinkins, not Koch, who in 1986 would sponsor a special meeting of elected minority officials to apprise them of the mounting and disproportionate toll AIDS was taking in their communities.

Moreover, the Koch administration consistently resisted implementing any AIDS curriculum in New York City's schools. It wasn't until 1991, under Mayor David Dinkins, that such education was mandated in the city's schools. (Dinkins brought down the wrath of many AIDS activists, however, with his appointment of Woodrow (Woody) Myers Jr. as commissioner of New York's Health Department; Myers had a conservative record on issues like quarantine while health commissioner in Indiana.) Koch did no better with regard to the adoption of a needle exchange program, an essential tool in any effort to lower the infection rate among intravenous drug users. Even Margaret Thatcher, the deeply conservative British prime minister, early embraced both needle exchange and AIDS education.

Given the mixture of hostility and apathy that characterized the public response to AIDS in general, it became clear to Mike, just as it had to the founders of GMHC, that the stricken would have to form their own organizations and rely on their own ingenuity to stay alive. GMHC was the only service agency in the city at a time when even

AIDS patients with health or disability insurance were unable to secure benefits. By the beginning of 1983, GMHC, remarkably, had put in place a hotline, crisis counseling, and a volunteer "buddy" system to visit and assist patients. Soon after came an array of additional services, including financial assistance and support groups—all of which Mike admired and applauded. Yet he continued to feel that GMHC's basic message to gay men to have sex with fewer partners and only "healthy" ones was both vague and dangerously misleading at a time when the HIV virus hadn't been discovered and "healthy" wasn't easy to spot or define.

Mike especially tangled with Mel Rosen, the first head of GMHC. In the fall of 1982, Rosen became GMHC's executive director—his "field placement" as a graduate school student in social work. Rosen's congressional testimony in 1983 to the effect that AIDS was "a steaming locomotive aimed at the general population" was in Mike's view a dishonest attempt to extract more money for research. Berkowitz reported to Mike that when one of Sonnabend's new patients contacted Rosen at GMHC, he'd warned the young man that "Dr. Sonnabend is not to be trusted." Mike himself readily acknowledged that Sonnabend had "the eccentricity of genius" and could sometimes come across as "bizarre," but that hardly meant that his scientific credentials weren't superlative or that his multifactorial theory shouldn't be taken seriously. The problem was that Rosen and the GMHC board had decided that they didn't want Sonnabend's theory taken *too* seriously. In the name of improving the public's attitude, GMHC had made the conscious decision to avoid or downplay any disclosure of gay male sexual "excess" for fear such behavior would be blamed as the "cause" of AIDS. They wanted to emphasize instead that it was *not* a gay disease but rather an imminent threat to everyone, regardless of age, gender, or sexual orientation. As Berkowitz reported to Mike: "They don't like what we're saying about promiscuity. . . . They're well-meaning but they're misguided. . . . It's like a club: you're in or you're out."

GMHC's first president, Paul Popham, was a former Green Beret, a decorated veteran of the war in Vietnam, a businessman, a Republican, and a person of traditional values who was trying to remain in the closet. He wanted GMHC to remain strictly a service organization and not to become entangled in political advocacy of *any* kind. Larry Kramer—who had scorned gay politics throughout the seventies as not "chic," denouncing the movement's "pitiful marches" as consisting entirely of "loudmouths, the unkempt, the dirty and unwashed"—now, ironically, was the person in GMHC most strenuously calling for aggressive advocacy. Kramer also believed—as he'd already emphasized in his novel *Faggots*—that gay men piggishly "fucking their brains out" would, if it turned out that AIDS was transmitted through a virus, further decimate the community.[13]

Kramer was essentially thrown out of GMHC, which had rapidly become the largest AIDS organization in the country. Ideologically, his insistence that promiscuous gay men change their behavior ostensibly aligned him with the Sonnabend-Berkowitz-Callen axis, but that wasn't an alliance either side particularly wanted. Kramer condemned *all* gay male promiscuity as unseemly and immoral, whereas Rich and Mike had celebrated sexuality, including sluthood, as a source of personal and political liberation—though fearing that the onset of the epidemic promiscuity had become too dangerous medically. Mike appreciated all that Kramer, who he personally knew, had done to alert the community and felt that "his heart's in the right place." But he also felt that Larry suffered from "ineptitude or tone problems" and that "ineptitude can actually be responsible for killing people. . . . The trust of a person is really a weighty thing." As he put it to Berkowitz, "what's making Larry frantic and sputter, is that no one is taking him seriously"—which was surely an exaggeration.

Mike wanted GMHC to pay for safe-sex posters to be put up in bathhouses and bars—posters that described in more detail which practices among gay men, like being the recipient in anal intercourse, were riskier than others. It should be remembered that in these early years of the epidemic Mike seemed to more established members of the organized gay community as a nobody who'd come out of nowhere—a legal secretary and part-time cabaret singer with no specific medical or scientific expertise (though he was in fact becoming far more knowledgeable than many of the self-proclaimed "experts"). GMHC did contribute a little money to the safe-sex posters but balked at the suggestion of explicit language warning against anal intercourse. The GMHC board feared it would be generally misread as "airing our dirty laundry in public" as well as interfering with individual decision making in particular. That didn't satisfy Mike. He was in favor of the revolution and of individual choice, but also in favor of staying alive and helping others to do so as well. He and Rich were friendly with Howard Cruse, the gifted gay cartoonist, and Cruse volunteered to do a poster with more concrete graphics.

Along with his other activities, Mike got involved with the AIDS Network—an umbrella organization made up of representatives from various groups, including GMHC—that formed in the summer of 1982 to deal with a variety of civil rights issues; it was headed by the gifted, forceful Virginia (Ginny) Apuzzo, current head of the National Gay Task Force. Mike thought that Ginny, an ex-nun and ardent feminist, had "tremendous political savvy" and regretted that the same wasn't true of the leadership at GMHC. He enthusiastically applauded GMHC's army of volunteers but thought much less of its public representatives.

In these first few years of the epidemic, causes and treatments alike were essentially unknown, and the sharply rising number of those afflicted paralleled a heightened increase of terror. One measure of the desperation that was becoming widely felt was the increased willingness to try any sort of nostrum rumored to be beneficial. It became commonplace, as fear mounted, to volunteer for a wide array of treatments. One doctor in San Francisco started giving his AIDS patients huge intravenous doses of vitamin C, based on a Linus Pauling protocol for cancer; another experimented unsuccessfully with using DNCB (a photochemical used on warts) for KS lesions.

As panic mounted, so did internal squabbling. As usual in such circumstances, raging helplessness found its most available targets close at hand. Mike was far more sensitive to people, and more generous about their apprehensions and actions, than either Berkowitz or Sonnabend. Both of them, for example, disparaged Dr. Larry Mass. Berkowitz—and Sonnabend still more so—insisted that Mass, in Sonnabend's words, "doesn't have the credentials to be writing in this area. . . . It's a highly technical subject. . . . He actually makes me angry." When Mass told Sonnabend in one long discussion that "there's so much epidemiological stuff for the single virus" theory, Sonnabend reported his own reaction as: "Well, like what? And we waited and he had nothing to say. Just silence . . . his intellect [isn't] working . . . his intentions are good . . . he wants to help . . . he's not a bad man." Mike told both Berkowitz and Sonnabend that they were being "arrogant" and predicted that "before it's all over with [Mass will] be on our side."[14]

Much as Mike admired Sonnabend, at this early point in the epidemic Mike felt it important to emphasize—adapting the view from feminist health manuals like "For Her Own Good"—that in truth "there are no experts," or if there were, then "*we* are the real experts. . . . We need to have forums on creative and medically safe ways to have sex: lovers, condoms, jerk-off clubs, closed circles of buddies are just a few of the creative and safe alternatives." A devout believer in self-empowerment and in political representation of the disenfranchised, Mike found it shocking that no members of the GMHC board were themselves PWAs (the first PWA wouldn't be elected to the GMHC board until 1987). Mike strongly disapproved of what he regarded as the organization's dishonest attempt to soft-pedal the truth about gay male sexual practices and to exaggerate the threat of AIDS to the general population; Larry Kramer had at one point declared that the epidemic could just as easily have happened to housewives in New Jersey. The attempt to mainstream AIDS based on the few cases that had as yet appeared among heterosexuals was in Mike's view mendacious. He was a consistent truth teller. He rejected the argument GMHC and others were pushing—in order to extract increased federal funding—that the spread of AIDS to the heterosexual world was imminent. (For complex reasons still not well understood, that did become true in Africa, but in the United States AIDS was and remains primarily a disease that disproportionately affects gay men.)

Sonnabend insisted from the beginning that the notion the country was on the verge of an explosion of AIDS into the heterosexual world was "rubbish." He predicted, moreover, that spreading such a notion would have serious consequences: a significant uptake in violence against gay men as the "originators" of AIDS, a bizarre spiral of accusations within the straight world, and a woeful neglect about the true cause of AIDS transmission. Joe told the story of a call he got one day from a man who'd been with a female prostitute three months before; he wanted to know if it was safe for his daughter to drink out of the same glass as he did. Heterosexuals who *did* come down with AIDS in the coming years by and large became infected through IV drug use, contaminated blood products, or same-gender "adventuring"; for women, through sex with an infected male partner (some bisexual men, in an effort to keep their male-to-male sex secret, would insist they were strictly straight); or, finally, a female passing the infection to a male, which would remain exceedingly rare. Since people often don't tell the truth about drug use or sexual activity, it would be many years before panic about a heterosexual epidemic could be laid to rest. In 1984, for example, there were exactly *four* purported cases of men getting AIDS from sex with women; in 1985, the figure went down to two; in the 1990s, about fifty such cases were claimed, but researchers and scientists came to agree that nearly all of them were men who injected drugs or shared hypodermic needles. Sonnabend—and Mike as his surrogate—were widely denounced for putting a damper on the notion of a heterosexual plague, but they went right on speaking the truth as they saw it. And science has largely validated their view.

In San Francisco, Bobbi Campbell ("Sister Florence Nightmare"), a member of the Sisters of Perpetual Indulgence, a gender-queer group that sported religious garb, was one of the city's first diagnosed cases of AIDS, and the very first to go public as a PWA. Early in 1982 Campbell began a column in the *San Francisco Sentinel* describing his experiences and offering recommendations to others. Like Mike Callen, Campbell had continued to believe that sexual liberation—sex as recreation and pleasure—should remain at the heart of the gay movement. Both men also agreed that sexual freedom had to include responsibility for one's own health and that of one's partners.[15]

As Mike said in a speech early in 1983: "Walking into the baths and backrooms with the delusion that you can check your responsibility at the door with your clothes is an act of personal and cultural suicide. Either you do not love life or you do not know death. What is over isn't sex—just sex without responsibility." What was now needed, he went on, was to "begin to formulate a long overdue sexual ethic. . . . The formulation of this ethic will require a change radical in its simplicity: We will have to talk to each other. Yes, even before sex and maybe even after. And we will have to learn to listen to each other. . . . Our challenge is to figure out how to have gay, life-affirming sex, satisfy our emotional needs, and STAY ALIVE. Hard questions for hard times, but whatever happened to our great gay imagination?"

Dr. Marcus Conant, a dermatologist in San Francisco who would become a leading figure in the struggle against AIDS, had a patient named Dan Turner who'd also been diagnosed early. Conant suggested that Campbell and Turner meet each other. Along with a few other PWAs, they gathered at Turner's house in the Castro hills, and out of that meeting emerged PWA San Francisco—the first organization "of, for and by people with AIDS." The principle was thus established that "people with AIDS themselves should be an integral part of AIDS service organizations," a principle not yet accepted at GMHC in New York, though a few board members (Paul Popham, for one) had already been diagnosed. The members of PWA San Francisco were asked to choose for themselves which boards to serve on. Bobbi Campbell went on the KS/AIDS Foundation's national board, and Dan Turner was elected to the board of the San Francisco chapter of the KS/AIDS Foundation.

In New York, as Mike told it, he and other PWAs had been feeling "growing frustration" at attending GMHC forums where they'd "sit silently in the audience" and hear assorted "experts"—from doctors and nurses to insurance and social work specialists—tell *them* what it was like to have AIDS. "It would be akin," he felt, "to having a conference on sickle cell anemia at which no blacks were asked to attend or participate." Mike himself suggested to GMHC that it hold a forum on the impact of AIDS on sexual behavior. Initially GMHC responded enthusiastically, and both Mike and Joe Sonnabend were asked to serve on the panel. Feeling strongly that GMHC and its board members had a "low consciousness" about feminism, Mike urged that women also be included. Ginny Apuzzo and Gloria Steinem were then added—but both Mike and Joe "mysteriously dropped." When Mike asked why, a GMHC spokesperson first denied that Mike had ever been invited and then told him that he'd "become too prominent lately." Outraged, Mike viewed the occasion as "the beginning of real war" with GMHC.

It apparently occurred to several PWAs at the same time— including Artie Felson and Tom Nasrallah, who were reasonably well known in the community—that *they* were the true experts on AIDS and that they should make their voices heard. In the fall of 1982, Mike and Rich Berkowitz formed a New York City group called Gay Men with AIDS (GMWA). Its stated goal was "to support each other by sharing our personal experiences, our strength and our hope," and it became oriented more toward therapy than politics. At the same time both Mike and Berkowitz joined the peer-run support group started by Dr. Stuart Nichols of Beth Israel Medical Center—possibly the first such group in the city. Another member of that group, Phil Lanzaratta, whom Mike adored and called a "sweetheart," had already done a number of TV and print interviews and is sometimes called the "granddaddy" of the PWA movement in New York.

At roughly the same time, Mike, Berkowitz, and Sonnabend began to work on what became a self-published forty-page pamphlet, *How to Have Sex in an Epidemic: One Approach*, which appeared in May 1983. Mike used the refund from his own tax return to pay for the publication; he found a typesetter on King Street who for a fee let him, Berkowitz, and Richard Dworkin use his IBM typesetting machine. They made it clear at the top of the pamphlet that their recommendations were based on the multifactorial theory of AIDS but claimed—accurately, as it would turn out—that the guidelines would prove equally valid for reducing risk of contagion even if a new, as yet unidentified, virus was discovered to cause the disease. Whichever theory you believed, they emphasized, promiscuity was central to the health crisis. The National Cancer Institute had itself reported that "AIDS is occurring in a specific subset of homosexual men, possibly but not exclusively defined by the number of lifetime sexual partners." Repeated exposure—whether to a specific virus or to an accumulation of infections—was at the heart of the matter. There were rumors of monogamous or sexually celibate gay men developing AIDS, but to date no such case had been produced. Nor was it accurate to say—as two articles in the left-wing Toronto-based gay paper, *The Body Politic*, had argued in 1982—that panic and "an anti-sexual sense of guilt" were blowing a minor health problem out of all proportion.[16]

As Mike put it, "I have tried to be a 'good gay' and 'wear my sexually transmitted diseases like red badges of courage in the war against a sex negative society,'" but as the numbers of those afflicted with AIDS steadily mounted, the stakes had simply become too high. Too many doctors, moreover—and, in some of its printed material, GMHC as well—were advising gay men to "cut down" on the number of different sexual partners and to have sex only with "healthy" ones. But as Mike asked with exasperation, what *specific* behavior was being advocated by the advice to "cut down"? Does that mean three partners a week instead of six? Does it mean going to the baths once a month instead of once a week? And were gay men being advised to *ask* their partners if they were healthy? Besides, some infections, at least initially, were asymptomatic, and the partner might not know himself whether or not he was "healthy." Even if he did know, "what does it say about our community that there are gay men having promiscuous sexual encounters knowing that they're ill?"

A fierce debate would soon spring up within the community about whether to close down the bathhouses. When it did, Berkowitz would turn out to approve closure, but Mike would argue strenuously against. He wasn't a believer, as he put it, in "legislating health risks; I have never and will never suggest such a thing." But that didn't mean that in the current crisis nothing at all needed to be done, and he tried to get safe-sex literature and condoms into the bathhouses. Most owners refused, arguing that "the atmosphere" would be "ruined." In *How to Have Sex*, Berkowitz and Mike argued that it was essential—this was the pamphlet's core recommendation—that one should avoid "taking in your partner(s) body fluids" (an injunction that resonates to the present day). That was the key to avoiding infection. The pamphlet emphasized that "sex doesn't make you sick—diseases do. Gay sex doesn't make you sick—gay men who are sick do." Mike and Rich wanted gay men to examine their lifestyles, but they discouraged "misplaced morality masquerading as medical advice." The sexual revolution of the 1960s and 1970s had made it clear that sex and love are not inevitably or ideally linked, but "the 1970s," they concluded, "are over. Taking ignorance to the baths and backrooms is not sexual freedom—it's oppression."

In the face of raging fears of contagion, the pamphlet gave lucid, detailed advice about what was or was not "safe" sex and also underscored the importance of talking openly with sexual partners (whether intimates or strangers) about which practices or behaviors were riskiest in terms of disease transmission. The guidelines Mike and Rich suggested are still largely followed: sucking your partner without a condom isn't 100 percent risk-free; fucking someone probably poses no threat, but one should always use condoms during anal sex for the bottom's protection, though they weren't designed for assholes and might rip during penetration; getting fucked without a condom posed the greatest risk; S/M practices almost never did; fist fucking, which could produce anal tears, could be "extremely dangerous." Bathhouses and back rooms were full of disease, but if one wanted to partake, the four "musts" had to be followed: talking, washing, light, and condoms. Safest of all were "creative" masturbation, closed circles of fuck buddies, and jerk-off clubs.

In a transcribed phone conversation, Mike told Berkowitz that the more he became involved in politics, the less he felt he understood it. Why did it seem so impossible to separate issues from personalities? He told Rich that he'd done a lot of reading in feminist literature and as a result began to understand that you can disagree with somebody about an issue without insisting that the other person was "gross and disgusting." He wished that more gay men would avail themselves of feminist insights: it would do wonders for cutting down the personal abuse that seemed to accompany the struggle against AIDS. He perhaps had in mind the comments made by Dr. Peter Seitzman, president of the New York Physicians for Human Rights, who'd written in the *Native* a few months before the publication of *How to Have Sex* about those people—naming Berkowitz and Callen—"whose guilt is shouted from the rooftops." Mike was probably thinking, too, of Dr. Larry Mass, who'd characterized the two men as "sex-negative propagandists" intent on "blaming the victim."

In general, though, *How to Have Sex* was well received, selling nearly all of the five thousand copies printed. "This is the sanest, most sensible advice I've read yet about AIDS," wrote Edmund White, the novelist and co-author of the liberatory *The Joy of Gay Sex*. Dennis Altman, the well-known Australian writer of many gay-themed books, including *The Homosexualization of America*, hailed the pamphlet: "At last: a response to the effect of AIDS on our lives that goes beyond fears and myths to suggest positive actions." Both GMHC and the state of New York flatly refused to distribute the pamphlet, but most people seem to have felt that in the face of conflicting dogmas, murky theorizing, and hysterically aggressive moralizing, Callen and Berkowitz had produced a pioneering, modulated, nonhectoring guide, and that it did *something* to assuage the confusion and anguish of those who'd considered celibacy as the only possible safeguard against death.

The pamphlet elevated the two men to the status of minicelebrities, and Mike, especially, received a host of invitations to speak and write. His careful, moving remarks to the New York congressional delegation so impressed Representative Geraldine Ferraro that on May 18, 1983, she had them read into the *Congressional Record*. Mike eloquently described to the delegation the process by which at least some gay people were being radicalized as a result of the epidemic: "The tragedy of AIDS has made many . . . take a new look at the situation of America's other disenfranchised groups. We are beginning to see that homophobia and racism are not, as some of us thought, totally unrelated. We are beginning to see that America's fear and ignorance of homosexuals and its hate and bigotry toward black and brown people are not just coincidental."[17]

Mike pointed out that in the few years since AIDS had first been recognized, it had killed more people than swine flu, toxic shock syndrome, Legionnaires' disease, and cyanide-laced Tylenol combined. Yet the federal government had continued to ignore the epidemic. After all, the disease had struck only "disenfranchised segments of American society: homosexual men, heroin abusers, Haitian entrants and hemophiliacs," plus some prisoners, sex workers, "and the children of high-risk groups who are also victims of poverty." Mike felt sure, he told the New York congressional delegation, that "if such a deadly disease were affecting more privileged members of American society, there can be no doubt that the government's response would have been immediate."

He ended the speech with these telling and poignant remarks: "Surely when you first dreamed of holding public office you did not, in the furthest reaches of your imagination, foresee that your duties would include having breakfast on a Monday morning with a homosexual facing a life-threatening illness. You can be sure that ten— five—or even one year ago, I could not have imagined the possibility that I, too, would be up here begging my elected representatives to help me save my life. But there you are. Here I am. And that is exactly what I am doing."

Within two weeks of giving that speech, Mike, on June 1, 1983, spoke to the New York State Senate Committee on Investigation and Taxation. He reiterated many of the same points he'd previously made to the New York congressional delegation but put more emphasis on the demeaning and legally incriminating sorts of questions that government researchers were commonly asking AIDS patients. In the current CDC questionnaire, for example, they were being asked if they'd had sex with animals, and if so, how often; asked, too, to detail sexual practices "which are illegal in a number of states"; and asked as well to list which illicit drugs they'd taken. The answers were then stored on government computers, and many patients rightly doubted if confidentiality could be ensured. As a result, most AIDS patients were *not* providing truthful or helpful information to researchers.

As Mike started to become better known, the media came calling regularly. His first experience with television in the fall of 1982 taught him much about the need to arm himself in advance for future encounters. That first trial by fire was an interview for CBS national news. It lasted a half hour, but when it aired that night the segment had been cut to twenty seconds. That was Mike's first lesson: master the art of the sound bite. He was a quick learner, and mischievous. From then on he'd decide in advance of an interview the one or two points he wanted to make—and would then *make* them, come hell or high water. At that first CBS interview, he'd been asked the appalling question that he'd hear repeated hundreds of times in the future by different interviewers: "How does it *feel* to know you're going to die?" He'd stumbled that first time around, unprepared for the callousness of the question. Thereafter, he learned to use the question as an excuse to make whatever point he wanted to; he would pause dramatically and then smoothly say, "You know, that reminds me of . . ." and then swiftly proceed to deliver his preplanned sound bite.

But though he learned how to steer an interview, Mike would never get over the discrimination and abuse that attended such sessions. At NBC, he became aware that the other guests for segments of the show were together in a guest lounge—but Mike had been asked to wait, by himself, in a different room. The others were taken one at a time for makeup; Mike wasn't offered any. When, eventually, they came to take him to the studio for his interview, a soundman "tossed a microphone at me and told me to pin it on myself. I noticed that he was wearing rubber gloves. I had never met a sound person who didn't prefer themselves to pin the microphone. I asked him to please do it for me. He refused. I was faced with a terrible choice. I could storm off the set, I could get angry on camera, or I could swallow my anger, pin the microphone on and use my minute of airtime to spread a little hope" (the segment was about long-term survival). Shaking with anger, Mike chose the latter course. But as soon as he left the studio he put in a call to the American Civil Liberties Union. The ACLU acted swiftly—and henceforth NBC was forced to educate its employees about AIDS.

As hysteria about AIDS continued to mount, irrational practices of various kinds were taking hold. One union of social workers threatened to go out on strike if forced to help AIDS patients fill out social security or welfare forms. When Sonnabend—who'd joined with Dr. Mathilde Krim and other colleagues to form the AIDS Medical Foundation (a precursor to amfAR) for coordinating research—tried to send a package to another colleague, the delivery company refused to handle it because the word "AIDS" appeared in the name of the foundation on the return address. Mike did his best in his public appearances to educate people about the fact that AIDS was the kind of contagion that develops within an individual over a period of time and was not readily or casually transmitted. He emphasized the point that to date not a single case had been reported of a health care professional developing AIDS solely from contact with patients.

Mike was fully aware that "conservative forces are attempting to use this tragedy for their own political ends." In Texas, for example, a group calling itself "Doctors to Wipe Out AIDS" had called upon the state legislature to recriminalize consensual sodomy. In New York City, the *Post* had printed several of Pat Buchanan's nationally syndicated and inflammatory articles calling AIDS "Nature's retribution"—the implication being that those with AIDS, having committed *unnatural* acts, were themselves responsible for their own suffering and death.

Joe Sonnabend may have had his "eccentric" moments, but he cared deeply about the stricken, terrified young men who clogged his waiting room. He cared as little about money as he did about surface appearances, and as the epidemic spread, he started to see patients who couldn't afford to pay. And so, out of his own pocket, he'd foot the bills for lab tests or the shipment of samples and other assorted treatment expenses that his patients couldn't afford. And he'd often spend hours with a single patient, as his waiting room overflowed, every chair taken, frightened young men standing against every wall. Had Sonnabend not had able assistants in Abby Tallmer, who often socialized with the patients while they waited, and Harley Hackett, the situation might well have become unendurable.[18]

Eventually it did become untenable. Sonnabend started actually to lose rather than make money. Hackett, an unsung hero of the epidemic, not only stopped drawing a salary, but dipped into his own savings in order to keep the bill collectors from closing down Joe's office. Others on staff drew only minimal salaries. Joe remained obliviously unconcerned, but the day came when Hackett ran out of money and had to take another job; even then, he'd come into the office every Saturday evening to do the bookkeeping and to check on medical test results. It wasn't masochism on Hackett's part. He simply shared Mike's belief that Sonnabend "was the perfect man at the perfect time." Not everyone agreed, of course. Among the dissenters were the members of the co-op board at 49 West Twelfth Street, the building that housed Joe's office. In a shock to him and his staff, the co-op refused to renew Sonnabend's lease, citing the "danger" and "unsightliness" of so many AIDS patients coming in and out of the building—even though it was a fact, if not widely accepted, that AIDS couldn't be casually transmitted. Joe fought the eviction in court—one of the first such cases challenging AIDS-related discrimination—but lost. He had to move late in 1983 to much less desirable quarters—to an office that lacked even a refrigerator.

3

Career Moves

By mid-1983, Joe Beam "had grown weary of reading literature by white gay men." One could read issue after issue of *The Advocate*, the national gay biweekly, without once encountering anything about black gay life. At the time, Beam worked at Giovanni's Room, Philadelphia's gay bookstore, and he longed to see more titles on its well-stocked shelves that spoke to black gay men like him. Beam also wrote for *Au Courant*, an alternative paper to the *Philadelphia Gay News* (which featured mostly white gay news). The same bias that Joe protested was true of the whole range of gay male publications—from porn mags like *Drummer* or *Mandate* to the highbrow literary magazine *Christopher Street*. Beam decided to do something about it. He sent out press releases through the black and gay media soliciting manuscripts for a black gay male anthology.[1]

Beam wasn't exaggerating or overreacting. The gay press, with its emphasis on the world of middle-class white men, accurately reflected the state of the gay political movement. The leading organization, the National Gay Task Force (belatedly renamed the National Lesbian and Gay Task Force), focused its efforts on trying to secure basic civil rights through the traditional devices of voting and lobbying—probably the most that could be hoped for at a time of deepening economic recession and conservatism (the columnist George Will, for one, denounced the efforts to pass gay rights ordinances as "part of the moral disarmament of society").

But the marginal status of the organized gay political movement and its pragmatic goal of trying to shrink the boundaries of *official* homophobia didn't explain the absence in its ranks of people of color. The first African American elected to the board of the National Gay Task Force, Jon L. Clayborne, resigned after a short time, complaining that racism within the movement wasn't being adequately addressed. The black writer Thomas Dotton angrily complained in a 1975 article, "Nigger in the Woodpile," that after five years of working in the movement he'd become fed up with "the endless apologies and excuses" for failing to deal with the absence of black faces. Pat Parker, the black lesbian writer, put it more succinctly: the white lesbian's foot might well be smaller than the white man's, she wrote, "but it's still on my neck."[2]

The Beam/Parker indictment certainly ties in with my own experience in the movement during those years. At a 1980 high-priced dinner at the Waldorf to celebrate Democratic presidential candidate Walter Mondale, I'd been struck at the near total absence of people of color, and two years later, when giving a speech at a Lambda Legal Defense Fund event, I referenced that fact and said that it seemed to me symbolic of the lack of representation of people of color in the agendas and personnel of our political organizations. As if in confirmation, a number of gay white men angrily walked out in the middle of my speech, and others later protested what one of them called my "inappropriate and offensive" remarks.

Beam had read the writing not only of Pat Parker, but of other black lesbians as well—Audre Lorde, Barbara Smith, June Jordan, and Michelle Cliff. Such works, he felt, had greatly informed his perspective, but he longed for comparable black gay male voices. There were certainly a number of prominent black gay writers in these years—preeminently James Baldwin and Samuel Delany—but none were active in the gay movement. Determined to repair the lack of representation, Beam set to work on the anthology he would call *In The Life*.

Essex saw one of the ads Joe Beam placed soliciting material, immediately decided that he "wanted to be a part of it," and submitted ten poems for Beam's consideration; ultimately Beam included four of them when *In The Life* finally appeared in 1986. By then the two men had long since become friends. According to Essex, Beam initially wanted a romantic relationship but Essex firmly told him, "Joe, that is not for us." But they became such close friends that Beam was the only man in the country who had keys to Essex's apartment.[3]

The two young men had much in common. They were roughly the same age (Joe was two years younger) and both had gone to college, although Joe had subsequently dropped out of graduate school at Iowa; neither believed in religion or in moneymaking as significant elements in their lives; both were handsome, smart, and full of natural charm; both were open and proud, yet wary, about their status as double-outsiders—usually angrier about being treated badly by white gays than by black straights; and both could be moody. Essex was the more passionate perfectionist and Joe the more easily given to depression ("I am so weary of my hopes being dashed against the rocks; after a while one (me) begins to internalize this sort of thing"). He was vulnerable, sensitive to slights, and deeply lonely. Unlike Essex, who'd started having sex (and writing poetry) at fourteen, Joe thought of himself as "asexual"—or, alternatively, as "androgynous"—and had his first experience at twenty-two.

Both men, too, were deeply reliant on the friendship and advice of black lesbian feminists. "Lesbians," Joe Beam wrote a friend, "appear to be so much more supportive of each other or am I just perceiving the grass as greener, but I am at a loss to find that quality of support from other gay men." Joe's particular mentor was Barbara Smith, founder of Kitchen Table Women of Color Press and author of the pioneering anthology *Home Girls*. Barbara gave Joe advice on issues ranging from literary agents and publishers to the wording of contributors' forms. He also turned, on an occasional basis, to Audre Lorde (*Zami*), Anita Cornwell (*Black Lesbian in White America*), and the Latina writer Cherríe Moraga (*Loving in the War Years*). Essex's special ally continued to be Michelle Parkerson.[4]

Essex had already self-published two chapbooks, *Diamonds Was in the Kitty* (1982) and *Plums* (1983), and at least one poem of his had been printed as early as 1977 (in *Obsidian*). Others appeared soon after in *Painted Bride Quarterly*, *Callaloo*, and *Black Scholar*. The biggest break yet in Essex's burgeoning career came in 1985 when he, Michelle Parkerson, and Wayson Jones performed for the first time at d.c. space, the most prestigious of all the outlets for the downtown arts scene. Located on Seventh and E Streets, and known to the cognoscenti simply as "the space," the club presented everything from performance artists like Tim Miller (later to become a good friend of Mike Callen) and Karen Finley (she did her infamous piece, "Yams Up My Granny's Ass" there), to progressive jazz like Sun Ra and the World Saxophone Quartet, to influential punk rock groups, to Cecil Taylor and Cassandra Wilson. "The place just glowed," according to one frequent attendee; it "was electric with talent and love. It's difficult for me not to weep remembering being there." Ray Melrose, who'd run the Coffeehouse, became a manager at d.c. space, serving as a kind of bridge between the two venues, and Bill Warrell, d.c. space's owner, proved particularly supportive, hosting an outdoor arts festival that took place right next to the National Portrait Gallery. Essex, Wayson, and Michelle also made strong connections at "the space" with those artists in the punk community who formed the social activist group Positive Force. By 1986 the three were regularly receiving favorable reviews from W. Royal Stokes, the jazz critic for the *Washington Post*, and word of their artistic promise had begun to spread beyond the borders of the District of Columbia. It was also in 1986 that d.c. space hosted a heralded monthlong performance series, "Four Nights of Music, Poetry and Disruption," that also featured the gay and lesbian artists Cheryl Clarke, Jewelle Gomez, Chris Prince, and the rock group Betty.[5]

Of Essex's published work to date, an article he did for *Essence* was probably his most significant. "I am a homosexual" was its dramatic opening line, and he elaborated with a series of provocative comments. He claimed to have known since age five "that I would love men," though he didn't know at that early age that " 'brother,' 'lover,' 'friend' would take on more intimate and dangerous meanings. I did not know a dual oppression, a dual mockery, would be practiced against me."

He went on to reveal in the article that when, at age nineteen, he told his parents he was gay, "they had trouble accepting the news." His mother (as is often the case) blamed herself, though Essex assured her that no blame was involved and that homosexuality was entirely "natural," as was "sensitivity"—it wasn't a "sissy" thing. "I have yet to understand," he wrote, "why emotional expression by men"—emotion other than anger, that is—"must be understated or under control when the process of living requires the capacity to feel and express." Essex claimed that he got some encouragement from his family "to aggressively pursue my human rights," though given his father's emotionally distant and at times violent temperament and his mother's ambivalence (at best) about his homosexuality, the human rights in question may well have been black, not gay.

Homosexuality *was* often accepted within the confines of a black family, or even within the black community as a whole ("everyone knew that the choir master at church was queer")—but what was not widely accepted was for the individual in question to "go public." It would have been highly atypical in the heterosexual black world to have urged a son or daughter to become active in openly fighting for the acceptance of gay people. The black gay essayist and poet Craig G. Harris, who died of AIDS in 1992 at age thirty-three, put it this way: "The strong tradition of the extended family holds a highly esteemed position for the bachelor uncle or spinster aunt. These are often the family members who, because they have lesser financial responsibilities, can assist in the rearing of their siblings' offspring. Afro-American families relate well to homosexuality—as long as they can turn their backs on the issue. But often when the homosexual family member decides to be political, or obvious in other ways, the family becomes confused, frightened, or disgusted by the display."[6]

In his *Essence* article, Essex withheld any specific details about his private life and instead spoke generally of not having "found loving a man easy," (while also saying that he didn't feel loving a woman would be any easier). His *Essence* piece was also noteworthy for the sharpness of its attack on the gay rights movement as "racist and sexist." It was a view common among black gays and lesbians. As Craig Harris put it: "The feelings of violation experienced by many gay white men when encountering heterosexist discrimination are largely due to an innate belief that, as white men, their civil liberties are a guaranteed birthright. This unconscious illusion of supremacy promotes racism and misogyny, rather than eliciting empathy for victims of discrimination based on race or sex." This sense of exclusion from the white gay inner sanctum had led to a number of separate black political formations, ranging from the consciousness-raising groups sponsored by the Committee of Black Gay Men to Salsa Soul Sisters/Third World Women, to the 1985 National Coalition of Black Gays (NCBG), whose letterhead slogan read: "As proud of our gayness as we are of our Blackness."

Among those who served on NCBG's board were Audre Lorde, Barbara Smith, Michelle Parkerson, and the Reverend Renee McCoy. Like most gay organizations at the time, NCBG was understaffed and underfunded. Yet it managed to convene a national gathering in St. Louis late in 1985. Both Joe Beam and Essex attended, though the convention was so hectic, they saw little of each other there. But both of them found the conference a pivotal experience. During the workshop on organizing, Joe was especially taken with Betty Powell's view that black lesbians and gays "are the current, forward-moving crest of the Black liberation struggle." He felt "more and more committed to that struggle each day," and he recognized that it would be a long one; but "if Nelson Mandela can spend a quarter of a century in prison then certainly I can learn to work when I am weary, but free to move as I please." For his part, Essex started negotiations with a D.C. club, the Brass Rail, to do a benefit performance for NCBG—and that wasn't the sole extent of his involvement. As Renee McCoy has put it, "he provided significant support and guidance when we were building the Coalition."

The essential accuracy of the indictment of the white gay movement as indifferently sexist and racist is, in broad outline, inarguable. Yet Essex's severe characterization of it "as an insincere human rights struggle" can be contested partially. In the 1970s and early 1980s the organized LGBT movement was small, fragmented, and largely middle-class and white. As someone involved in forming the National Gay Task Force and the Gay Academic Union of those years, I know that serious efforts were made to include women and people of color. These efforts were somewhat successful in regard to women but largely ineffective in regard to people of color. Obviously more, much more, outreach was needed before blacks and Hispanics could comfortably feel ownership in those organizations. Yet some effort is different from none.

Essex's indictment of the white gay movement and community was encompassing. "When I first came to the life," he wrote, "I would go to these gay clubs here [D.C.], like the Lost & Found, and those white sissies would give me fever for not having thousands of pieces of I.D. before they'd let me in. I watched white queens sail through the door with barely a nod, and they weren't asked for I.D. but I had to fish around in my pockets for numerous pieces. . . . Now, none of those white sissies sailing through the door would ever stop on my behalf or on the behalf of any other brother being hassled at the door and ask, 'Why are you demanding I.D. of him, but not of me?' Your only chance of avoiding those ugly scenes was to show up at the door with a white boy on your arm or in a racially mixed group. . . . I was humiliated constantly." Yet he found that at the baths, "undressed and in my towel, white boys would chase me around and around the place, wanting to suck my dick, wanting me to fuck them, and basically being goddamn nuisances."

Essex was speaking for many black gay men (and women, for that matter), and his indictment was unquestionably on the mark, if perhaps too totalizing, *too* sweeping to acknowledge the effort, both pre-Stonewall and in the mid-1980s, of some white gays—though certainly nothing close to a majority—to confront their own racism and that of the organizations to which they belonged. The pioneering (and tiny) D.C. Mattachine had attempted to recruit members at Nob Hill, the popular African American gay bar, and even devoted one of its evening discussions to "How Can We Bring the Negro into the Homophile Movement?" Such efforts were undoubtedly minor, and the inability to enlist more than a very few blacks may well have been due to a lack of understanding that sexual orientation can often be concealed, but skin color only rarely—which made the black struggle, not the gay one, of necessity the primary emergency for most blacks.

The most prominent gay organization in the immediate aftermath of the 1969 Stonewall riots had been the radical Gay Liberation Front (GLF). Its agenda was broader than gay rights; it wanted to fight against all forms of oppression and made overtures to both the Black Panthers and the Puerto Rican Young Lords. But the macho orientation of both groups militated against any combination of forces with "faggots"; only Huey Newton (so far as is known) responded sympathetically to the GLF initiative. One could also cite the fact that when Lost & Found opened in the fall of 1971 in D.C., the popular disco was immediately picketed by the newly formed and multiracial Committee for Open Gay Bars in protest over its racist and sexist carding policies. The well-known gay Regency Baths in D.C., which started in 1968 (and in 1985 was the first to close during the AIDS epidemic), had an entirely open membership policy. Similarly, the Black Panthers'

Revolutionary People's Constitutional Convention in 1970, held at the All Souls Unitarian Church in D.C., was an event staged with GLF's strong support.

Those instances can arguably be dismissed as the marginal residue of the radical decade of the 1960s. In New York City, after all, the hugely popular disco the Ice Palace, despite a long-term campaign against its carding policy in the early eighties, never capitulated to the protesters—and few whites ever withdrew their patronage. Similar failed campaigns against racist door policies were tried without success against a number of prominent New York City gay and lesbian bars from the 1970s through the 1990s. After the early seventies, the gay movement pretty much shed its radical origins and impulses and started on a trajectory that has veered ever closer to the nonradical goal of mainstream assimilationism. Yet at least at the fringe of the movement, white gay radicalism has persisted down to the present day. When Essex wrote his 1983 *Essence* piece, the organization Black and White Men Together did exist, as did the influential radical anti-racist publications *Gay Community News, Conditions*, and *Fag Rag*. But they were marginal to the mainstream gay movement. Essex's allegiance, in any case, was clear-cut: his priorities understandably and overwhelmingly focused on the well-being of black gay people, not gays in general. Throughout his poetry the anger he felt about white bigotry often surfaced:

> I live in a town
> where pretense and bone structure
> prevail as credentials
> of status and beauty—
> a town bewitched
> by mirrors, horoscopes
> and corruption . . .
> ("Family Jewels: For Washington D.C.")

> I could leave with no intention
> of coming home tonight,
> go crazy downtown and raise hell
> on a rooftop with my rifle.
> I could live for a brief moment

on the six o'clock news,
or masquerade another day
through the corridors of commerce
and American dreams.

("Cordon Negro")

In the country as a whole, Ronald Reagan's 1980 election on a wave of white popular support had seen a host of mounting ills for the working class as unionization declined, technology replaced workers, and corporations moved increasingly overseas—where the Reagan administration backed regimes, especially in Central America, notorious for their dictatorial brutality. Yet in regard to wars at home against poverty, racism, and AIDS, the federal government managed to remain passive and indifferent. The Omnibus Budget Reconciliation Act of 1981 made massive cuts in social services and wiped out most of the gains won against poverty initiated by Lyndon B. Johnson two decades earlier. As the number of AIDS cases aggressively mounted, topping three thousand by the end of 1983, Congress began to vote larger, though still not adequate, budgets for research and assistance—only to have the administration fail to spend all the funds allotted.

The cities of San Francisco and New York suffered most. Washington, D.C., still had the comparatively low figure of eighty-nine cases, and the response there had been minimal. The gay STD clinic Whitman-Walker, in existence for a decade, was a comparative hub of activity, all but uniquely trying to do *something*. It had launched an Education Fund for AIDS, hired its first AIDS program director, and issued its first AIDS education pamphlet. Yet the candlelight march and memorial service that marked Gay Pride Day in D.C. on June 19, 1983, saw a turnout of fewer than a thousand people.

Essex would later describe the black men who availed themselves of Whitman-Walker's services as usually requiring "more than medication. . . . [They had] an almost common set of symptoms that blatantly spell out the oppressive conditions black males endure in American society. Some of the men coming into the clinic need job training, marketable skills, improvements in their reading comprehension, pills, if there were such, for self-esteem and confidence, and surely, they desperately need to know they are loved. . . . By the time they walk through the doors of the clinic . . . keeping their bodies alive is often in sharp contradiction to the suffering of their souls, the suffering they endure for simply being black and male regardless of sexuality. They need a healing requiring more than medicine, education, jobs, and T-cells."

The racial division in the D.C. gay community was further heightened when the organizers of an AIDS vigil chose an office space above Badlands, a Dupont Circle gay bar that discriminated against blacks. Only after pressure from the recently formed group Black and White Men Together was the office location changed. In the early years of the epidemic, the Whitman-Walker clinic, with limited financial support, built a variety of services for its clients. But over the years blacks would come to regard it less favorably, accusing it of essentially serving a white clientele. Several small minority AIDS agencies arose to fill the gap, including the Abundant Life Clinic run by the notoriously homophobic Nation of Islam. By 1993, more than 60 percent of D.C.'s AIDS cases would be among blacks, but the bulk of D.C.'s AIDS funding had continued to go to Whitman-Walker, with only 20 percent earmarked for minority agencies. The disparity in wealth and services between white and minority organizations was true across the country, meaning that communities of color were generally underserved—and rightfully resentful of the fact.[7]

The political scientist Cathy Cohen has provided an unusually subtle analysis of the differences in how AIDS impacted white gay male and poor black communities. "In most communities of color," she points out, "AIDS interacts with other crises, such as the lack of health care and education, homelessness, drug addiction, poverty, racism, sexism, and numerous other ills." Some white gay men, Cohen fully acknowledges, have to deal with similar issues, perhaps poverty and lack of health care especially. Yet at the least one can say that such concerns are on the whole of greater magnitude in communities of color, just as (to quote Cohen) "the general resources afforded to each community for political struggles are also in no way equal." This is not to say that African Americans are utterly powerless, but rather to emphasize that in the white world many more people of economic and political privilege exist capable of contributing individual resources to the AIDS struggle.

This was true not only on the individual level, but also in regard to how governmental agencies—preeminently the Centers for Disease Control (CDC)—perceived the nature of the crisis. Put most simply, the CDC, at least initially, treated AIDS as a disease of gay white men, and, as counterpoint, minimized its impact on women, poor people, children, sex workers and their partners, and IV drug users (where, we now know, AIDS appeared at least as early as the 1970s). The poor and marginalized, to the extent they had access to medical treatment at all, had to rely—much like today—essentially on Medicaid mills and the emergency rooms of hospitals for their care. Until the women in ACT UP (founded in 1987), many of them lesbian, pressured the CDC to revise its definition of AIDS to include pelvic inflammatory disease and other markers, women were not officially classified as "having AIDS" and were thus denied access to federal disability benefits.

For black gays in D.C., an artistic community had decidedly emerged, but no political organizations had taken deep enough root to serve as cohesive rallying points for dealing with the emerging epidemic. Sexual behavior and medical services alike continued to be the preserve of the individual. Besides, many blacks (even some who were gay) commonly dismissed AIDS in the early eighties as a white affliction—in parallel to the way the black church dismissed homosexuality itself, arguing (falsely) that it had been unknown in precolonial Africa. As a result, in the early years of the epidemic, the sole acknowledgments in the African American D.C. community of the new health threat were a forum at the African American bar Nob Hill and the September 1983 AIDS discussion held at the Clubhouse dance club, which was managed by Rainey Cheeks, who later found Us Helping Us.

In 1984, Reginald G. Blaxton, a young ordained black pastor, became a special assistant for religious affairs to Washington's mayor. Soon after Blaxton started work, Jim Graham, administrator of the Whitman-Walker clinic, approached him for help in identifying local black clergy who might join an advisory panel designed to stimulate the religious community's involvement in the AIDS crisis. The idea was certainly appropriate, given that D.C. was the oldest majority-black city in the country, with no fewer than eight hundred congregations, and that it contained some of the black community's most prestigious churches—including the National Cathedral of African Methodism and the Metropolitan AME Church. The Howard University School of Divinity also lay within the city limits, rivaled only by Atlanta University in the number and quality of black theological leaders it produced.

It was already clear in 1984–85 that white church leaders would lead the howling pack in denouncing gay sinners who'd contracted AIDS. There was some expectation that the black church and black people in general, given their own history of suffering, would respond less venomously. In fact no black church person would ever match the Jerry Falwells of the land for sheer rhetorical viciousness. Considerable anecdotal evidence further suggests that many black churches (and families), however profound their homophobia, never "threw away" their gay members with comparable ease; for some a silent compact existed instead: the doors to church and home would remain open so long as the closet door remained shut.

This comparatively softer edge may have reflected the black community's awareness of the alarming fact that the rate of infection among African Americans was much higher than their 12 percent of the population: of the roughly thirteen thousand Americans who had died from AIDS by the end of 1985, some 3,500 were African Americans. Yet formally, the black church in the early days of the epidemic was less forgiving than were black families. To Reginald Braxton, it had already become clear that the religious community's response to those afflicted with AIDS was "a harsh public piety unmixed with compassion." Braxton gave Jim Graham of the Whitman-Walker clinic the names of fifteen black clergymen in Washington who might join its advisory panel on AIDS. Fourteen of the fifteen refused any involvement to any degree with the work of the clinic. The one pastor who did agree to assist deserves noting: the Reverend J. Terry Wingate, pastor of the Purity Baptist Church in Northeast Washington.

A few years later, when public health authorities were pushing for more AIDS education in schools, including making condoms available, the Reverend Willie Wilson, black pastor of Union Temple in D.C., publicly denounced the suggestion: "This policy teaches the wrong values in a society already crippled and dying from a lack of morals and values." When D.C. officials suggested that condoms be made available in prisons, the Reverend D. Lee Owens, black pastor of the Greater Mount Zion Missionary Church, argued vehemently against the proposal: "Perhaps the fear of AIDS is just what is needed to scare these men straight." White religious figures, of course, were no less—and arguably more—unforgiving in their attitudes.

In reaction to the stark homophobia of the black church, Dr. James S. Tinney, the white Pentecostal church historian and theologian—who was himself gay and would die of AIDS in 1988—decided as early as 1982 to found Faith Temple in D.C., a predominantly black lesbian/gay institution. A few months earlier, another black gay church had been started in New York City but had soon lost its struggle to survive. Determined not to be dismissed as a mere cult, Faith Temple announced it "would not use the term 'Christian' loosely enough to include anything outside the essential, fundamental, orthodox beliefs that had identified most Christians through the ages."[8]

The black church's predominantly hostile attitude toward homosexuality has too often been equated with that of the black world in general. Though the evidence is somewhat contradictory and limited, at some periods in regard to some issues, it can in fact be argued that blacks on the whole are somewhat *less* homophobic than whites. A *New York Times* poll in 1993, for example, found that 53 percent of blacks supported equal rights for gay people but only 40 percent of whites did—and a Gallup poll that same year found that 61 percent of blacks favored lifting the ban on gays serving openly in the military, while only 42 percent of whites approved. The African American writer Cheryl Clarke has persuasively argued that the issue hasn't really been well studied but that "the poor and working-class black community, historically more radical and realistic than the reformist and conservative black middle class and the atavistic, 'blacker than thou' (bourgeois) nationalists, has often tolerated an individual's lifestyle prerogatives even when that lifestyle was disparaged by the prevailing culture."

The black writer and TV commentator Keith Boykin, further, has pointed out that with "a few high-profile exceptions," a significant number of black leaders—including Jesse Jackson, Joseph Lowery, Coretta Scott King, Julian Bond, and David Dinkins—have been strong and public supporters of civil rights protections for gay people. In the House of Representatives, moreover, the Congressional Black Caucus has led the fight against gay discrimination. In 1998 the Black Radical Congress adopted Principles of Unity that included the statement "Gender and sexuality can no longer be viewed solely as personal issues but must be a basic part of our analyses, politics and struggles." Fighting heterosexism is coming to be seen as a deeper problem than fighting homosexuality.

But back in the early eighties, support from the black leadership was much harder to come by. Gil Gerald, who headed the NCBLG, has provided a telling account of the group's effort to join the planned march celebrating the twentieth anniversary of the historic 1963 March on Washington. The NCBLG's board of directors voted unanimously to endorse the 1983 march—at the time, the only national gay or lesbian organization to do so. The established black leadership initially greeted the endorsement with dismay, not delight. D.C. congressional delegate Walter Fauntroy, who chaired the administrative committee of the march, scornfully compared lesbian and gay rights to "penguin rights"—though later, under pressure, he denied having made the remark.

Gil Gerald decided to contact the march coordinator, Donna Brazile, directly about getting the NCBLG listed among the endorsing organizations and to suggest as well that a gay or lesbian speaker—probably the well-known writer and activist Audre Lorde—be added to the roster. Initially Brazile was reassuring, but she then began ignoring Gerald's phone messages. Unable to get a response from Brazile, a frustrated and angry Gerald left word with her office that he saw no alternative but to "declare war." He consulted with Ginny Apuzzo, the progressive executive director of the National Gay Task Force, and the two decided to apply pressure on individual members of the march's steering committee.

Apuzzo ultimately did manage to get the cooperation of Judy Goldsmith, then president of the National Organization for Women (NOW), with the result that NOW let it be known that it might pull out of the march if an agreement wasn't reached with the gay and lesbian community. By then a half dozen national gay organizations had joined in the campaign for inclusion and both the *Washington Post* and the *Washington Times* carried stories about the ongoing struggle. Donna Brazile finally picked up the phone and asked Gerald if he'd be available for a conference call with the march leaders. Backed by Apuzzo and Ray Melrose, Gerald's closest confidant, he agreed. But he felt it was "ironic that I, a beneficiary of their struggles with racism in the 50s and 60s, should now be attempting to teach them something about oppression and civil rights."

Among the march leaders participating in the call that day were Walter Fauntroy, Coretta Scott King, Dr. Joseph Lowery, Benjamin Hooks, Donna Brazile—and both Ginny Apuzzo and Judy Goldsmith. Gerald's voice cracked when he tried to convey his "feelings about the devastation that AIDS was already having on the Black Gay community," and to convey as well the poignant need of the community for affirmation. The two-hour conference call was successful in the sense that agreement was reached to have a gay or lesbian speaker during that part of the program called a "Litany of Commitment"—but not during the time allotted for major addresses. It was further agreed that *individually, not as a group,* the black leaders would announce their support for the pending—and even now still pending—National Gay Rights bill in Congress.

After the conference call Gerald contacted a number of gay leaders—Essex was not yet well enough known to be among them—for their opinions, including Melvin Boozer, Ray Melrose, Dr. James Tinney, Billy Jones, Barbara Smith, and Audre Lorde, and got mixed reactions. Some felt additional pressure should be applied, others were satisfied with what had been accomplished, even though it wasn't ideal. At the press conference preceding the march, Joseph Lowery introduced the scheduled speakers and made the unauthorized, matter-of-fact—and memorable—comment that "twenty years ago we marched, and one year later, the 1964 Civil Rights Act was passed. It is now time to amend that act to extend its protections to Lesbians and Gay Men." Audre Lorde was listed in the official program as representing the gay and lesbian community, and from the steps of the Lincoln Memorial, twenty years after Martin Luther King Jr.'s "I Have a Dream" speech, she spoke these resonant words:

> We marched in 1963 with Dr. Martin Luther King, and dared to dream that freedom would include us, because not one of us is free to choose the terms of our living until all of us are free to choose the terms of our living. . . . We know we do not have to become copies of each other in order to work together. We know that when we join hands across the table of our difference, our diversity gives us great power. When we can arm ourselves with the strength and vision from all of our diverse communities then we will in truth all be free at last.

Back in 1982, Mike and Rich Berkowitz had helped form a small support group called Gay Men with AIDS, where those who were ill could share personal experiences and coping mechanisms with one another. They became aware, the following year, of the New York AIDS Network—formed by Harold (Hal) Kooden, Ginny Apuzzo, and Dr. Roger Enlow of the Office of Gay and Lesbian Health—with a different agenda: to serve as a political forum for sharing information and ideas. At one of the Network's meetings, discussion turned to an upcoming national AIDS gathering called for May 1983 in Denver. Bobbi Campbell and others in San Francisco urged major service organizations like GMHC to sponsor one or more people actually diagnosed with the disease as delegates.

The idea enthralled Mike. He may have been a self-described "bottom" but had never confused that with being temperamentally passive. "I knew," he once said, "I was going to live or die by my wits and by my knowledge." He believed deeply in self-empowerment in all areas and had already expressed anger at GMHC for failing to give those with AIDS a direct voice in its deliberations even as it provided them with immensely important services. As Mike saw it, GMHC had been treating them as "clients" and themselves as ladies bountiful, dispensing charity to the afflicted. Among other criticisms, he thought GMHC showed a racist disregard for less educated, poor black and Hispanic youth, "who cannot reasonably be expected to read between the lines of the white persons' [vague] double-speak."

For its part, the majority of GMHC's board was uncomfortable with Callen's and Berkowitz's determination to speak plainly about gay male promiscuity and the hazards of specific gay male sexual practices, regarding both as upstart radicals lacking the needed clout (and common sense) to court the white establishment. Though GMHC had refused Mike's earlier request to help distribute copies of *How to Have Sex in an Epidemic*, its board did accept his suggestion for a local forum on "AIDS and Sexuality"—but then kicked him off the panel because, as Mike saw it, he "lacked the proper professional credentials" and was too controversial to boot.

Mike and Rich both made it to the Fifth National Lesbian and Gay Health Conference in Denver in June 1983, thanks to a wealthy donor with AIDS who paid their way. Once there, they caucused with others from around the country who were now insisting on being called

"People With AIDS" (PWAs)—*not* "patients" or "victims"—and together this group of about twenty drafted a manifesto that became known as the "Denver Principles." At its heart was the feminist health movement's credo that "there are no experts on peoples' lives except those people themselves."—which Mike would later come to see as an overstatement. According to him, they "stormed" (Mike's word) the closing session of the conference and asked the nearly four hundred delegates (mostly health care professionals) that PWAs henceforth be regarded as having the "right to control their lives, their healing and their own destinies." According to one newspaper account, there wasn't a dry eye in the house, and the keynote speaker, Ginny Apuzzo, had to wait ten minutes before the audience was able to compose itself. The PWA self-empowerment movement had been born.[9]

An ecstatic Mike and Rich returned to New York and, once back in the city, placed an ad in local gay papers calling for the formation of "a rabble-rousing group of PWAs"—this was a full four years before the formation of ACT UP, with a comparable goal. As a result of the ad, PWA–New York came into existence, though due to a combination of deaths and internal dissent, it soon transformed into the PWA Coalition (PWAC). From the start, the coalition's mission was in line with the goal earlier laid out in the historic "Denver Principles": PWAs were entitled to full explanations from the "experts" so that they could make "informed decisions" regarding *every* aspect of their own treatment. It wasn't till 1987, when GMHC began putting *publicly* identified PWAs on its board of directors, that the two organizations would work together much more harmoniously.[10]

Mike and his San Francisco ally Bobbi Campbell had disagreed about one matter during the intense discussions in Denver. Mike had urged the inclusion of the principle "People with AIDS have an ethical obligation to apprise potential partners of their health status." Campbell believed that the foundational axiom of gay liberation had been the separation of love and sex: "Hey, if you're here in this bath house, that's your business. You want to suck my dick, that's your business, and I don't have to tell you anything that's going on with me." Besides, Campbell insisted, people in a bathhouse or in a jerk-off session typically don't talk, and "it's silly to say you have an obligation to wave your hand and say, 'Hello, everybody, I have AIDS.'"

Mike argued that at the very least, one had the moral obligation to be truthful about one's health in a dating situation, where the possibility existed not only of sex but of some sort of future relationship. He didn't press the matter in Denver, not wanting to jeopardize the PWA group's unity, but he continued to feel strongly that while gay liberation *was* based on sexual freedom, it was also based on bonds of brotherhood, on emotional concern for and connection to one's fellow gays—even during brief, "anonymous" sexual assignations. "Affection is our best protection" is how Mike phrased it on a 1984 poster, a phrase he would repeat in many speeches.

The debate about the separation of love and sex has a long history and was but one example of how AIDS came to represent a host of political issues and values that emerged from and yet transcended the disease itself. The very notion of self-empowerment was another. Many gay men—and particularly those more affluent white gay men who'd had no involvement with the liberation movements of the 1960s and 1970s—had often internalized deference to authority (including submission to the psychiatric view of homosexuality as "pathology"). Moreover, in a society that worshipped science, including medical research, some gay men had trouble believing they could or should play an active role in determining their own health.

According to Mike, many of the women involved in the AIDS movement "got it instantly"; they immediately understood that scientists made real contributions but weren't the ultimate authorities. Starting in the 1960s, feminists had established the view that patients should be partners in any policies or decisions relating to their own health and that women being in control of their own bodies *was* a political issue. (Later on in the AIDS movement, many focused on getting "drugs into bodies," buyers clubs proliferated, and with the formation of ACT UP in 1987, the Food and Drug Administration came under direct attack for failing to accelerate the research process.)

But Mike understood much earlier the underlying principle that people, especially the disenfranchised, had to become active on behalf of their health. After the Denver conference, he and Campbell spearheaded a self-empowerment movement that took the organizational form of PWA coalitions, culminating in the National Association of People with AIDS. Speakers went out to various venues, including colleges, to spread reliable information about how to *continue* to have sex, but to have it safely. The San Francisco AIDS Foundation headed up the movement on the West Coast, and in New York Mike had the inspiration for PWAC to sponsor a new publication, *Newsline*, which became widely read and kept readers up-to-date on a myriad of developments. Mike became both *Newsline*'s editor and the president of PWAC. He understood that most gay men remained closeted, unaffiliated with any movement organizations, and therefore unlikely to be abreast of the latest information. To reach them, he saw to it that *Newsline* was surreptitiously photocopied after hours in an unsuspecting law office and left anonymously in a wide variety of bars and public places.

As the issue of whether or not to close down the gay bathhouses started to heat up in 1984, Mike agreed to become a member of the Safer Sex Committee chaired by Dr. Roger Enlow, director of the New York City Office of Gay and Lesbian Health Concerns. Mike thought Enlow self-important and defensive but felt the committee might itself prove influential. The controversy over the baths flared first in San Francisco, then in New York. On the West Coast, public demonstrations against closure (one protester carried a sign that read "Today the Tubs, Tomorrow Your Bedroom") failed to stop the San Francisco Department of Public Health's decision in October 1984 to close down the city's bathhouses.

To prepare himself for the debate in New York, Mike decided to give himself a tour of the bathhouse scene, marking the first time in two and a half years that he'd entered one. At his first stop, the Club Baths, he saw no one having unsafe sex but noted that its bulletin board had no risk-reduction information on it, even though by that point GMHC and the Safer Sex Committee had produced and distributed posters and brochures to dozens of establishments. He also noted that most of the customers were black or Hispanic and reminded himself that the Coalition's materials needed to be translated into Spanish.[11]

The East Side Sauna was his next stop. He had a West Villager's "chauvinistic disdain for anything even vaguely 'Upper East Side,'" but he did his "totally demoralizing" duty. The sauna was packed, but he saw none of the spontaneity and abandon that had previously characterized the bathhouse/back-room bar scene. A way of life was over. The expressions on the patrons' faces reminded him of "the endless

Life magazine photos of children of war." An image stuck with him "of little boys lost—each wandering around aimlessly . . . holding on to his penis for what small comfort might be left in this hostile, frightening world." Once again he found a bulletin board with various announcements tacked to it—gay Front Runners, tickets to an Alvin Ailey concert, and so on—but once again nothing at all relating to precautionary measures in regard to AIDS. And this time he did see some unsafe sex—men fucking other men without condoms.

A similar scene awaited him at Everard's, the oldest and best known of the city's gay bathhouses. It was filthy and Mike could smell mildew and mold everywhere. "The management" had put up a number of signs: "No Drugs"; "We Reserve the Right to Refuse Admission to Anyone"—even one that urged the patrons to "Shower Between Contacts." But nothing at all was posted about AIDS and safe sex.

After his grim tour of the bathhouses, which had proven utterly lacking in AIDS or safe-sex information, Mike launched into the debate about the pros and cons of closing the bathhouses. He understood the civil liberties issues involved and disliked the notion of authorities of any kind dictating permissible individual behavior. He also recognized that the bathhouses, ideally at least, represented a place where a cross section of individuals could meet: "I don't want to make too much of the democracy of gay life," he wrote in notes to himself, but where else but in a gay bathhouse "could you find a Park Avenue doctor and a Puerto Rican delivery boy, stripped of all outward appearances of social rank, naked in mutual need." He knew, too, that the baths were among the few places where closeted or married men would allow themselves to go.

Mike had also long advocated lots of sex as a necessary antidote to society's erotophobia. He stood by the view that "bathhouses potentially promote healthy abandon"—but "potentially" was of course the sticking point. If the baths promoted disease as well as abandon and barred safer-sex information on the premises, weren't they then a liability? Abandon could be achieved elsewhere. Then again, it was also true that it was safer—in terms of violence, not disease—to have sex in an indoor bathhouse than, say, in an outdoor parking lot prey to violence-prone homophobes.

Mike insisted that in the original 1982 article he'd written with Berkowitz ("We Know Who We Are"), they'd "never suggested closing down the baths"—as their critics had claimed; rather, they were the first to warn about the threat of the government doing so. "Ultimately," they'd written, "it may be more important to let people die in the pursuit of their own happiness than to limit personal freedom by regulating risk." But that was in 1982. Mike's recent tour of the bathhouses apparently led him to shift the balance and come down on the side of closure. "These men are too nice to die," he now decided. The few patrons he'd talked to directly during his tour did *not* seem well informed about how AIDS might be transmitted or about how to protect themselves and their partners. And the bathhouse owners were obviously not going out of their way to enlighten them; they were, predictably, far more concerned with maintaining their margin of profit than with the health of their clients.

Throughout the 1970s, Mike had believed that having lots of sex was the equivalent of being a soldier in the sexual revolution. And he continued to believe that partaking of sexual abundance was far preferable to the alternatives of monogamy or abstinence. He knew, too, that closing the bathhouses was unlikely to make more than a slight dent in the spread of the epidemic, since alternate venues were no safer. Besides, in 1984 it was commonly believed—a notion pushed by GMHC—that AIDS was *not* a gay disease. IV drug users, hemophiliacs, heterosexual women, and children were among those already known to be infected, and many activists insisted that it could only be guessed how the disease might be distributed in the future. Mike was not among them. He remembered "cringing when I heard the executive director of the Gay Men's Health Crisis compare AIDS to a steaming locomotive roaring down the tracks" toward the general, that is heterosexual, population. As a tactic for prompting a more active response from federal research institutions and increasing support and sympathy from the public—who'd shown indifference to a disease confined to gay men and drug users—depicting the epidemic as an equal threat to heterosexual people can be considered a somewhat successful political ploy, but the depiction was an inaccurate one for the United States and Europe.

Sonnabend was particularly incensed by the argument that AIDS would soon spread widely into the heterosexual world. He and Dr. Mathilde Krim (who was married to Arthur Krim, a leading Democratic fund-raiser and head of Orion Pictures) had been colleagues in interferon-related research in the 1960s. In April 1983, Sonnabend and Krim co-founded the nonprofit AIDS Medical Foundation (amfAR) to raise private funds for research, and hired Mike and Rich to advance safe-sex education. They were grateful for the opportunity, having been turned down repeatedly for grant proposals, often, according to Berkowitz, "by panels that included GMHC board members who sat on funding committees."

Berkowitz further claims that after Krim hired them, two GMHC board members threatened that "they would turn the community against her unless she got rid of Sonnabend, Callen and Berkowitz." As a compromise, she held on to Sonnabend but let Rich and Mike go. Rich spent the next year (until the end of 1985) reporting weekly on AIDS and safe-sex-related issues for Lou Maletta's cable TV show. But Maletta couldn't afford to pay him, and Rich decided to accept an invitation from a former client to move into his oceanfront apartment in Miami Beach; he continued to do safe-sex education at South Florida bathhouses and bookstores, but returned to New York City and to hustling in 1986. As for Sonnabend, his history with Mathilde Krim would be marked by alternating cycles of friendly cooperation and angry disaffection. This was especially true in the mid-1980s, when Joe became incensed at the continuing insistence of some amfAR representatives that the epidemic would soon engulf the heterosexual world.

By 1985, Mike felt compelled to conclude that going to a bathhouse seemed like "a highly suspect act of suicide." Didn't police (the state) have the right, or even the duty, he asked, to interfere if someone was about to jump off the Brooklyn Bridge, to coax someone down with smooth arguments about how different tomorrow might look, how hopeful new options might present themselves? Yet he doubted if that was a true equivalent. Suicidal moods can pass, but a fatal disease doesn't cease to be a killer over time. If people could be informed about the deadly risks of the baths and make their own decisions, that would be one thing, but what if you couldn't disseminate the pertinent literature, or if people chose to ignore it?

Earlier, when Mike had asked one of the men he encountered at the Club Baths if he wasn't afraid of getting AIDS, the man had calmly replied, "No, I can tell by looking at someone if they've got it." With foolish attitudes like that around, Mike for a time went back and forth in a painful internal debate about the tricky issue of bathhouse closure. He felt it was a judgment call for which no simple answer existed. In the upshot, the city decided that bathhouses could remain open—but only if they complied with strict regulations about the availability of condoms and information. Only four out of fifteen were still operating at the end of 1985. Mike blamed the bathhouse owners in New York (in contrast to those in San Francisco) for failing "to take any initiative in educating their patrons" and also held GMHC accountable for conducting fund-raising events—but not educational forums—in the notorious orgy bar the Mineshaft.[12]

As early as 1983 the French scientist Luc Montanier had announced his discovery that a virus—for a time referred to by various names, but which by 1986 had consolidated into HIV—was the likely culprit in depressing the immune system and opening the body to the multiple "opportunistic" infections known as AIDS. The noted and controversial American retrovirologist Dr. Robert Gallo soon after named himself as the discoverer of the virus and a series of complex charges and countercharges followed, with most scientists giving the palm to Montanier. In any case, the discovery of HIV would, on its face, seem to put an end to Sonnabend's multifactorial theory about the origin of AIDS. Gallo in 1988 denounced the notion of co-factors as "cock and horseshit . . . baloney," and Dr. Anthony Fauci, head of the National Institute of Allergy and Infectious Diseases (NIAID) at the National Institutes of Health, acknowledged that co-factors "might enhance the expression of HIV" but unequivocally insisted that "HIV is the answer."

Neither Joe Sonnabend nor Mike agreed. As Sonnabend later put it, "I'd been trained in a view of health and disease that had gone out of fashion by the time this hit. In my day, we were taught to look at disease not simply as something caused by a germ—there are many other factors that affect one's immunity and the ability to handle infectious diseases." Not only did Sonnabend feel that ascribing *the* cause of AIDS to a single virus was simplistic, but he also felt that the readiness to believe in a sexually transmitted "killer virus" was due to the theory's political and psychological appeal to many different constituencies: "People who like 'family values,' people who hate gay men, prostitutes and junkies, people who love to think that extramarital sex can kill. Some gay men liked it, too, because it deflected attention from all the sex taking place in the bathhouse scene." Of course the fact that a particular theory "appealed" to many people has no bearing on its validity, only on the degree to which it is widely accepted or rejected.[13]

Nearly a decade later, Mike conducted two interviews with Sonnabend for the declared purpose of trying "to pin him down about where he stands on the question of HIV." But Mike found him "as usual . . . slippery . . . certainly he's been more willing lately to at least speak the language of HIV" and to agree that it might well be *a contributing factor.* But Sonnabend was also insistent that in Europe and the United States (Africa is another—still not well understood—matter) "it's very hard for a man to get this disease from women. Women *are* at risk—not from heterosexual men who aren't drug users, but from bisexual men and from men who use intravenous drugs." Sonnabend also contended that there was no convincing evidence of woman-to-woman transmission, and the scientific data bore him out: of the seven reported instances in 1993, mitigating circumstances—usually IV drug use or sex with men—were present in all cases but one. And the scientific and community data verified that "VERY, VERY few lesbians practice safe sex with any rigor," which theoretically should have led to many more cases of AIDS among them.

Sonnabend continues to this day to insist on "the complexity of what causes disease." In his view, "there are many more people infected with HIV than people who have AIDS"—as well as some AIDS patients who don't test positive for HIV. Thus, "genetic factors, genetic susceptibility does exist, even with HIV. . . . [Also,] the presence of other diseases can influence it. . . . All infectious disease, including HIV, is multifactorial." In his words, "infection may have a single cause—HIV causes HIV infection. Measles virus causes measles infection. Polio virus causes polio infection. Once infected the next step is the disease. Not everybody infected . . . becomes sick. It's called the attack rate. Whether you get sick seems to depend on the organism, the dose, the way it gets into you, the presence of other diseases and also on environmental, nutritional and genetic factors. The only disease that I'm aware of that has an attack rate approximating 100 percent is rabies." Sonnabend has never said that there wasn't a new agent at work in producing the disease of AIDS, nor has he ever said that the purported new agent was harmless or didn't exist. "I have no doubt that HIV plays a role in this disease," he acknowledges; "it's the necessary but not sufficient cause insofar as cause is defined as a single agent." As regards disease, he continues to believe (as do others) that AIDS is "the outcome of a constellation of factors acting simultaneously"— which in essence is an alternate description of the "multifactorial" position. In sum, Sonnabend's view was, and is, that not everybody who is exposed gets infected, not everybody who is infected gets sick, and not everybody gets sick at the same rate.

For his part, Mike pointed out that in regard to HIV "there is a correlation with AIDS; but it used to be accepted in science that correlation was not the same thing as causation." He believed, following Sonnabend, that there was no one specific cause, that getting infected with HIV was not the equivalent of getting AIDS. He made an analogy with a heart attack or stroke: genetics, diet, exercise, and stress all play a role. In the same way, he argued, HIV is more likely to progress to AIDS if other immunosuppressive co-factors—like multiple infections from multiple sexual partners—were also present. Yet in 1998 Sonnabend would himself acknowledge that he'd been wrong to believe at the beginning of the epidemic that the *only* gay men who came down with the disease had "a history of multiple STDs"; he later encountered some people who didn't fit that model and yet did have AIDS.

As for Mike, he emphasized back in 1984–85 that we still "cannot explain why Person X with under 200 T-4 [cells] develops pneumocystis and Person Y with under 200 T-4s doesn't. We simply don't know very much about the natural history of AIDS." He suspected that both competing theoretical camps would eventually turn out to be right—"that some role for HIV in causing AIDS may indeed one day be proven . . . [but] there are probably multiple causes, of which HIV might be one important element." Neither Mike nor Sonnabend ever came close to being an out-and-out "denialist"—that is, a follower of the University of California molecular biologist Peter Duesberg, who believes that HIV is not the cause of AIDS, not even in a contributory sense. In 1984–85, Mike did believe that Duesberg's arguments deserved serious consideration and needed refutation. He thought Duesberg was "dead wrong about there being no infectious process," as well as in his suspicion "that it was toxins INTERACTING with pathogens" that produced AIDS. "Why don't tops," Mike asked, "get AIDS if there isn't an additional infectious component involved?" As for the book *The AIDS War*, by John Lauritsen, another denialist, Mike found it a "tedious, flip reduction of complex and subtle statements."[14]

Sonnabend separated himself even more emphatically from Duesberg. It was one thing to say, as Sonnabend did, that he didn't believe HIV had been "adequately demonstrated to be the sole cause of AIDS," but quite another to say—as Duesberg did—that he'd completely ruled out the possibility that HIV could be the cause. Sonnabend hadn't ruled it out. He considered it a hypothesis, not a proven fact. When Mike specifically asked him, "So, unlike Duesberg, you do not rule out the *possibility* of a role for HIV in the etiology of AIDS?" Sonnabend replied, "Certainly not." He even went on to say that in stating that HIV *cannot* be the cause of AIDS, Duesberg was making "categorical, dogmatic statements which I don't feel ought to be made." When Mike then asked Sonnabend whether he felt "on balance, that Duesberg has been more good than bad in keeping the debate about the etiology of AIDS open?" Sonnabend said flat out, "I think he's been bad. . . . It's easy enough to discredit all skepticism about HIV because of Duesberg." On another occasion Sonnabend was even more pointed: "Duesberg has no credentials whatsoever to have an opinion—he's out of his depth." The strongest evidence in favor of HIV as the cause, Sonnabend went on, is the association of HIV seropositivity with AIDS—"that is a powerful argument which cannot be dismissed lightly or ignored."

When Mike questioned why other pathogens in the patient besides HIV were dismissed as playing no role in the progression of the disease, Sonnabend suggested the possibility that the presence of HIV antibodies might actually be the opportunistic *result* of whatever is truly suppressing the immune system. He felt it was also plausible— that is, "completely consistent with basic virologic principles—for some unknown percentage of people to be carrying HIV . . . without having ever formed HIV antibodies."

Could Sonnabend imagine a proof that would ever satisfy him that HIV was in fact *the* cause of AIDS? "Certainly," Sonnabend responded. "HIV has been found in people who don't seroconvert [from negative to positive] over the long term. The way to prove the theory would be

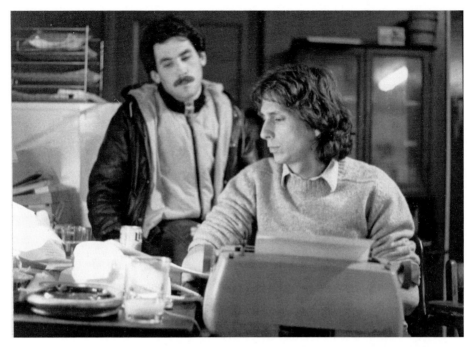

Richard Berkowitz and Michael Callen writing *How to Have Sex in an Epidemic*, New York, 1983 (photo courtesy of Richard Dworkin)

SAFER SEX GUIDELINES
One Approach

Limit what sex acts you choose to perform to ones which interrupt disease transmission. The key to this is modifying **what** you do—not how often you do it nor with how many different people.

★ **Affection Is Our Best Protection**
   If you care about the person you're having sex with, you will want to protect his health and your own.

★ **Common Sense**
   Proper diet, rest and reduced stress are necessary for good health.

★ **Talking**
   Discuss your health concerns with your partner. Find a partner who will be reassured by your concerns—not put off by them.

★ **Shower Thoroughly Before and Immediately After Sex**
   Examine your partner while showering. Don't be clinical. Make it a part of foreplay.

★ **Stay In Control**
   Safe sex requires you be sober. Avoid the use of substances which may impair your decision-making ability.

★ **Avoid the Exchange of Semen, Urine and Feces (Fecal Matter)**
   These bodily fluids may contain high concentrations of cytomegalovirus (CMV) and other infectious agents.

★ **Use Condoms (Rubbers)**
   Condoms provide the best protection against CMV and other infectious agents.

The first safe-sex poster, 1983

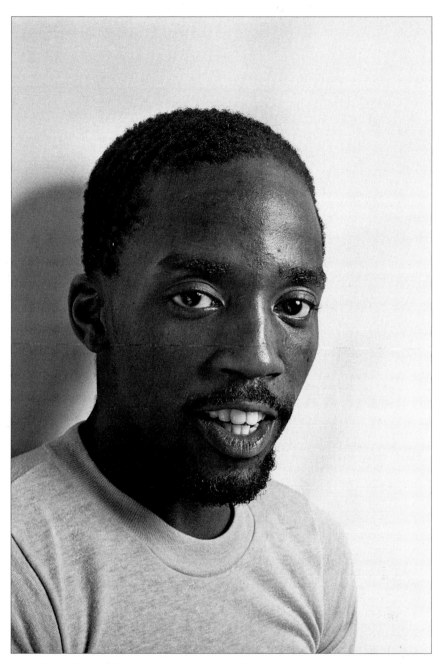

Essex Hemphill, the young poet (photo © Sharon Farmer/sfphotoworks)

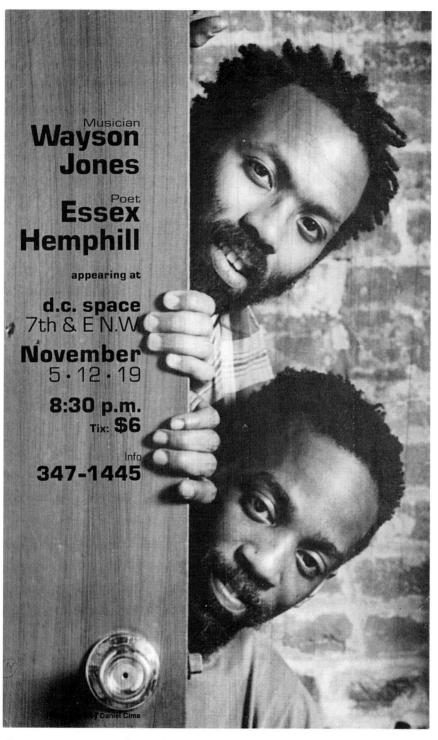

Musician
Wayson Jones

Poet
Essex Hemphill

appearing at

d.c. space
7th & E N.W.

November
5 · 12 · 19

8:30 p.m.
Tix: **$6**

Info
347-1445

Daniel Cima

Poster announcement of an early gig at d.c. space (courtesy of Michelle Parkerson)

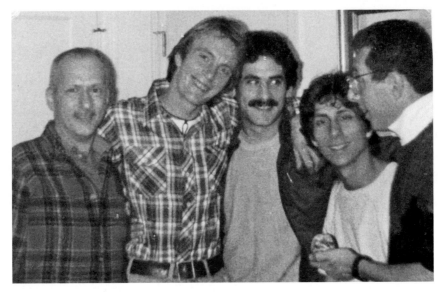

Denver Conference, 1983—left to right: Tom Nasrallah, Bobbi Campbell, Rich Berkowitz, Mike Callen, and Artie Felson (photo courtesy of Richard Dworkin)

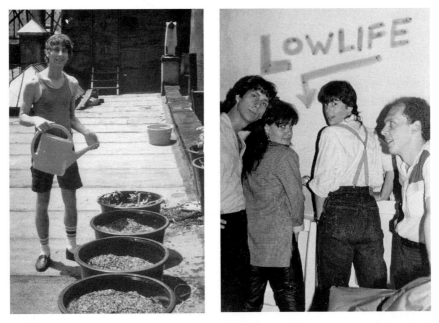

(Left) Mike the city gardener, circa 1984; rooftop on Duane Street in New York (photo courtesy of Richard Dworkin)

(Right) The band Lowlife using the men's room, circa 1984—left to right: Mike Callen, Pam Brandt, Janet Cleary, and Richard Dworkin (photo courtesy of Richard Dworkin)

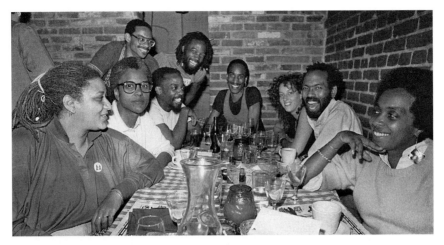

"Poets, Artists, Musicians, Friends" having dinner at the Iron Gate Restaurant in Washington, D.C., May 6, 1986—left to right: Jewelle Gomez, Cheryl Clarke, Colin Robinson, Essex Hemphill, Ray Melrose, Craig Harris, Elizabeth Ziff, Wayson Jones, and Joyce Wellman (photo © Sharon Farmer/sfphotoworks)

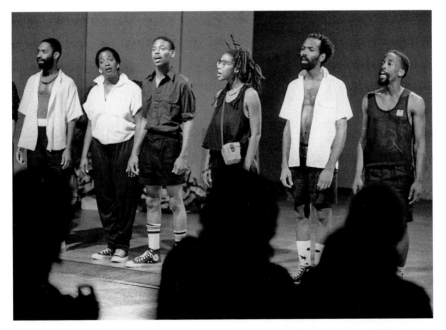

A performance at the Painted Bride Art Center, Philadelphia, August 9, 1986—left to right: Brenda Files, Larry Duckett, M'lafi Thompson, Chris Prince, Michelle Parkerson, Wayson Jones, and Essex Hemphill (photo © Sharon Farmer/sfphotoworks)

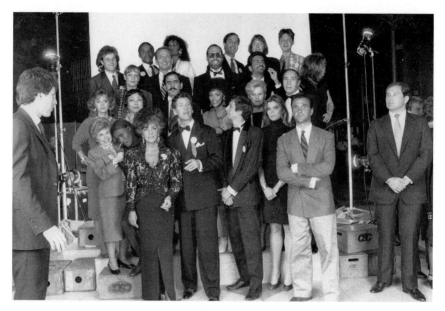

AmFar benefit at the Javits Center, New York City, April 29, 1986—left to right (front row): Dr. Ruth Westheimer, Grace Jones, Elizabeth Taylor, Calvin Klein, Michael Callen, Mariel Hemingway, and Michael Vollbract (photo by Richard Corkery)

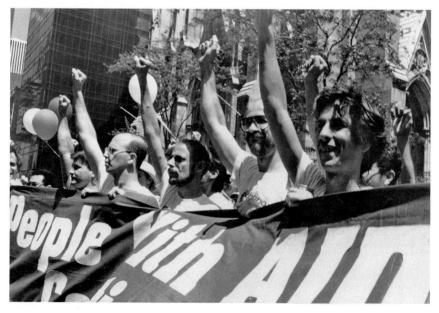

Gay Pride March, New York City, June 6, 1986—left to right, unidentified man, Michael Hirsch, David Summers, Sal Licata, and Michael Callen (photo by Jane Rosett)

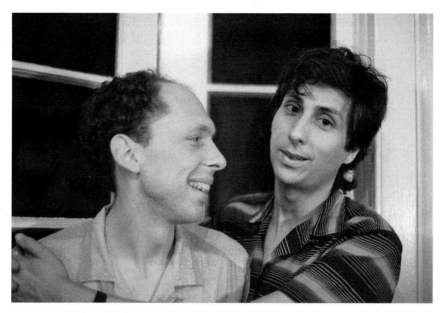

Richard and Mike, 1988 (photo courtesy of Richard Dworkin)

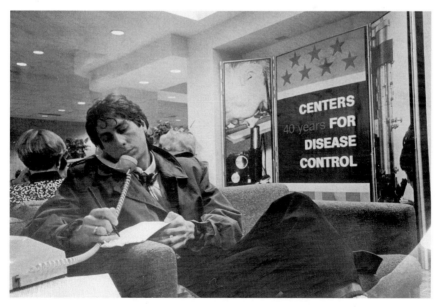

Michael Callen at the Centers for Disease Control, Atlanta, 1988 (photo by Jane Rosett)

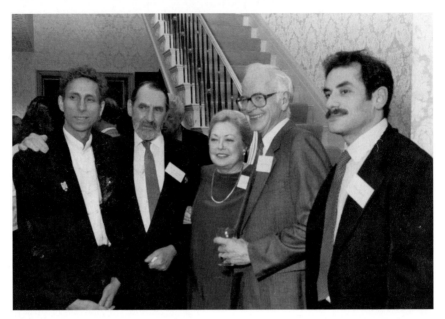

A party at Mathilde Krim's house honoring Joe Sonnabend, 1988—left to right: Michael Callen, Joe Sonnabend, Mathilde Krim, Harley Hackett, and Richard Berkowitz (photo courtesy of Richard Dworkin)

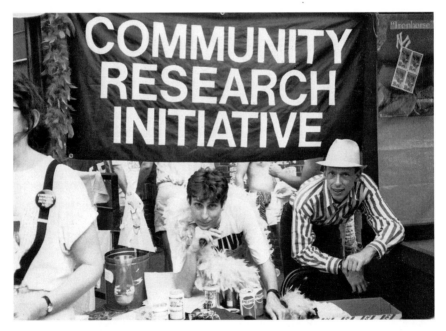

Michael and Richard under the CRI banner at the Christopher Street celebration following the 1989 New York City Gay Pride March (photo courtesy of Richard Dworkin)

to find HIV in seronegative people by taking specimens at autopsies of thousands of people and looking for HIV in tissues. . . . Also, if an anti-retroviral therapy were to 'cure' AIDS, that would largely settle the question as well." Mike's skeptical mind objected to speculation being presented as established fact, since that excluded the fair consideration of other possibilities. That was precisely Sonnabend's bottom line as well. Both of them felt that the multifactorial explanation had its own problems, and one major criticism leveled at Sonnabend was that he'd never devised a model to test his own multifactorial theory—a criticism he didn't deny. What both men required, above all, was an open-minded approach that *invited* diversity of opinion.

Mike also required a rest. He'd been going nonstop, writing, organizing, arguing, petitioning, testifying—as well as demanding every step of the way, as one interviewer put it, "that we [gay people] see beyond our own needs to include women and the poor and health care issues of concern to every American." Homophobia and racism, he insisted, were not unrelated: "We are beginning to see that a Haitian infant dying in poverty in the South Bronx and the death of a middle-class gay man in Manhattan are sadly but undeniably interconnected."

In August 1984, he let Richard Dworkin persuade him that they could squeeze just enough pennies together to jump off the New York fast track and take a brief holiday in Europe. It proved a restful break overall, though Mike preceded Dworkin by a few days and those proved somewhat difficult for him. Along with periodic fever and exhaustion, Mike had a cyclical history of depression, going back ten years, which usually occurred in late summer. True to form, when he was alone in Wales in late August, the weather penetratingly cold and wet, "an incipient depression"—as he wrote in the occasional diary he kept during the trip—"imperceptibly began to gather. I had that most dreaded feeling: racing mind, dry throat and cough, queasy anxiety." He'd learned from past experience that "the key is control and distraction." He took some Valium and talked quietly to himself about how he'd "survived worse depressions in the past" and how Richard would soon be meeting him in London. It worked. The depression was aborted short of the "lethal momentum" of past episodes. Once he and Richard were together, travel became easier, though Mike's exhaustion periodically resurfaced, along with abrupt alternations between sweating and freezing.[15]

Struck at how full of children England was, Mike realized, as he put it, "how absolutely sequestered from reality I am—living in NYC in the USA as a queer man." He didn't want children—quite the contrary: he thought that "surely if hets [heterosexuals] knew before hand—truly knew—the horrific responsibility of raising kids, there'd be no more of them." He felt that one aspect of straight resentment against gay people was precisely their freedom from child rearing, freedom to focus on their own needs and pleasure. His feminist sensibility rebelled at the sight of all those mothers traveling with kids: "Most engineer collapsible strollers and Kleenex and diapers and harnesses and candy and toys." In awe, he watched them patiently tell their offspring, "No. Don't bite Mommy"—leading the kid "to increase his screaming several decibels, while the father sits willfully oblivious reading the paper." Little could Mike have guessed at the wave of gay parenting that would soon occur.

The feminist in him delighted in the discovery of a portrait of Mary Wollstonecraft in a museum—but he then became appalled when he spoke to the guide and she knew of Wollstonecraft only as "the mother-in-law of Shelley." Mike the tourist was taken most of all with English botanical gardens. He thought them "spectacular" and couldn't quite figure out "why verdure makes me so *calm*"; he thought maybe it was the smell. At one point they passed a couple of apple trees and Mike the cook was transported by the idea of "baking lard-crusted pies out of fresh apples. . . . I'm sure I could change Richard's mind about fruit pies!"

From London they went briefly to Paris. Richard spoke French, which was helpful, though verbal Mike hated being stripped of communication through language. But he loved being with Richard—"my sweetest man," he called him—and he romantically picked wildflowers to press into a book to give him. Mike decided that what frightened straight men most—and he didn't think "gay politicos" understood this—wasn't the notion of sex between men, but rather *affection*. "Two men fucking they might understand—as aggression, as competition. But two men kissing? I would say that the average het male would be less offended watching one of Berkowitz's S/M sessions than watching a loving and affectionate pairing of two men."

Throughout the trip, he and Richard succeeded in accommodating each other's very different pace and style. Once awake in the morning, Mike quickly showered, brushed his teeth, and wanted to *eat*—breakfast was his favorite meal. Besides (as he put it), "I need focus, a goal, I can't hang loose"; he was "no good at wandering aimlessly." Richard was very nearly the opposite. He liked to take things slowly, especially in the morning: "Have a cigarette or two and read. Then, shave, then shower, then another cigarette, then maybe breakfast." Mike, a non-smoker, nonetheless sympathized. "I wouldn't want to travel with me," he wrote. He realized that he and Richard were "oil and vinegar" but thought they made "a delicious if exotic salad dressing in these salad days. . . . We're getting along amazingly well." Mike only wished he had his health: "I feel I could move on and lead a good life."

"What does fate have in store?" he wrote sadly in his diary. "My pressing sense of my fragile mortality."

4

The Mideighties

Joe Beam's ad soliciting manuscripts for a black gay male anthology initially produced only a few responses, and it made him more aware than ever that "the path I'm on is basically an untrodden one." Cherríe Moraga and Gloria Anzaldúa had published the pioneering anthology *This Bridge Called My Back* for women of color in 1981, and Barbara Smith had put out a similar collection of writings for black feminists, *Home Girls*, in 1983, but nothing comparable existed for black gay men. Both Smith and Audre Lorde were supportive with their advice to Joe Beam both in terms of the specifics of contributors' contracts and by way of general encouragement to persevere. And despite his discouragement at times, he did. By the spring of 1985, he'd collected about a hundred manuscripts from which to make his choices. In the end, he'd include twenty-eight contributors, several of them (including Essex) appearing more than once.[1]

Part of Beam's discouragement while putting the anthology together related to matters peripheral to it. Two of the contributors died of AIDS before Joe could fully edit their work, and in Philadelphia, where Beam lived, came the additionally horrifying news on May 13, 1985, that the police had bombed the building in which the black urban commune MOVE had long lived. The action destroyed sixty-one homes in the Osage Avenue neighborhood, killing eleven residents—

five of them children—and leaving 250 people homeless. The only known adult to escape the fire, Ramona Africa, was sentenced to prison. Though MOVE had had a long series of conflicts and confrontations with its neighbors, it was inconceivable to many that Philadelphia's first black mayor, Wilson Goode, would approve such violent and repressive action. The bombing produced a national uproar and a plethora of conflicting testimony and theories.[2]

Essex was outraged at the bombing and wrote a poem to add to the new version of *Voicescapes*—a stripped-down version, without the elaborate slides and film that had been part of the original piece—that he, Wayson, and Michelle were performing in 1987:

> What will be bombed today?
> What will be bombed today?
>
> What will be bombed today?
> American café at noon
> A playground full of nappy heads.
> Do you dread your house will cinder
> and firemen stand ground
> watching the block burn to the
> ground like a Salem witch, a nigger
> in a tree?
>
> Do you see?
> Do you dread?
> Do the papers panic you?
> Do you sleep with a gun under your pillow?
>
> What will be bombed today?
> The A uptown?
> Another funeral in Soweto?
> An abortion clinic?
>
> What will be bombed today?

A critic for the *Philadelphia Inquirer* who interviewed the trio after their performance told them that she felt their work "has no deliberate desire to unsettle, disorient and provoke audiences, [that] engagement comes from identification and understanding rather than confrontation." Essex laughingly replied that he didn't think you had to say, "I want to make this audience walk out of here with their minds in shatters, tatters, they'll be recuperating next week." "Valiums for everybody," Michelle interjected. "Right!" Essex added, "a nurse at the door. Nurses in the bathroom. Nurses at the stage." But, Michelle added, "we need a bigger budget to hire nurses." On a more serious note, Essex told the interviewer that "I may, at the point of starting out, be heavily moved by something, something that I may have seen on the news or on the street or heard on the phone or in a letter or in a conversation. That may be the stepping stone, but where I wind up after that, I'm as amazed as everybody else because I'm just following the flow of what's being unleashed."

Joe Beam was no less horrified by the MOVE bombing, by "the madness of the incident." It heightened the moody sense he often had of feeling "real weary" or, as he put it succinctly to Isaac Jackson, his friend and managing editor of *Blackheart*, "Underneath this strong, efficient exterior is a man easily devastated." And the horrors of the MOVE episode continued to have lingering effects on him. He felt that if it wasn't for the anthology, "I'm sure I'd go into hiding. I just feel too vulnerable" and "I [am] weary of being misunderstood."

He wasn't simply referencing the hostile power of the white world, which was real enough, but also the sense that he didn't have a community: "You have to fight Black people for inclusion on grounds of sexuality; you have to fight white people for inclusion on grounds of race; you have to fight with other Black gay men on the grounds of age and jealousy. All I really want is a place where I can be all of who I am at the same time, a place where it's not necessary to check parts of myself at the door." Above all, he wanted a steady lover and, handsome and gifted as he was, seemed mystified at his inability to connect with one.[3]

Temperamentally, Essex wasn't nearly as anguished as Joe, nor as lonely. Until recently, moreover, he'd been living for three years with a partner ("Mel"), who ended up giving primacy to his career in the navy and broke off the relationship. Essex missed "the domestic repetition of beauty that is found in caring for and being cared for by a lover." He thought it would console Joe to know that he, too, has "calendars of months that have gone by without so much as a hint of love. Or either love has come to me disguised so perfectly I have not, in all my haughtiness, seen it." But Essex didn't want to dwell on his own complaints. He wanted simply to tell Joe "quite frankly, I love you, for the man you are, which is why I believe our friendship will be forever. . . . A friendship tied to concerns that when galvanized will [help] us all. . . . Please stay well in spirit, and believe love will come to you and make you stronger, but be strong, now, while it seems love is not near. And please know, we're brothers."

Essex did, unlike Joe, later enter into another relationship that again lasted for about three years. Several of his friends thought he made bad choices in his partners, and one of them felt Essex was in general attracted to men who mistreated him, the attraction a product of his early experience with his own abusive father. When word leaked out that the current lover had actually threatened Essex's life, an alarmed Joe wrote to remind him that "you weren't put on this planet to leave on the end of a jealous lover's gun." Essex himself referred to the dangers he risked in that relationship in a poem entitled "The Tomb of Sorrow":

> I was your man lover,
> gambling dangerously
> with my soul.
> I was determined to love you
> but you were haunted
> by Vietnam.
> taunted by demons.
> In my arms you dreamed
> of tropical jungles,
> of young village girls
> with razors embedded in their pussies,
> lethal chopsticks
> hidden in their hair,
> and their nipples clenched
> like grenade pins
> between your grinding teeth.
> You rocked and kicked
> in your troubled sleep,

as though you were fucking
one of those dangerous cunts,
and I was by your side,
unable to hex it away,
or accept that peace
means nothing to you,
and the dreams you suffer
may be my only revenge.

Despite Essex's best efforts to bring him some solace, Joe's dejection remained deep-seated. He could only briefly shake the sense that to the extent he was loved at all, it was "for what one does as opposed to who one is. . . . No-one wants to touch this baby. He writes well and does wonderful things, but don't touch him." Though he'd been motivated to do *In The Life*, he wrote Essex, "in an effort to create community, yet I've alienated much of the community in which I wish to belong. The book isn't even out and I've been transferred to this league of folks who are idolized but not dealt with." So sensitive was he that "a single shard from a cutting remark is enough to wound deeply, so I keep myself safe, at home: the door locked, phone off the hook. . . . Rejections like mercury accumulate in the body, in the heart. I have had more than my share. Initially I could dodge the rebuffs, discount individual reactions, but the cumulative effect is shattering."

Joe was fortunate in that at least his immediate family, his parents, Sun and Dorothy Beam, supported, if warily, his lifestyle and his literary efforts. His father, born in Barbados, was (in Joe's words) "kind and gentle . . . but we are not friends. . . . We are silent when alone together. I do not ask him about his island childhood or his twelve years as a janitor or about the restaurant he once owned where he met my mother. He does not ask me about being gay or why I wish to write about it. Yet we are connected. . . . His thick calloused hands have led me this far and given me options he never dreamed of."

With his mother, Dorothy, Joe had a much deeper connection. He showed her everything he wrote, though he felt that "somewhere along the line she has either stopped reading it or simply doesn't comment upon it." Yet in one letter to him, Dorothy Beam warned him that "the world is a cruel place to live," and she worried that his open acknowledgment of his homosexuality would bring him harm. "Joe," she wrote, "gay people have a long way to go before society will truly accept them." Over lunch one day, Joe kidded his mother about starting a meeting of parents of black gay activists, where they "could sit around exchanging horror stories about their crazed children." Dorothy laughed but seemed as if she might actually be interested. "We are putting them through changes," Joe wrote Essex, "forcing them to grow as we are doing."[4]

Joe also felt lucky in his job at Giovanni's Room. He considered the bookstore "a warm, supportive, nurturing place to work." The money wasn't great, but he felt he was making "a contribution to the gay community, and the community at large." To him, Giovanni's Room was a wonderful "vestige of the 1960s." The store used a toolbox for a cash register, let people sit as long as they liked on the sofa to read books they might not be able to afford, and posted free of charge a wide variety of community announcements and flyers. In many ways, Giovanni's Room functioned more like a community center than a business.

Yet the time came when Joe felt he had to devote himself full-time to the anthology, and on July 12, 1985, he left his job at the bookstore. Ed Hermance, its co-owner, knowing about Joe's project, had all along been generous about letting him take time off, and Hermance now gave him a large enough severance check to free him to work solely on the anthology till at least the end of the summer.

All of which gave Joe a needed boost of confidence: "I am more sure each day," he wrote a friend, "that this is precisely what I should be doing. Everything that has needed to happen for this book to become a reality has happened." He was nearing a final decision about which essays and poems to include and he'd lined up a group of strong contributors. They included many of the prominent and promising black gay male writers of the day—the poet and novelist Melvin Dixon; Gil Gerald, the executive director of the National Coalition of Black Lesbians and Gays (which was headquartered in D.C.); Essex (four poems); the essayist and poet Craig Harris; the Haitian-born poet Assotto Saint, who also wrote musical theater pieces; the well-known science fiction writer Samuel Delany; and Sidney Brinkley, the founder of *Blacklight*—and Joe had left space as well for a significant number of unknown newcomers.

By mid-September, though, he was so low on finances that he couldn't afford the bus fare from Philadelphia to D.C. to pay Essex a surprise visit. Not that Essex was doing much better; at one point his phone service was cut off for lack of payment. Both men were living the lives they wanted to, and they treated financial hardship as an inescapable aspect of the choices they'd made. Essex self-published his latest chapbook of poetry, *Earth Life*, in 1985, and then turned it into a performance piece with Wayson—who in Essex's view was "becoming such a fine musician and a willing adventurer." Joe, too, was nearing completion of the manuscript for *In The Life*, though toward the end he gave in to necessity and took a part-time sales job at a Barnes and Noble bookstore, while also moonlighting as a part-time restaurant waiter to make ends meet. He finished the manuscript in early November 1985, and the prominent gay press Alyson accepted it for publication.

By way of celebration, he and seven others, including Essex, drove out to St. Louis in a rented fifteen-passenger van for the NCBLG weekend-long convention. For Joe it was an "absolutely fantastic" event. He renewed old friendships with people like Pat Parker and for the first time met face-to-face with people he'd talked with on the phone countless times, thus initiating new friendships. To top off the excitement, he was elected to the NCBLG board of directors and asked to edit its new newsmagazine, *Black/Out* (*Blackheart*, Brinkley's earlier journal of writing and graphics by black gay men, had ceased publishing after its third issue); Essex, Barbara Smith, and Audre Lorde all joined *Black/Out*'s publications committee. Essex, too, had been stirred by the convention. The NCBLG's "Statement of Purpose" tied in closely with his own values. Its emphasis on "Black Pride and Solidarity" concurred with his own primary commitment to creating "positive attitudes between and among Black non-Gays and Black Gays."[5]

But if racial solidarity took primacy over gay liberation for Essex, the former didn't invalidate or cancel out the latter. Multiple ingredients based on race, class, gender, sexual orientation, education, income, and so forth contribute to forming an individual "identity," rising and falling in comparative importance depending on immediate circumstances. Just as the NCBLG statement declared the need "to work cooperatively with other national and local lesbian/gay organizations in the pursuit of human/civil rights," so Essex the individual would himself acknowledge a few years later that "a lot of my recognition is attributable to support from the gay and lesbian community," particularly but not exclusively from the black gay community.

The St. Louis convention also set in motion plans for holding the first National Black AIDS Conference for "some time late in 1986." Essex also planned what he called "the Membership Cabaret," a series of performances that included his friends Wayson and Michelle and was designed to extend the rolls of NCBLG's membership. Joe Beam knew the owners of the Allegro café in Philadelphia and organized one of the events there.

Unexpectedly, Essex had to cancel the performance at the last minute, a cancellation that he mysteriously and somewhat ominously attributed to "circumstances related to my health." He went into no detail, nor was Joe Beam forthcoming about some of his own proliferating physical symptoms. In a letter to Joe, Essex made an oblique reference to "believing this period of my life to be a test," and Joe similarly acknowledged in a letter to his parents that "I am so tired and troubled all the time." But beyond that, both men seemed to keep matters relating to their health primarily though not entirely to themselves.

When asked by an interviewer for the publication *Network*, "What's your sense of the toll that AIDS has been taking on the Black gay creative community?" Essex bluntly answered, "It's just been cutting it to shreds." He thought "a fundamental mistake" had been made in the early 1980s: because the initial AIDS deaths seemed to be largely of gay white men, black gay men had felt they had little to worry about— "and that had been crazy." It had led, Essex felt, to a dangerous passivity in regard to the epidemic. The myth of AIDS as a white disease, Essex believed, continued in 1986 to encourage inactivity within the gay people of color community. The writer Craig Harris was among those who broke through the barriers erected within and without the black gay community to emphasize publicly the havoc that AIDS was wreaking on their lives.

Harris had been a classmate of Abby Tallmer's (Sonnabend's assistant) at Vassar, and she describes him as "whip smart, witty, a sweetheart and while bold had a very, very shy side. He also had no tolerance for stupidity or bigotry of any kind." Soon after graduating, Harris had become active with Gay Men of African Descent (GMAD) and was one of the organizers (others included Gil Gerald, the Reverend Carl Bean, Suki Ports, and Amanda Houston-Hamilton) of the July 18, 1986, National Conference on AIDS in the Black Community held in Washington, D.C. Some four hundred educators, health care providers, and activists attended.

When it came time for Harris to give his speech as conference coordinator, he spoke of the "need for culturally sensitive risk education in the Black community. We must consider how people at risk perceive themselves and address that. For example, black bisexual men tend not to identify themselves as bisexuals, so they may exclude themselves from information targeted to gay men." Harris was well aware that as of 1986 the crisis of AIDS in the black community had reached staggering proportions. Although African Americans comprised 12 percent of the population, 25 percent of the diagnosed AIDS cases were among blacks—with only 30 percent of them self-identifying as gay and 42 percent as IV drug users. Moreover, the mean survival time for blacks after diagnosis was eight months—compared to eighteen to twenty-four months among whites: this differential reflected, among much else, that blacks avoided and/or couldn't afford to seek health care until they'd reached the end stage of the disease. Later in the conference, a number of its organizers talked for more than two and a half hours—the meeting had been scheduled for fifteen minutes—with Surgeon General C. Everett Koop, then in the midst of preparing what would be a historically important report on AIDS.

Soon after, in October 1986, Harris daringly disrupted the American Public Health Association's first session on AIDS. Not a single person of color had been invited to participate in the event, but Harris was determined to be heard. He stormed the stage, grabbed the microphone away from San Francisco health commissioner Dr. Mervyn Silverman, shouted, "I will be heard!" and proceeded to lecture the audience on the specific challenges AIDS posed in communities of color. The following year, Harris and other activists formed the National Minority AIDS Council "to build leadership within communities of color to address the challenges of HIV/AIDS"; Patti LaBelle became one of its spokespersons.

Neither Essex nor Joe Beam felt equipped to match Harris' public activism. The two were intensely private people who disliked and avoided speaking about their own health issues, even with friends, preferring to focus on staying busy with their writing and with black gay cultural activism. In the 1990s Essex *would* occasionally speak out openly, and eloquently, about "being a person with AIDS," but in the mid- to late 1980s his poetry rarely referenced AIDS. "O Tell Me, Brutus," published in 1986, was among the few:

> O tell me, Brutus,
> With corpses decomposing
> In the river,
> Loved ones keeping fevers
> Quiet in city hospitals,
> The backrooms, locked and chained,
> The police with new power to seize
> And search our hearts, our kisses,
> Our mutual consents around midnight . . .[6]

Late that same year, Alyson published Joe Beam's anthology *In The Life*, with an initial printing of 7,500 copies. Giovanni's Room threw a book party for him, and within the first three weeks of publication the store sold 120 copies. Although the anthology was ignored in the straight black world, it garnered considerable attention in the gay community. Several black gay reviewers offered searching evaluations rather than perfunctory praise, though they differed with one another over the book's strengths and weaknesses. If any of the contributors came off unscathed, it was Essex. One reviewer praised his "open dark, ruminating glimpses of the human condition" and his "deceptively plain, visceral use of language." The somewhat well-known black gay novelist Larry Duplechan wrote in the national gay publication *The Advocate* that he found the anthology "an uneven reading experience"—yet he singled out Essex's poems as "more finely wrought than the short stories" in the anthology.

Both Joe's parents attended the book party, and he felt "so pleased and thrilled that my father had the courage to come out and support his gay son. Those few moments with me made up for so much in the past, so much." Joe started to get letters almost every day from black gay men around the country telling him "how heartened they've become from reading the book." Within a month, the glossy new thirty-six-page issue of *Black/Out* appeared, and a nonprofit foundation, the Chicago Resource Center, simultaneously renewed its annual $10,000 funding of the publication for another year. Alyson and Joe were soon discussing a sequel to *In The Life*, tentatively titled "Brother to Brother." Joe found all this "exciting but overwhelming."[7]

He hoped that his writing would eventually afford him "an actual living, perhaps not a great one, but a living nonetheless." But in the meantime, he still had to pay the bills, and he again took a job as a waiter in a Philadelphia restaurant. With editorial help from Barbara Smith, he also began work on collecting his essays, some old, some new, for publication, probably with Essex's Be Bop Books (publisher of his own earlier chapbooks, including *Earth Life*, which had two sold-out printings). Be Bop Books also had in the works a collection of Michelle Parkerson's prose and poetry and a volume of Assotto Saint's poetry.

An incident involving New York City's preeminent gay publication, the *New York Native*, helps to illustrate why Essex, Joe Beam, and most of their circle gave primacy to black over gay liberation. In celebration of Black History Month in February 1986, the *Native*, unlike other white-dominated gay publications (like *The Advocate*), did publish a special supplement, "Heritage of Black Gay Pride," edited by Craig Harris. It was an excellent collection, and Sidney Brinkley, the pioneering founder of the Blacklight Press in D.C., sent Harris his congratulations. But Brinkley went on to point out that in the very same issue of the *Native*—and typical of "their hypocrisy, their racism"—was an ad in the employment section which they'd been running for several weeks: a lawyer was advertising for a legal assistant, preferably a "WM in mid-'20s." That, as Brinkley put it, "blatantly breaks discrimination laws in 3 categories: race, gender and age." And this wasn't the first or last time, though the discriminatory ads varied, sometimes explicitly barring replies from "fats and femmes," sometimes "people over 30," sometimes nonwhites. Was this a free-speech or a hate-speech issue? Well, one might say, free for whites, hate for blacks. Legally, the racial references in the employment ads were blatantly discriminatory.[8]

Colin Robinson, who lived in New York City and was an influential Blackheart editorial board member, sent his own response directly to the *Native*'s editor, Chuck Ortleb. Robinson graciously began by congratulating Ortleb on the supplementary section "Heritage of Black Gay Pride," and did so even though "in the Black gay community, it is considered by some leaders impolitic to praise white gay publications, by some unprincipled even to work with you." Robinson then went on to deplore the "WM in mid-'20s" ad and further to point out that the *Native*'s record on racial issues had been at best spotty. The *Native* had never, for example, published a review of any of the three issues of *Blackheart*, or covered any of the frequent literary readings in the city by black lesbians and gay men. The oppression most black gays shared with white gays, Robinson pointed out, "is much less often mitigated by socioeconomic status," making it even more critical that white gay publications and institutions make room for addressing and expressing minority points of view. Robinson was neither soliciting nor advocating white paternalism; he was simply registering the fact that the black gay community lacked the organizational and financial resources readily available to many within the white one.

Essex often had to live close to the margins. In 1984–85 he'd worked for a time as a graphic artist with the Potomac Electric Power Company (PEPCO). According to Wyatt O'Brian Evans, a friend Essex made at PEPCO, the "racist, demoralizing" higher-ups "worked overtime in attempts to subjugate [him] but to no avail. . . . Although he was a sensitive, caring guy, 'Es' took no crap. From anybody." He simply quit his job with PEPCO.

Like many other low-income writers, white and black, Essex tried to piece out an income from grants. He first applied to the National Endowment for the Arts. Turned down, he tried again the following year, but again failed to win support. On both occasions he'd been entirely circumspect about his sexual orientation. But that didn't come naturally to him; as Evans, his buddy at PEPCO, has put it, "confident about and in who he was, 'Es' was firmly grounded and rooted in his sexuality. He was unabashed about it. His affecting smile and that mischievous twinkle which danced in his eye—both 'slightly corrupting' in a good kind of way, of course—could win you over in no time flat. The 'bruh' had swagger, and exuded raw sexual appeal."

And so in 1985, when Essex next applied for a grant, he decided, "Fuck it. I'll send what *I* want to send, not what I think they want to read," and he included gay-themed poetry from his current chapbook, *Conditions*, that he'd been compiling (he'd been self-publishing his chapbooks—five in all—since 1982). This time, the application was approved—a major surprise. Over the course of time, Essex would go on to receive four additional grants from the D.C. Commission on the Arts and Humanities, and later, he'd be awarded a Pew Charitable Trust Fellowship, an Emery Award for community-based activism, and a visiting fellowship at the Getty Center in Santa Monica. By living frugally, he was usually able to avoid taking on any additional work.

The grants he received were sometimes accompanied by attempts at censorship, but Essex invariably bucked all efforts to dictate how and where he expressed himself. At the ceremony for the Washington, D.C., Mayor's Arts Awards in the fall of 1987, for example, Essex (along with Wayson) was invited to perform his poem "Family Jewels," about a young black man unable to hail a taxi because of his race. The black executive director of the D.C. Arts Commission asked Essex, just hours before the show, to omit the word "corruption" or not perform the poem at all, the implication being that it might embarrass Mayor Marion Barry, whose administration was then famously under investigation.

To placate the executive director, Essex agreed to drop the poem—or said he would. But once he got onstage he read it anyway, and without omitting "corruption." He followed the poem with a short speech in which he specifically detailed the Arts Commission's attempt to censor him and his work. After a brief silence, the crowd reacted with thunderous applause, and Essex completed the performance with another poem. A *Washington Post* reporter subsequently interviewed the commission's executive director, who confirmed her effort to remove "corruption" from the poem. "I considered it inappropriate for the event," she said in her defense, which was designed as a "celebration of artists—a light, upbeat evening. There's a fine line between saying what's appropriate and censorship." She likened Essex to "a spoiled child who has reprimanded us publicly." She might more accurately have referred to him as a consistent defender of free speech.

The following year, a nonprofit progressive radio station in D.C., WPFW, a member of the Pacifica broadcast network, invited Essex and Wayson to be part of its ongoing "The Poet and the Poem" series, hosted by Grace Cavalieri. No suggestion was made to them about cutting, editing, or substituting material to bring it in line with FCC guidelines about what might be "offensive." Yet when they subsequently heard a broadcast of the program, they discovered that not only had "seven dirty words" (as Essex called them) been edited out, but the "progressive" station had also edited various ideas and concepts—and without prior consultation.

Early in 1987, Essex jumped at the chance to leave such hassles behind him for a bit and welcomed an offer to do a set of readings in London and environs, after which he planned two weeks of travel through the Netherlands "to visit relatives and to spend some time in Amsterdam." The trip "turned out to be a very fine experience" for him, one that he felt sure he'd be "synthesizing for many months" thereafter. In all, he presented twelve readings—mostly from *Conditions* and *Earth Life*, along with a few unpublished poems—in the space of six weeks, and in his opinion the work "went over very well with audiences there." Additionally, he met the black gay filmmaker Isaac Julien for the first time. The meeting came about after Julien had called Michelle Parkerson to talk with her about his forthcoming project on Langston Hughes and Michelle had suggested Julien contact Essex, about to leave for England. The two men did meet in London, got along well, and would do important work together in the future.

The reading Essex did in Manchester—a city outside of London with a large black population—exemplified the growing impact of his poetry and person on the upcoming generation of younger blacks, as typified by the reaction of one young man in an audience of some forty people. He'd been familiar with only a few of Essex's poems before attending the performance, which was held in the city's small black community center. Those few poems had put him, like others in the audience, in a state of "high anticipation." Nor was he disappointed: the reading, he felt, was "absolutely brilliant"; Essex touched him "deep inside," so much so that he mustered up his courage after the reading and introduced himself. Essex kindly answered the young man's many questions: "He really allowed me to feel free to probe and discover who he was."

Essex told him that he was taking the train back to London the following morning and spontaneously asked his new fan if he'd like to accompany him. The answer was an enthusiastic yes, and the train trip proved memorable: "Essex was so revealing, considering that neither one of us knew much of the other. I felt I could quickly trust him." They had a "great conversation"; Essex left the young man "with questions and answers that sparked in him new ways of thinking." Years later he still regarded the trip as having been "memorable": Essex had "helped influence me in a positive way about accepting myself as a dignified black gay man."

His is but one of the many tributes that would accumulate over time attesting to Essex's seminal influence. "The first time I saw him read," another black gay man would write, "was a revelation . . . accomplished, funny, heartbreakingly honest." Another man found him "SO down to earth." A third spoke of his "generosity," yet a fourth about how he "usually brought the house down wherever he performed," and a fifth about how the reading Essex did in Detroit "was the most powerful thing that [had] ever happened in Detroit's black gay community." And so on. Essex was decidedly becoming a writer to reckon with.

Yet on his return to the States, among the first things he learned was that he'd lost his part-time job—the company had decided to move to San Diego. And jobless the sage of Manchester would remain for a number of weeks before finding just enough work to keep him in food and to pay the rent. "Times are lean, pretty baby," he wrote Joe Beam.

Mike Callen's black and Latino friends also provided him with evidence of how subtle omissions could cause hurtful consequences for people of color. Emilio, a Puerto Rican friend of his, had been diagnosed with KS in 1984, but had ignored the brown lesions that began to develop on his skin because GMHC and the gay papers kept saying that KS lesions were purplish-pink, failing to note the fact that in brown or black people they were likely to appear brown. A.J., a black friend of Mike's, told him that when he visited San Francisco he was impressed with how much more the city was doing about AIDS than New York—every day some item about the disease appeared on television. But then A.J. realized that the reports *always* showed white men, even when the stories were about volunteers at the AIDS agencies. Mike agreed with A.J. that (as Mike put it) "in a better world, white gay men who have themselves experienced the bitter sting of oppression for being gay would make an effort not to oppress others."

Not that Hispanics and blacks did much better in their relations with each other. By 1985, New York's Health Department had still not developed AIDS prevention material in Spanish, though it was the city's second language. Late in that year, with the formation of the Hispanic AIDS Forum and the New York chapter of the Minority Task Force, an opportunity seemed at hand for cooperative efforts to do more in reaching minority communities. But when suggestions were made that the two organizations merge in order to better utilize the limited resources available, the Hispanic group refused on the grounds that past experience in mixed minority groups showed that African Americans ended up setting an agenda that ignored cultural differences. Proceeding on separate paths, both agencies experienced slow growth. What many of the heterosexual members of the two communities did share was the view that homosexuality was shameful and that an AIDS diagnosis should be concealed.

By the end of 1985, more than twenty thousand cases of AIDS had been reported in the United States—with a startling 50 percent of them African American. By then, the scientific community had pretty much unified around the theory—despite some stubborn dissenters who persist to the present day—that HIV causes AIDS. Until then, many in the black community, gay and straight, had dealt with the disproportionate numbers of African Americans affected by telling themselves that AIDS was a white or IV drug user disease and that only black men who slept with white men became infected; some even insisted, with the Tuskegee experiment in mind, that AIDS was a deliberate plot by the government to decimate the black community.[9]

By the mideighties such views had subsided, replaced by an awareness among black gay men and lesbians that they had to rely primarily on their own organizations to provide services to those afflicted and preventative information to the community in general. GMHC was doing a heroic job—but mostly for whites. Its brochures contained no black images, which meant that people of color had difficulty identifying with its message. That realization led to the formation in 1986 of, among other groups, the Minority Task Force on AIDS (MTFA), which promptly issued its own brochure, *AIDS in the Black Community*.

Mike Callen and some other PWAs in New York City saw GMHC as essentially parental in its attitudes—*we* know what is best for *you* and will provide it—and they had decided to take matters into their own hands. In April 1985, Mike and eight others founded the People with AIDS Coalition (PWAC), declaring in its by-laws that "people with AIDS are the experts on the subject of the epidemic." (Mike later came to regret the implied dismissal of scientific and medical expertise.) To that end, the group had started a monthly newsletter, *Newsline*, with Mike Callen as editor and Jane Rosett as co-editor; from an original print run of two hundred, it had developed a national readership. Under Mike's editorship, the contents came to include everything from mainstream medical findings to the dangers (for PWAs) of eating raw oysters. By 1987, the print run had reached fourteen thousand.[10]

PWAC—all but ignored in the standard histories of the AIDS epidemic—came along at a point in time when spirits in the gay community had sunk to a low ebb. In the summer of 1985, the American Hospital of Paris formally announced that Rock Hudson, a patient there, had been diagnosed with AIDS. President Reagan—who had yet to utter his first public word about the epidemic—put in a call to his old acting friend offering encouragement. But instead of Hudson's illness (he died a few months later) leading to more aggressive federal action against the disease, what followed was a frightening spate of invective against gay people and a host of brutal suggestions for spreading further terror among them.

The Reverend Jerry Falwell insisted that the time had come to institute a quarantine of gay people as "a threat to public safety." No fewer than twenty states in the mideighties mulled over propositions for the kind of concentration camps inflicted on Japanese Americans during World War II, and Congressman William Dannemeyer offered a resolution to that effect on the floor of the House. The well-known psychologist Helen Singer Kaplan published a letter in the *New York Times* in which she expressed the view held by many that gay people had the *obligation* to the general population to submit to blood tests for HIV (the ELISA test was used for preliminary screening, the Western Blot, for confirmation—but both tended to produce a disturbing number of false-positives). Since no viable treatment for AIDS was then available, the knowledge of one's status could for some have a debilitating psychological effect, including suicide. "So what?" seems to have been the reaction of Singer and others: if no benefit followed for gay people themselves, knowing who was HIV-positive would facilitate the roundup for quarantine. As I wrote at the time in my diary,

Singer and those who shared her views showed "no awareness of the moral hypocrisy inherent in treating gay people like scum for generations and then demanding that they behave like saints."[11]

During this same time period, the *New York Post* ran a series of lurid, inflammatory articles *purportedly* about gay life; in one, the *Post* reported that nurses in hospitals were having trouble policing AIDS patients who kept insisting on having sex with each other—though no such instance has ever come to light. At roughly the same time, New York Governor Mario Cuomo ordered the state's health department to study whether all bathhouses should be shuttered, while in New York City, Mayor Ed Koch waited until after his reelection and then directly ordered the gay bathhouses—but not straight sex clubs like Plato's Retreat—closed, pompously declaring "you can't sell death in this city and get away with it."

Meanwhile, the *Wall Street Journal* had raised a "bemused" question about the "curious" lack of public debate over possible quarantine measures—thereby helping to provoke them. On the West Coast, all gay foreigners were being detained—not merely deported. The cry to force gay men to submit to the new blood test for HIV mounted. The vote in Houston went four to one against a gay civil rights bill. Terror and paralysis seemed to be descending in tandem over the gay population. In a poll at the time, 57 percent of Americans surveyed answered yes when asked if gay and lesbian relations should be declared illegal. Then, in 1987, came an incident in Arcadia, Florida, which gave bigotry a whole new dimension. The three HIV-positive hemophiliac young sons of Clifford and Louise Ray were denied the right to attend local public schools. When the courts ordered the schools to admit the boys, the Rays' house "mysteriously" burned to the ground. The family decided to leave town.

The low point of the deepening demonization came in June 1986 when the Supreme Court in its *Bowers v. Hardwick* decision upheld a Georgia law outlawing sodomy. The law had been used to arrest Michael Hardwick and another adult man for having consensual sex in the privacy of Hardwick's bedroom. Homosexuals, in other words, were—unlike other citizens—subject to government intervention and regulation of their private lives. In an eloquent dissent, Justice Harry Blackmun wrote that "depriving individuals of the right to choose for themselves how to conduct their intimate relationships poses a far greater threat to the values most deeply rooted in our nation's history than tolerance of nonconformity could ever do." Spontaneous protest demonstrations took place in many major cities, and Mike Callen and some six hundred or so other gay men and lesbians (including Michael Hardwick) protested the *Bowers v. Hardwick* decision on the steps of the Supreme Court— Mike, along with others, was promptly arrested. The policeman who fingerprinted him wore latex gloves. Mike stared at him in disbelief, and the officer shot back, "Yeah, I'm wearin' gloves. If you don't like it, tough shit. You could all have AIDS for all I know." Mike thought that the real contagion the cop feared was queerness.[12]

The *Bowers* decision angered and mobilized the gay community. On the night it was announced, three thousand demonstrators blocked traffic in Greenwich Village, and a small group of activists began to lay plans for what would become a massive March on Washington in 1987. Essex's poem "The Occupied Territories" gave further voice to the community's outrage:

> You are not to touch other flesh
> without a police permit.
> You have not privacy—
> the State wants to seize your bed
> and sleep with you.
> The State wants to control
> your sexuality, your birth rate,
> your passion.
> The message is clear;
> your penis, your vagina,
> your testicles, your womb,
> your anus, your orgasm,
> these belong to the State.
> You are not to touch yourself
> or be familiar with ecstasy.
> The erogenous zones
> are not demilitarized.

A friend of mine, the gay ACLU lawyer Tom Stoddard, told me that the *Bowers* decision was in his view "our *Dred Scott* case"—the reference being to the 1857 Supreme Court decision in which blacks were declared to be property without any rights of citizenship. Ironically, Tom had himself recently been a victim of discrimination—and by the New York Civil Liberties Union (NYCLU) no less. I'd been a member of the NYCLU board since 1981 and was present throughout the discussions about whether Tom or a rival candidate should be chosen for the post of executive director. The decisive meeting lasted seven and a half hours, without a food break, which conveys some sense of the tension involved. Twice during the debate—for that's what it was—board members referred to Tom as "a magical creature," a third called him "a whiner," and a fourth thought him "too emotional." Since Tom wasn't flighty, and certainly not a "whiner," I took those references as code words for gay—especially when yet another speaker warned against making an "unsafe" choice. The vote went against Tom and I felt deeply dismayed to have heard so much covert homophobia from members of the NYCLU board, that presumed bastion of decency. Tom agreed with my analysis and was furious about it—he'd expected to win. But he landed nicely on his feet, becoming executive director of Lambda Legal Defense and Education Fund and—before dying of AIDS at age forty-eight in 1997—a major player in the gay civil rights movement.[13]

The general climate in the mideighties was a gloomy one for many gay people, a decided low point in morale. More and more people in Mike's circle began to fall ill and die; he felt as if he "was living in London during the blitz, except not everybody seemed to know that bombs were raining down on our heads." He wrote a song called "Living in Wartime" and said it was "sort of a call to arms." Back in the fall of 1984, for the first time in two years, he'd again been in the hospital—at St. Clare's in Manhattan, named, as Mike drily noted, for a Catholic saint, not exactly his choice of benefactors. "My breakfast grew cold outside my room on the floor where it had been left," he wrote. "As I rang for the nurse, a middle-aged black man, wearing a surgical gown, gloves and a mask, skittered nervously across my room (keeping close to the far wall). He flipped a switch which turned on the rental TV and fled."

Mike recovered well, but then in 1986 he had to be hospitalized on three separate occasions for pneumonia, with attendant fevers and weight loss. "AIDS is about bed pans and respirators," he wrote. "It's about loss of control—control of one's bowels and bladder, one's arms or legs, one's life. Sometimes the loss is sudden; sometimes tortuously gradual. It's about the *anticipation* of pain as well as actual pain itself. . . . It is horror." Five years in, he thought of himself as a long-term survivor, but one day in the hospital he turned to his lover Richard Dworkin and said something about it maybe being time to put down some of those songs that had been going through his head and that he'd been threatening to record. Dworkin was delighted with the idea and suggested they make an album. One side would be more "produced"— twenty-four tracks, overdubs, multiple musicians, several takes; the other side would be "live to two track," like the live cabaret performances Mike used to do, "quieter, sadder, more contemplative," Mike at the piano singing, and no editing—though they could do several takes and choose the best one.

After Mike's release from the hospital, the idea of a record stayed with them. But so did AIDS. He soon found himself flying out to Las Vegas to give a talk to the American Public Health Association. He told them that "AIDS is the moment to moment management of uncertainty. It's a roller coaster ride without a seat belt. Once this ride begins, there is never a moment when the rush of events that swirl around you stops long enough for you to get your bearings." Yet he did manage to get his bearings—managed it over and over again.

When feeling well, he put much of his energy into expanding PWAC's offerings, motivated above all by "a desire to put a human face on AIDS." He had the strongly held faith—*not* religious in origin, yet perhaps owing something to midwestern optimism—that if the general population could be shown that "AIDS was happening to real people, not faceless 'risk groups' . . . an all-out war against this disease" would be mounted.

One of Mike's guiding principles was "prepare for the worst and then hope for the best. . . . Decide how and under what circumstances you want to die. . . . Then, forget about it. Turn your attention to the formidable task of staying alive and living life to its fullest. Be hopeful and optimistic—even cheerful. Surround yourselves with others who support your hope." And so PWAC began to sponsor potluck dinners, a "Laughter Lab" (Saturday night comedy films), support groups (for women with AIDS; for mothers of PWAs, etc.), teas for singles, even a weekly class in how to apply makeup to cover KS lesions.[14]

As editor of *Newsline* (as well as president of PWAC), Mike opened its pages to all sorts of contributors, including "inspiring" stories and strategies from long-term survivors of AIDS (then defined as more than three years, which meant only one patient in ten; in 1987 only one in thirty-three stayed alive five years or more) and advocates of a wide variety of theories about the disease's origins, including such far-fetched ones as African swine flu. "My ruthless commitment to seeking out diversity of opinion," Mike wrote, "meant that with these fingers I typed things that made my skin crawl."

Sonnabend had initially dismissed the view that HIV "caused" AIDS. He told one TV interviewer that the claim was "absurd," another that "I don't believe there is any such thing . . . as a novel agent," and yet a third, less certainly, that the HIV theory was "a conjecture, a hypothesis, not an established fact." He soon modified somewhat his early position, but both he and Mike essentially stuck with Sonnabend's earlier multifactorial explanation. "I still believe," Mike wrote,

> that repeated infection by common sexually transmitted diseases that had reached epidemic levels is a more plausible explanation [than simple onetime exposure to HIV] for the epidemic. . . . There is, of course, a lot of *circumstantial* evidence implicating HIV in the etiology of AIDS. But it is by no means conclusive. . . . One important challenge to the assertion that HIV could explain AIDS that has never been answered is this: Instead of being the cause of AIDS, why isn't it just as likely that HIV is merely another opportunistic infection that has been reactivated from a latent state after whatever is *truly* causing AIDS has left out the possibility that HIV antibody . . . is the *effect*, rather than the cause, of immune deficiency.

In Mike's view, regardless of which theory you chose to believe, exposure to sperm through receptive anal sex with multiple partners was central to the present health crisis: "If you believe the single virus theory, promiscuity is how this unidentified, killer bug is being 'spread.'" For a time, Mike's own immunosuppression began slowly to reverse itself, and he credited the improvement to having "stopped promiscuity completely and . . . allow[ed] my body to recover from the abuse it has suffered." What still remained unanswered, Mike felt, was precisely how HIV caused depletion of the critical CD4 cells.

Mike continued to work closely with Sonnabend, though in Mike's view they "had a very tortured relationship." They had a doctor-patient relationship, a personal friendship, and a political alliance. Mike had a subtle and deep intelligence—and a writing style of absolute clarity— yet he considered Sonnabend "the most brilliant person I've ever met. He is completely eccentric. He thrives on chaos." And though basically tender and caring, he could be prickly, irritable, and uncommunicative. But Mike never doubted that Sonnabend was the reason he was still alive.

Sean Strub—the founder and publisher of *POZ*, an important source of information about AIDS research and treatment—was also a patient of Sonnabend's and also credits him with keeping him alive. Recently, Strub conducted a series of interviews with Sonnabend at his home in England, where he's retired. Throughout the long sessions, Sonnabend made it clear that he's continued, with some adjustments, to hold to the theory he'd outlined in the early 1980s. Emphasizing that infection and disease are not the same thing, Sonnabend did, and does, believe that every disease (as opposed to infection) is multifactorial in nature in the sense that one passes into the other depending on a variety of factors—the way the infection enters the body, the immune response of the host, varying genetic susceptibilities, the presence of other diseases in the host, nutritional factors, psychological states of mind, and so on. In Sonnabend's view, the course of *all* infectious diseases is in that sense dependent on a wide variety of factors.

Many questions about the role of HIV remained unanswered. Some people were getting sick in the apparent *absence* of any trace of HIV. Ironically, Mike himself was, as he put it, "an HIV factory. One of the cell lines for HIV antibody tests comes from me. . . . I'm notorious among researchers in the city. Whenever somebody needs to culture active, live virus, they come to me." Duesberg claimed that there were four thousand AIDS cases in which HIV was absent, but others found only 299 HIV-seronegative individuals with AIDS, and even that figure was subsequently lowered to 168. Other questions—perhaps inevitable in the early stages of research for any disease—that the skeptics raised included: Why isn't HIV found in many of the T cells it purportedly kills? Why do some HIV-positive people suddenly test negative—without any intervening treatment? Why do so many spouses of HIV-positive people remain negative, even when safe-sex techniques aren't used? Does the "AIDS test" measure antibodies or the virus itself—and can one test positive for antibodies without having the virus?

It was a sign of Mike's sophistication that he wondered what reasons, other than scientific ones, led someone to prefer one explanation for AIDS to another. What might be the political or psychological advantages to the choice made? He decided that, in his own case, the "killer virus" theory was too "disempowering." He found the notion that those with HIV were " 'timebombs'—that all that matters is having or not having HIV—that once one is infected, nothing one does matters much since HIV is a conveyor belt leading inevitably to sickness and death"—too frightening for someone like himself, "a control queen." He was also a temperamental skeptic with a knee-jerk distrust for "experts" and "authority"—in contrast, he felt, to the many "religious" gay men willing to suspend reason and logic and genuflect before "revealed truth." Further, Mike believed that most gay people preferred the HIV theory because it held a virus rather than particular sexual practices responsible for the transmission of AIDS. He recognized, though, that putting the blame on a multiplicity of sexually transmitted diseases played into the hands of all the right-wing crazies who held the behavior of gay men itself responsible for their plight—and thus deserving of neither compassion nor adequate research funding.

Mike was even more adamant (as was Sonnabend) about rejecting the antiretroviral drug AZT when it first became known in 1985. Sonnabend read the study reports on AZT and was immediately suspicious of it. Among other things, he was struck by the number of deaths during the trial of participants who were on the placebo, not on AZT. What had in fact happened was that some participants in the study—by now sophisticated about trials—had been able to discern the difference between the AZT pill and the placebo, had sent their pills to commercial labs for analysis, and had gotten those taking the actual medication to share it. Despite the unreliability of the trial, the FDA proceeded to approve AZT in 1987.

Hailed for its ability to prevent HIV from replicating, AZT was widely prescribed and earned millions of dollars for its manufacturer, Burroughs Wellcome. Along with having potentially disastrous side effects, like anemia, it showed a short-term increase in T-helper cells for some—but did not extend life. Mike read deeply in the medical literature and concluded that the Phase 2 trials of AZT had been inept, the research conducted by "amateurs." He pointed to a French study published in 1988 that concluded that the benefits of AZT were limited at best to a few months of additional life, and also to a Veterans Administration study that suggested AZT actually *shortened* life span.

Besides, Mike had begun to deplore the slogan—and actuality—of "drugs into bodies, meaning any drug into any body." It was predicated, he felt, on what he called "the conveyor-belt conceptualization of AIDS"—on the cruel (and, he felt, unsupported) notion that once a person is infected with HIV, death became inevitable and therefore any experimental drug was worth taking even if the odds of it having any efficacy were low. To Mike that was the "equivalent of resorting to thermonuclear warheads to rid their homes of roaches, rather than starting first with less extreme measures"—like reducing risky sexual behavior.

Mike welcomed the birth in 1987 of the group ACT UP. "The blunt truth," he felt, was that up to that point "the familiar cast of AIDS buffoons in charge of the federal AIDS response are third-string scientists: lethally arrogant, ignorant and inept; and in several cases, probably actionably corrupt. Those in charge of AIDS . . . have botched it hopelessly." ACT UP, through militant direct-action protests, Mike felt, might well force the powers that be to speed up the drug approval process. Nonviolent direct action was decidedly in the American grain; it had been successfully employed both in the black civil rights struggle and in the protest against the war in Vietnam, and it had been a staple during labor struggles as far back as the late nineteenth century. During 1987–88, ACT UP's first year of existence, it managed to mount some two dozen civil disobedience actions that effectively mixed anger and theater, put direct pressure on NIAID and the FDA—and achieved some notable results.

But Mike's active opposition to the use of AZT put him at odds with many of the most prominent members of ACT UP, as well as several other notable figures in the AIDs struggle: the federal AIDS czar, Dr. Anthony Fauci, who predicted that eventually all of the 1.4 million Americans with AIDS would need to take AZT; John James, the prestigious editor and publisher of the San Francisco–based newsletter *AIDS Treatment News*, which was the bible for many in the AIDS community; and Martin Delaney, founder of the respected Project Inform, who acknowledged "some problems" with AZT but nonetheless stood by it. As early as the May 1986 issue of *AIDS Treatment News*, James had written, "The general public, and even most AIDS organizations and activists, do not yet realize that we already have an effective, inexpensive, and probably safe treatment for AIDS"—namely, AZT.[15]

The controversy over the drug would drag on for years. When Mike published his book *Surviving AIDS* in 1990, his publisher, Harper-Collins, "begged" him not to include the chapter titled "The Case Against AZT," but Mike held out against the pressure. It would only be with the rigorous "Concorde" study in 1993 that the efficacy of AZT for extending life was disproved and the position taken by Mike and other dissenters validated. When the results of the Concorde trial reached him, Mike deplored the "nauseatingly shameless recent attempts to rewrite history" and reminded people that "a majority of AIDS activists joined with federal researchers in brutally suppressing doubts about AZT and *aggressively* promoting so-called 'early intervention'"; their advice had been to "get tested, and if you're HIV antibody positive, and if your T-cells happen to fall below 500, *get on AZT right away!*"

The troubling questions that Mike, Sonnabend, and others had raised from 1987 to 1993 about whether AZT might actually *shorten* survival by destroying bone marrow and causing lymphoma had been shunted aside and those raising the questions denounced as uninformed fools. Mike's detractors included those he called "key AIDS activists"— his allusion was to those members of ACT UP's Treatment and Data (T&D) Committee who vigorously defended AZT and to its "star," Mark Harrington in particular. The T&D Committee members had coalesced around the need to develop additional AIDS drugs but who in Mike's opinion had settled "for being near the center of power instead of questioning whether the powerful person's scientific output justified the power in the first place." Mike had come to believe that "the obvious and simple notion of PWA self-empowerment" had "mutated into the absurd belief that one opinion was just as good as another. Desperate and confused people with AIDS," he wrote, "facing life and death treatment choices have been duped into believing that the opinion of a Marty Delaney, a Mark Harrington or a Michael Callen is just as good as the opinion of someone who has spent 20 years tending the sick and studying virology."

As Mike himself came to acknowledge, his own early insistence on self-empowerment and his view that AIDS patients were *the* experts on the disease "had a hand in fomenting rabid anti-expertism," had helped to influence the Harringtons and Delaneys to highlight their own considerable expertise and to emphasize getting "drugs into bodies." As he put it, "I realize, looking back over my collective writings, that by excoriating establishment AIDS-think, I created the impression that there wasn't any such thing as true expertise." He felt that somewhere along the road, "the self-evident truth that the opinions and experiences of people *with* AIDS had value got twisted into the absurd notion that all opinions are of equal value," whereas in fact the typical PWA could not evaluate complex pharmacological and toxicological questions.

In the years before the release of the 1993 Concorde study, Mike took a great deal of abuse—not only for his early stand against AZT but also for his disparaging reaction to what had become a burgeoning number of New Age nostrums. Given the lack of viable treatments for AIDS, it was understandable that some patients, most of them young and desperate to go on living, would resort to magical thinking and clutch at the robes of assorted spiritual gurus. The most prominent of these was Louise Hay, the self-proclaimed "author, lecturer, and metaphysical teacher." She originally established her Church of Religious Science in New York City but then moved to the more receptive environment of Santa Monica, where she established Hay House. It came to have a staff of twenty-two, an office complex for which she paid $11,000 a month rent, and a storage warehouse for her books and materials that extended for several blocks.[16]

Hay's philosophy centered on the two-prong doctrine of "positive thinking" and "personal responsibility," and her substantial group of followers took weekly "Hay Rides," a mix of colonics, reflexology, nutritional supplements, and "visualizations." She also wrote and sold pamphlets and audiocassettes in which she urged people to forgo self-criticism of any kind and to substitute self-love and responsibility. In 1984 she published a full-length book, *You Can Heal Your Life*, subsequently appeared on countless national radio and television shows, and held seminars across the country. Central to Hay's "philosophy" was the insistence that those who had a terminal illness had self-consciously *chosen* that illness—and needed to learn how to *un*-choose it. One prime technique was "mirror work": seated before a mirror, one repeated over and over, "I love you."

All of which made Mike (in his words) "curl my lip uncontrollably." With Western doctors frequently sending their AIDS patients for radiation and interferon injections—all of it harmful, none helpful—Mike had enough contempt for Western science to at least sympathize with those AIDS sufferers who believed that at a minimum Hay's techniques made them feel more hopeful and relaxed. He had been, after all, one of the earliest advocates of "self-empowerment."

Yet he found Hay unbearably pretentious and mocked Hay House as "The Church of the Happy Face." He also thought it outrageous for anyone to preach about "keeping the right attitude." The implication of such an injunction was that those who got depressed about the death sentence hanging over them had only themselves to blame if they fell ill and succumbed. The further implication was that the thousands (it would soon be millions) who'd already died somehow hadn't lived "correctly." Not that Mike advocated whining—far from it. When he heard someone bemoan their fate—"Why me? Why me?!"—he was more likely than not to say "Come on, *girl*! You had to *work* to get this disease. It's not like it tapped you on the shoulder one day while you were standing in line at the grocery store. Yeah traumatic, but let's get on with it."[17]

From his many conversations with other long-term survivors, some of them taped, Mike concluded that the one characteristic common to all of them was *grit*. As he put it, "These people were all fighters, skeptical, opinionated, incredibly knowledgeable about AIDS, and passionately committed to living." He was of course describing himself as well. Like most long-term survivors, Mike was all but uniformly skeptical about experimental drugs—and they kept surfacing, both in the underground and in doctors' prescriptions. Year by year, as the number of those infected multiplied and then multiplied again, one "miraculous" drug or treatment after another was invested with magical healing power: interferon, AL-721, rifabutin, catnip enemas, horse urine therapy, amino acid combos, Ayurvedic medicine, carrot juice, quinolinic acid, macrobiotics, NMDA, intravenous penicillin or ceftriaxone, Compound Q, trichosanthin, suramin—the list went on and on, as did the mounting desperation. By the early 1990s, various studies showed that 52 percent of all HIV-infected patients were on one kind of "unapproved" therapy or another.[18]

Mike himself wasn't entirely unsusceptible to a bit of experimentation. Tired of the government's limited response and the sluggish bureaucracy that required seemingly endless lines to join a treatment trial, he and a friend, Tom Hannan, decided they couldn't "wait any longer in the hope that good old corporate greed will speed up finding treatments," and they co-founded, with Sonnabend, the PWA Health Group. At the moment, the AIDS grapevine was abuzz with rumors that an egg yolk lecithin extract had shown "remarkable" benefits for many AIDS sufferers. Unable to obtain the substance commercially or through research trials, a number of people started whipping up homemade versions in their blenders. The PWA Health Group found a company, the American Roland Company, on Long Island, willing to sell them large quantities of an egg yolk lecithin substance. Mike and Tom made it absolutely clear that the Health Group was "not making any claim for efficacy. . . . We are merely acting as middle-persons to make available a safe *food substance* which many PWAs and researchers believe could extend" their lives. Mike himself tried the egg lecithin mixture for some three months, but when he failed to note any improvement he gave it up.

Mike understood that behind the widespread grasping at straws was really a grasping at hope. And he shared the belief that hope was necessary to survival. When he learned that his Methodist mother had organized a prayer group that met regularly to pray for his recovery, he was "simultaneously deeply moved and horrified." He had no use for religion, or for any form of belief that referenced a "higher power." Yet he was intrigued enough to research the literature on psychoneuroimmunology and found a few double-blind studies that fascinated him without producing any sustained conviction. "The idea that I'm alive," he wrote, "because a well-meaning group of Midwestern housewives include me in their prayers just makes no sense to someone as rabidly, rigidly rational as I am. I'm more comfortable just calling it luck—the atheist's noun of choice to explain the unexplainable."[19]

Mike's outspoken opposition to alternate therapies, and his general stance as a maverick—in his criticism of GMHC's "paternalism," for instance—turned him into a target for criticism, and even abuse. Early on, the first head of GMHC, Mel Rosen, had been anonymously taped referring to Mike as "a loony, and part of some cult, and not to be taken seriously." GMHC had resented his disapproval of fund-raising based on the premise that AIDS was "a threat to everybody," gay or straight. Accusations against him accelerated after he openly advised people against taking AZT. Even those who agreed with him about the drug's ineffectiveness nonetheless attacked him for "stealing people's hope." If anything, Mike was "guilty" of encouraging people with AIDS to believe that "survival probabilities are expected to double by 1993." More than one gay man even berated him for talking about survival "because it was bad for fund-raising."

The longer Mike survived, the more the rumors spread that he didn't "really" have AIDS. Even as early as his 1982 hospitalization, three doctors had gotten into a shouting match—in front of Mike—about whether he *really* had AIDS. One of them insisted that he "only" had "crypto" (cryptosporidiosis)—not yet PCP or KS (which he eventually did get)—and therefore didn't qualify. The second doctor insisted that "technically" he did, since crypto was on the CDC list. The third suggested that if he *died* from the crypto, he would posthumously qualify.

The charge was further leveled that Mike was an "AIDS carpetbagger," in it for the glory, and not "really" ill, an indictment that caused him (and his friends) great anguish. He ascribed the smear campaign to a number of factors: the controversial stands he'd taken (about AZT, for example), the fact that he was still alive, and the way in which he'd openly talked from day one about his, and by inference many other gay men's, sexual practices. Fed up with the accusations, Mike finally wrote a piece for *Newsline* in 1989 to say "once and for all, I have AIDS," and "by whatever definition you want to propose." He'd decided, he wrote in the article, to retell his story *one last time*, and proceeded to itemize his history—from the high fevers and bloody diarrhea in 1982, to landing in the hands of Joe Sonnabend, to his recent diagnosis of KS. He even included a photocopy of his biopsy report. He concluded with a signed statement from Sonnabend to the effect that "Michael Callen has AIDS." Sonnabend expressed his dismay "that people say he's lying about a matter as serious as an AIDS diagnosis, and I hope this ends such speculation." Sadly, it did not.

Mike viewed the debate over his status as an interesting conflation of epidemiology, a sporting match, and astrology. He took some comfort from reading the history of other movements, deciding "it was ever thus: Charges of personal aggrandizement, turf battles, personality clashes, in addition to profound, legitimate, philosophical disagreements over strategy and purpose." Mike may have looked like a "sissy" to some, but he had a forceful personality. Exceedingly articulate, his rational views were often unpopular but always stated clearly and cogently, and difficult for opponents to counteract.

If "I *had* died that summer of 1982," Mike mused, "no one would have questioned my 'right' to an AIDS diagnosis. It is the fact that I *refused to die* that makes me suspect; and the fact of my survival apparently threatens some people's image of AIDS as invariably fatal." But he didn't die, and the hurtful rumors continued. After Mike returned to music, the attacks would expand to include the view that he was an egotistical poseur eagerly glamming on to the AIDS crisis in order to further his singing career.[20]

I was born more than a generation earlier than Mike, had sown my wild oats before the onset of the epidemic (a heart attack in 1979 had put something of a period to that part of my life), and in 1986 had met the man with whom I've been living ever since. Mike—and Essex, too— had started to lose friends to the disease within the first few years after it surfaced, but the epidemic was nearly five years old before I knew someone well who died of AIDS. "Davey" was only twenty-eight years old. We'd originally met in a hustler bar, where he'd picked me from a lascivious circle of admirers to take him home.

We hit it off on a level beyond the cash nexus pretty quickly, and we saw each other with some regularity. Not only was Davey a beauty, but he also had a shrewd intelligence and was actively involved in gay politics. Following my heart attack, severe enough to require a six-week hospital stay, Davey visited me in my Greenwich Village apartment. After catching up on this or that, he nonchalantly announced that a blow job would do my sagging spirits a world of good, and promptly fell to the task. To my own surprise, it worked. I'd lost confidence in my body, and my libido had hiked off the map. Davey's ministrations—a product of his generosity, not lust—did wonders to revive it. We lost track after a few years, but when I learned that he'd succumbed to AIDS, I was horrified. He'd been such a gifted, sweet-souled person that I felt the loss as if I'd been recently and steadily in touch with him. As I wrote in my diary when hearing the news of his death: "What is there left to say about this gruesome, senseless killer? Except that the wrong people are dying, those who gave themselves incautiously to experience, to life: the risk-takers, the inventive ones. The fearful ones who literally sat on their asses still sit."

Mike Callen, himself a risk taker, kept saying over and over again in the mid- to late eighties (including in a 1986 speech to the American Public Health Association) that if he could challenge one assumption about AIDS, it would be that it's "an automatic death sentence—that AIDS has a 100 percent mortality rate. There are a handful of us—estimated variously at ten to eighteen percent—who happen to be quite alive more than three years after our diagnoses and who intend to be alive for many more years." But Mike's percentages might have been somewhat inflated, and besides, three years of survival was hardly the equivalent of a normal life span, never mind the quality of life involved. Even for those who'd managed to get through three years, as one researcher would later conclude, "there might be nothing 'special' about long-term survivors . . . [it] could be pure luck."

Mike himself included "luck" whenever asked for an explanation—that is, "Luck, classic Coke, and the love of a good man." Richard Dworkin hated it when Mike cited him as crucial to his survival because that implied that if he ever left Mike, he'd die; or, if Mike died, that Richard hadn't loved him enough. In the spring of 1988, Mike wrote a piece for the *Village Voice* in which he insisted that "the best-kept secret of the epidemic" was that not everyone died (by then it had been six and a half years since Sonnabend's original diagnosis). Mike argued that "there are very few infectious agents with a mortality rate of 100 percent for the simple reason that, from an evolutionary standpoint, any disease that killed all its hosts would die out itself." A *New England Journal of Medicine* study concluded that the rates of survival varied with different risk groups. The worst prognosis was for female IV drug users, most of whom were black and Hispanic.

Mike himself did some two dozen interviews with long-term survivors and concluded that what they had in common was that they were all fighters; passionately committed to living, they worked hard to stay alive. And they were all involved in the politics of AIDS—an involvement, Mike felt, that "can be an antidote to the self-obsession that comes with AIDS." One finding that surprised him in his study of long-term survivors was that a majority of them had experienced a rekindling of religious sentiment. He explained it as part of the will to live, "when rational systems offer no hope, we turn to those systems that do. In our culture that means religious systems that speak of life after death" and of "a caring, paternal god who will take care of you." As for himself, he wrote that he'd filed away a signed, notarized document indicating "that any request I might make for religious assistance is to be taken as prima facie evidence of dementia."

Mike also argued that the definition of "luck" needed to include one's race, income level, and access to health care. As the number of people infected continued to rise throughout the 1980s, it became ever more clear that minority groups, particularly blacks, Latinos, and IV drug users, were significantly underrepresented in federally sponsored clinical drug trials—despite the fact that at least some gay activists had been calling more and more attention to the social demographics of access. In 1989, for example, blacks and Latinos accounted for 42 percent of adult U.S. AIDS cases, yet were only 20 percent of the participants in current research trials. The same disproportion was true of women and children of all races.[21]

Late in 1987, Mike's prominence had led to his being appointed to the newly formed New York State AIDS Advisory Council, and he used his new position to make a special effort to arouse sympathy and treatment for IV drug users, whom many viewed as willfully self-destructive. Writing directly to Dr. David Axelrod, New York State's commissioner of health, Mike expressed his concern that the state was "completely unprepared for dealing with the complex problem of AIDS and IV drug use. . . . If sympathy cannot be generated for the IV users themselves, then sympathy must be extended to the sex partners and children of IV users, many of whom are at risk for AIDS." Given the disproportionate number of people of color among IV drug users,

Mike put the blame for government indifference squarely on racism. He denounced as "nonsense" the argument many officials used to reject the call for free, clean needles on the grounds that such a program would encourage or suggest approval of illegal IV drug use.

Along with four others, Mike even traveled to Albany to plead directly with Governor Mario Cuomo for a clean needle exchange program. Cuomo opposed the idea, citing the same tired argument about not wanting to send a message that drug abuse was acceptable. When Mike said something about Cardinal O'Connor's "mean-spirited" attitude toward people with AIDS, Cuomo responded, "I think you misread him. . . . In terms of helping people and reaching out to them, I think he has been extraordinarily generous." Realizing that Cuomo was a Catholic, Mike decided not to respond to what he viewed as a gross misreading of the cardinal's character.

A year on the New York State AIDS Advisory Council was enough to convince Mike that he could better use his energy elsewhere. He thought individual members of the council, like Episcopalian bishop Paul Moore, worked hard—usually behind the scenes—to get more accomplished, but as Mike said in his letter of resignation, "We've certainly *said* many of the right things; but I'm not sure we can take much credit for delivering." New York State, after all, had the largest concentration of people with AIDS in the United States, yet had dragged its feet in funding AIDS education, prevention, and clinical trials. Had it not, Mike felt, "we might now have treatments that would keep me and others like me alive." The root problem, he concluded, was that neither Commissioner Axelrod nor Governor Cuomo had ever taken the council's recommendations seriously; AIDS policy was "formulated elsewhere and where it comports with what the council may decide, good; but where it does not, too bad."

While most white gay men were clamoring for admission to experimental drug trials, some African Americans were reluctant to enter them. Thanks to the notorious Tuskegee experiment (1932–72), distrust of government was deeply entrenched—to say nothing of its prior historical support or indifference, on both the federal and state levels, to slavery and its successor, segregation. Just as some white gays feared quarantine, some blacks feared that AIDS was a deliberate genocidal plot—"just as the introduction of heroin had been"—to decimate minority communities.

But as the mortality figures for AIDS mounted, black gays and lesbians increasingly formed their own organizations to deal with the heavy toll on their communities. The CDC reported that by 1987 the incidence of HIV in African Americans was twice that in whites. Across the country, but particularly on the two coasts, a number of new groups started to emerge—the Black Coalition on AIDS in San Francisco, the Kupona Network in Chicago, GMAD (Gay Men of African Descent) in New York City, Black Gay Men United in Oakland, Unity and ADODI in Philadelphia, the multiple chapters of the Minority Task Force on AIDS, the National Coalition of Black Lesbian and Gays, and so forth.

GMAD in New York stood out for the rapid growth in its ranks. Founded in the summer of 1986, it initially met in private homes, but as membership swelled the group began meeting in the LGBT Center on Thirteenth Street in Manhattan. It remained a volunteer organization that provided both social space and public advocacy. By the late 1980s GMAD had developed into a structured organization, replete with officers and a board of directors, centered on providing information and consciousness raising to its members. It did not, unlike the Community Research Initiative, enter directly into medical research and trials.

In some cases, white gay activists lent information and support—more often, it should be said, than did traditional heterosexual black leaders and organizations. As late as 1988, for example, the Reverend Calvin Butts, executive minister of Abyssinian Baptist Church—the most prestigious church in Harlem—publicly denounced drugs and homosexuality as "against the will of God." On the other hand, Manhattan Borough President (and later Mayor) David Dinkins fought to get more money allotted from the city budget for AIDS programs.[22]

In Washington, D.C., a good deal less activity was apparent. A group called Best Friends was formed in 1986 to help provide social services to PWAs; Howard University sponsored a forum on "AIDS and the Black Population"; and the organization Spectrum came into existence to spread information about AIDS to the black community. By 1987, the Whitman-Walker clinic had considerably expanded its operations, but the Reagan administration—though the president had finally managed to say the word "AIDS" out loud in 1986, five full years after the epidemic began—kept budgeting only modest sums for research (which Congress several times raised, as did Mayor Marion Barry for D.C.). Yet Chief of Police Maurice T. Turner was unashamed to say publicly that he wouldn't want to be in a room with a person who had AIDS, and D.C. police continued to wear surgical masks and yellow gloves when dealing with AIDS patients—leading to the creative ACT UP chant: "Your gloves don't match your shoes / they'll see it on the news!"

Essex was entirely aware, as he put it, that "a mysterious agent was invading our bodies, hiding traps and explosions in our sweet cum and virile blood." And the agent was continuing to spread. "A generation," Essex wrote, "passes before my worn out, grieving eyes. An outlaw community is being decimated without remorse. The scythe swings back and forth, back and forth, random, wild, unpredictable." He himself still felt relatively well, but he did confide to Wayson Jones that he'd experienced some of the symptoms—fevers and night sweats—typically associated with the onset of AIDS. Wayson felt uneasy about how committed Essex was to using safe-sex practices; Essex had told him about "a night of fucking and, almost bragging, had said, 'and we didn't have no safe sex!'"

The black artistic community had continued its vibrant expansion at venues like d.c. space and the Painted Bride Art Center. The latter awarded a two-week New Works Residency grant from July 28 to August 9, 1987, to Essex, Michelle and Wayson, and the product was *Voicescapes: An Urban Mouthpiece*, staged for one night and reviewed favorably in the prestigious *High Performance* magazine. In essence, the piece was an extension of the performance style that they'd previously worked on in *Cinque* and *Murder on Glass*, continuing the exploration of oral traditions, especially the techniques of call-and-response and recitation in unison. Essex described *Voicescapes* as "choral arrangements . . . chants and music were employed to express new meanings from the poetry." Or as Chris Prince, one member of the cast of seven, put it, "a layering of the spoken word, the same way you would layer singing voices. . . . One would speak in a regular speaking voice, another person would talk in a higher range, and a third in a lower one—and you would get this choral effect." (*Voicescapes II*, with just

Essex, Wayson, and Michelle, followed later.) The evening was a success, and in the mayor's prestigious Arts Awards of that year, Essex was nominated in the category of Outstanding Emerging Artist. He then began work on what he hoped would be his third collection of poetry, *Soft Targets*, and he and Wayson continued a collaboration that they hoped would eventuate in the release of their first cassette recording.[23]

They were very conscious, as the number of experimental events accelerated, that the black gay community was involved in a wave of creativity, a much-talked-about "Second Harlem Renaissance." D.C. "was just bubbling," as Chris Prince put it, "politically, artistically, and socially. . . . [It was] an amazing, amazing time in Washington." Following *Voicescapes*, they did a piece called *Dear Motherfuckin' Dreams* at the Kitchen, the well-known experimental venue in New York City. No director was used. When needed, Essex or Michelle came up with the blocking, which Chris Prince, at least, felt was "one of our flaws," since an "outside" perspective might have been helpful at certain points and could have served as a "filter."

But by the late eighties, an almost imperceptible lessening in energy could be detected. AIDS had begun to make significant inroads in the black gay artistic community, to ensnare a growing number of the creative spirits that Essex counted among his friends. The *Washington Post* published an appallingly callous article entitled "Black Gays Evade Reality"—appalling because it seemed ignorant of the horrors that the black gay community had been regularly enduring. Essex wrote a furious rebuttal. The *Post* article had suggested that afflicted blacks were relying medically and politically on the "charity" of the white gay community—meaning primarily the Whitman-Walker clinic. Essex knew there was some truth to that, but in fact he and his friends had participated in fund-raisers and performances to raise money for AIDS-related causes in the Washington area and had gathered artists together regardless of their sexual identity to benefit a homeless shelter.[24]

Besides, the *Post* article declared that "AIDS messages developed by white gays for white gays have not worked for the black gay community" because of "vast differences in language and culture." In his response, Essex sharply asked, "We are speaking of English, aren't we? I am writing this letter in English. Are we to believe that black gay men speak another language? If so, what is that language? Does it have a set of symbols that can be learned for the sake of writing more effective AIDS alerts or newspaper columns?"

Essex had himself claimed on occasion that "a black gay identity is separate from a gay identity," but he also hoped "to meld those identities into one being." The irreducible element in his anger—at the *Post* in particular, at the white gay world in general—was the knowledge that "I can go anywhere in the country and I'm going to be dealt with as a black man—whether I'm flaunting my faggotry or being discreet. The first thing they see is a black male, and that is a constant and ongoing confrontation." The term "gay" had for him "always implied white and middle-class," and he applied it to himself simply because it was "expedient . . . it is what popular culture uses to identify a homosexual." But he did wish that there was "another word that would more aptly affirm not only our sexual, but our racial identity and heritage. Maybe it is a word that we have to put into being." He didn't feel that his sexuality was "so big a thing that it's going to overwhelm my desire to see us [blacks] live and survive."

Long-standing white detachment from black suffering provided the subsoil of Essex's anger, but it had probably been further aggravated by the recent news that Joe Beam had fallen seriously ill. The year 1987 had started out triumphantly for Joe. The D.C. gay newspaper the *Washington Blade* listed *In The Life* as the number one selling gay male book in the country, and he got a host of invitations to speak, including a short tour of California that included San Francisco, Los Angeles, and San Diego. He'd also gotten a prized letter from Audre Lorde telling him that the book "gives me a lot, the pieces themselves, and a lot of hope & satisfaction, too, that it exists. The ending of one kind of isolation. I think it represents an incredible piece of work." As well, Joe began talks with the gay British filmmaker Isaac Julien about collaborating on a new work. On top of all that, Joe continued as editor of *Black/Out*, and the journal's sponsoring organization, the National Coalition of Black Lesbians and Gays, got yet another $10,000 grant.[25]

So far as is known, Joe hadn't told anyone that he was HIV-positive, not Essex, not even his mother, Dorothy. He'd fallen ill several times with respiratory and intestinal ailments during 1987 and 1988 but hadn't put a public name on his assorted afflictions. When he died late in 1988, three days before his thirty-fourth birthday, the obituary in the *Philadelphia Inquirer* read—as did so many AIDS obits then—that "he is believed to have died of natural causes." Essex was quoted in the obit as saying that "he has to be remembered for helping to lead us out of our silence—and by us, I mean black gay men, who heretofore had not been speaking out through literature."[26]

Essex put his deepest feelings about Joe into his poetry. One of those poems has never been published:

> There should have been
> More letters between us.
> In later years it will be difficult to ascertain
> The full meaning of our relations.
> Most of us will not be here
> To bear witness.
> There should have been
> more letters hastily written
> or carefully typed,
> long-winded scripts
> or short, cryptic messages.
> Volumes of letters
> should have gathered
> over time, but we leave
> hastily scrawled postcards,
> outrageous, long-distance
> phone bills,
> and in rare instances
> evidence that some of us
> were more than brothers,
> we were intimate,
> loyal, companions.[27]

The Toll Mounts

The number one killer of people with AIDS by the mid- to late eighties was Pneumocystis pneumonia (PCP). As far back as 1977—before the AIDS epidemic began—Dr. Walter Hughes of Tennessee and his colleagues had conducted a placebo, double-blind study that definitively proved the effectiveness of Bactrim in preventing PCP, and they'd published their findings in the *New England Journal of Medicine*. Joe Sonnabend knew about the Hughes article, had corresponded with him, and shortly after Mike's diagnosis in the summer of 1982 had put him on two double-strength Bactrim tablets a day. After AIDS proliferated, Dr. Michael Gottlieb of Los Angeles and his colleagues, in a 1984 article in *Lancet*, strongly recommended long-term prophylaxis for PCP, but their recommendation had been ignored.[1]

During the 1987 International Conference on AIDS in D.C., Mike and several other activists met with Anthony Fauci, director of the National Institute of Allergy and Infectious Diseases (NIAID, a subsidiary of the National Institutes of Health) and ultimately the head of the AIDS Clinical Trials Group (ACTG)—the AIDS czar in all but name. They tried to persuade Fauci to issue federal guidelines recommending Bactrim or, since some people couldn't tolerate the drug, the lesser alternative, aerosol pentamidine, as preventatives against PCP. Fauci rejected both on the grounds that no controlled studies of their efficacy and safety existed. Yet a year later, under oath before Congress, Fauci said, "If I were an individual patient [with AIDS], I would probably take aerosolized pentamidine if I already had had a bout of pneumocystis. In fact, I might try, even before then, taking prophylactic Bactrim. If I were unable to tolerate that, I might go to aerosolized pentamidine . . . be it available in the street or what have you." Fauci the fantasy patient, in other words, would illegally buy a drug on the street that Fauci the head of NIAID refused to otherwise make available. In other words: "Do what I do, not what I say." Some went further: governmental intransigence on approving Bactrim, they claimed, very nearly approached criminal neglect.

Eager to provide an alternative to the needlessly slow procedures of federally sponsored research, Mike, gay activist Ron Najman, Joe Sonnabend, and Mathilde Krim (co-founder of amfAR) decided in November 1986 to set up the Community Treatment Initiative. Its aim was to hasten the discovery of new treatments by bringing trials to the community and to expand access to them. In May 1987, the project was renamed the Community Research Initiative (CRI). Originally spawned by PWAC, CRI quickly took on a life and identity of its own. It embodied a self-reliant initiative, reached out to minorities, and brought together PWAs, community physicians, and clinical researchers in collaborative efforts to discover viable treatments. Community physicians tended to distrust the new organization (and amfAR as well), and the New York Physicians for Human Rights—a group of gay physicians—declined Sonnabend's request for support. They sometimes supplied patients for trials, but most came of their own initiative.

It was a remarkably bold, though not unprecedented, move. In San Francisco, community-based cancer research had existed for some time, and in 1985, the Community Constituency Consortium (CCC) had formed on the West Coast. It consisted of a group of doctors connected with San Francisco General Hospital who initially banded together with their AIDS patients to disseminate information and, subsequently, get involved in organizing community-based trials; amfAR, too, had started community-based trials.

A multitude of cynics and detractors scorned the notion that community-based research could possibly match the high-tech, costly procedures of traditional trials. They couldn't completely, though CRI did hire statisticians and contracted with specialist labs to study samples. What they could do superlatively well was to gather the relatively untapped resource of on-the-ground data represented by the patients of physicians in private practice, and further, they could establish a program for the controlled testing of promising treatments. At the time, the federal Public Health Service was sponsoring five experimental drug treatments at fourteen medical centers across the country, with an overall goal of enlisting two thousand participants. This represented a tiny fraction of those who might benefit from such participation. Similarly, a number of substances were being investigated at nongovernmental medical centers or administered by private physicians—but in both cases without formal protocols, which meant that data from such informal trials could not be properly evaluated. At the same time, a large number of individuals with AIDS, or at risk for it, yearned to volunteer for drug trials—far, far more than were being accommodated into the few trials that existed.

To conduct additional trials, CRI proposed an Institutional Review Board (IRB) to pass on all proposed protocols in accordance with federal regulations, as well as a scientific and medical committee "to seek out, suggest and evaluate promising interventions." The population for such trials would be drawn from the patients of private physicians in New York—ideally suited for testing experimental treatments because "they are highly motivated, geographically stable, and in many instances have expressed a strong desire to participate in research studies."

Launching CRI, Mike would later write, "was the most difficult, bloody, heart- and back-breaking project I ever attempted." When he initially floated the project, everyone said it couldn't be done, that it was too ambitious. Yet as CRI—and also CCC in San Francisco— soon demonstrated, it *could* be done. Protocols were designed that were as highly sophisticated as any put together by government health officials or university researchers—and far more speedily. NIAID, for example, spent a full year writing and rewriting its protocol for testing aerosol pentamidine.

There were, of course, problems along the way. From the first, CRI had announced—with a sensitivity to race, class, and gender issues that was unprecedented—that it aimed at "making the demographics of CRI trials roughly reflect the demographics of AIDS in New York." They did make slow and steady progress to that end, but the goal was never fully achieved. Still, CRI's demographics were better than those of any federally conducted trial. CRI included populations heavily affected by AIDS but heretofore rarely among the subjects of study—IV drug users, African American and Hispanic people, prisoners, and women. By 1990, approximately 10 percent of the subjects in CRI trials were people of color, and the figure sometimes approached 25 percent. CRI also advertised its trials both in English and in Spanish and its representatives visited drug rehabilitation programs and community health centers further to publicize their protocols. Moreover, the group went to great lengths to ensure that in its work—as Vanessa Merton has documented in her important article "Community-Based AIDS Research"—"every precept of classic clinical research [was] either meticulously observed or else deliberately and rationally departed from." Both CRI's Review Board and its scientific advisory committee were staffed with distinguished clinicians and scientists.

Despite these remarkably valiant efforts, CRI ultimately failed to produce any major treatment breakthrough. Of course, neither did anyone else during the decade that roughly spanned the years 1985–95. CRI, it can be argued, had a better record than other researchers simply because it continued to press the FDA on PCP prophylaxis. Again in 1988—more than a decade after the Hughes study—Dr. Margaret Fischl and colleagues proved that Bactrim could prevent PCP in an immune-compromised individual. But since some people couldn't tolerate Bactrim, and since the AIDS establishment was discouraging its use, the need to win approval for aerosol pentamidine as an alternate prophylaxis seemed crucial. Yet in Joe Sonnabend's opinion, pentamidine proved "a huge distraction." The pharmaceutical company Lyphomed held the patent on pentamidine administered by aerosol, and paid CRI (and CCC in San Francisco) to do a trial, with Sonnabend as chief investigator. Because Fauci had dismissed Bactrim, Joe agreed to lead the pentamidine trial, since it was better to have an alternate, if inferior, choice than none at all. Ultimately, the use of pentamidine as a PCP prophylaxis more or less stopped in the 1990s.[2]

What made this entire struggle all the more maddening was the contrast with the approval process for AZT. The trial that led to the expedited approval of that drug had been hailed by the FDA and other organizations as the gold standard of how proper AIDS research should be conducted. Yet one of the FDA reviewers, Dr. Harvey Chernov, had recommended *against* the approval of AZT—for exactly the same reason Fauci had turned down the superior drug Bactrim: "The available data are insufficient." Yet the data for both Bactrim and pentamidine were in fact fuller and more persuasive than those for AZT.

At a Columbia University forum in November 1988, Edward Bernard of Memorial Sloan-Kettering made this comparison: "Eighty percent of people on AZT not receiving [PCP] prophylaxis had a recurrent episode of pneumocystis. Among patients receiving aerosol pentamidine, only 5 percent in the 15-month period . . . developed a recurring episode. . . . This is a 16-fold reduction." Earlier that same year, Mike had read in *People* magazine that the fifteen-year-old hemophiliac Ryan White—at that point probably the most famous person with AIDS in the country—was again in the hospital with PCP. Somehow Mike managed to track down Ryan's family and discovered to his astonishment that Ryan's doctor had never mentioned—or heard of—PCP prophylaxis. After Mike put Sonnabend in touch with the doctor, Ryan went on prophylaxis. The episode illustrated for Mike the different levels of access available to different segments of the population. As he put it, "ethnic minorities, IV drug users and the poor" lacked not only crucial information but also the money to afford private physicians with substantial expertise. The nonaffluent, as usual, were bearing a disproportionate burden of deaths. To Mike, this was "a scandal of unspeakable magnitude."

In the late eighties, the indifference of the Reagan administration meant that no coordinated AIDS program existed through which the exchange of data on the disease could be facilitated. Nor were the media focused on treatment issues. Some concerned health officials tried to alert various newspapers to the growing enormity of the AIDS crisis and to the resistance of the government to a more sustained effort to deal with it. Gossip, not protocols, entranced the media, who centered most of their limited attention span on whether the disease threatened heterosexuals or on speculation about which closeted celebrities had already come down with AIDS. After Rock Hudson's death in 1985, the focus shifted between Perry Ellis, Roy Cohn, Michael Bennett, and Liberace. The *New York Times* obits almost never mentioned AIDS as the cause of death.

After Mike returned to New York from his frustrating meeting in 1987 with Fauci, he told the CRI board members that they themselves would have to come up with supporting data sufficiently full and technical to persuade NIAID to take action on pentamidine. Mike's long-standing advocacy of self-empowerment was about to find new applicability. CRI, along with CCC in San Francisco, proceeded, in a precedent-setting move, to effectively demonstrate through community-based research what NIAID proved unable to do itself. Mike was rightly furious at the federal response, denouncing it as "sluggish, inhumane and frankly, third-rate."[3]

His anger went up another notch when he learned that Fauci had been forced under oath to admit to a congressional oversight committee that the Office of Budget and Management had approved only eleven of the requested 127 new full-time staff positions for AIDS research during fiscal year 1988. The lack of personnel, Mike felt, had undoubtedly contributed to the fact that out of twenty-four AIDS drugs identified by a NIAID Selection Committee as "high priority," eleven were still not in clinical trials.

Why couldn't the government understand, Mike justifiably raged, that they were living in *wartime*. Most of the citizenry, he wrote in one article, "don't hear the bombs dropping and shells whizzing past your head, don't have to step over the bodies of friends and loved ones." For those "scratching and clawing in a desperate attempt to stay alive," the national indifference amounted to "passive genocide." As early as 1987, Mike had testified before a House Energy and Commerce subcommittee on Health and the Environment—called by Representative Henry Waxman, one of the few people in Congress who seemed to care—that the "U.S. government's track record in terms of *treatments* for AIDS is nothing short of scandalous." A full six years into the epidemic, only about three thousand people had ever been enrolled in trials and a paucity of compounds had been tested. And most of the few trials that had been conducted had continued to focus almost exclusively on gay white men, though more than half of all AIDS cases were by then occurring in people of color. Federal research priorities were largely being set by academic scientists devoted to endless bureaucratic protocols and review boards. The federal trials claimed to have run into great difficulty in finding patient populations willing to participate; in contrast, community physicians had a plethora of patients lining up to volunteer.[4]

Two months later Mike, in the name of PWAC, called a press con-ference to announce that "for the first time in the human history of epidemics, a group of people with a disease have banded together to sponsor top-notch treatment research in an effort to save our own lives and the lives of those who may eventually be diagnosed with AIDS." The NIH, he declared, not only was obsessed with the notion that it alone knew how to run proper clinical trials, but was also hog-tied by "the placebo fixation of federal treatment research de-sign"; such double-blind trials might be the "cleanest" way to get good data, but they weren't the only way, and "given the reality of AIDS, it is unreasonable to expect us to participate in placebo trials." What CRI proposed was nothing less than "the creation of a Manhattan Project for treatments which would essentially pursue every reason-able lead with all due haste."[5]

Mike was also able to announce at that press conference that CRI had signed a $400,000 one-year contract with Lyphomed, the pharma-ceutical company, to conduct a trial involving two hundred subjects to determine—yet again—the efficacy of inhaled aerosol pentamidine in preventing PCP. Within the AIDS activist community in general, there was considerable criticism of Lyphomed for the price increases that it claimed were necessary to fund research (research, Mike felt, that the federal government should have paid for). He didn't claim to know if Lyphomed's argument for hoisting prices was justified, but he did know that Lyphomed was "the first company to put their money down in a gamble on an experimental approach to AIDS treatment research."

In preparing the trial, CRI followed standard state and federal regulatory procedures: it established its own IRB (Institutional Re-view Board), and staffed it with experts from medical ethics, law, and medicine, as well as PWAs (including Mike himself), to ensure that research subjects were protected from undue risk. CRI also made sure that its clinical trials would be open to all, irrespective of race and gender. As well, it set up a scientific advisory board of AIDS medical experts (chaired by Sonnabend), which included Dr. Donald Armstrong, head of infectious diseases at Memorial Sloan-Kettering, Dr. Michael Lange of St. Luke's-Roosevelt Hospital Center, Dr. Mathilde Krim, co-chair of amfAR, and Dr. Bernard Bihari, director of Kings County

Addictive Diseases Hospital. The scientific advisory committee would review and revise all protocols as well as generate protocols of its own. Mike made it clear that CRI did not view itself as in competition with federal research efforts, but rather "as a creative addition to AIDS treatment research. . . . Surely in a crisis of the magnitude of AIDS, there is room for creative solutions."

True to Mike's feminist orientation, CRI fought aggressively for the inclusion of women in its clinical trials; when a drug company submitted a protocol on a "hot" drug that excluded women entirely, CRI's IRB demanded a counterproposal that unconditionally included women—and won. In several other protocols, CRI got the age limit lowered to twelve, though it didn't attempt any pediatric trials. Its initial trial for aerosol pentamidine, moreover, proved conclusively that it was a successful prophylactic against PCP. One year later, the FDA sent a team to CRI to inspect its procedures and results and issued a report that concluded that the group was engaged in "good science." Thereafter, the FDA formally approved aerosol pentamidine. CRI had pulled off an astonishing feat of self-empowered scientific rigor—and saved many lives.[6]

Yet community-based research lacked the resources of NIAID and other federal agencies. Rumors continued to multiply about the many possibly effective drugs that were languishing on the shelves due to the apathy of the Reagan administration and the FDA's traditionally slow protocols and drug approval process. By 1987, there was a notable uptake in demonstrations against the stalling and red tape that had characterized the testing of potentially useful drugs—and against the appalling focus of the drug companies on the profit motive above all other considerations.

Some of these unruly and defiant direct-action protests preceded the formation of ACT UP and sprung up in a variety of locales. Several protests involved only a few participants, who the police easily dispersed. But others—like those organized by the Lavender Hill Mob in New York City—involved hundreds of angry protesters in a series of scattered demonstrations and "zaps." Desperation and rage were unquestionably building—and early in 1987 exploded at New York City's Gay Community Center when Larry Kramer gave an emotional speech (which Mike admitted and applauded) demanding that the gay community take action. Tim Sweeney—GMHC's associate director—

then encouraged a follow-up meeting. From that meeting, ACT UP came into being. Its series of media-savvy demonstrations and actions began with a sit-in on Wall Street and expanded rapidly thereafter. By spring 1988, ACT UP chapters existed across the country and for nine consecutive days protests were mounted on a set of issues ranging from the global impact of AIDS to the plight of those in prison.

Fortunately, an unexpected ally from within the Reagan administration arose in the person of C. Everett Koop, the surgeon general. Koop had an impeccably conservative background, including strenuous opposition to abortion, and his appointment in 1981 as surgeon general had horrified liberals across the country. But Koop proved to be his own independent man. Throughout 1986, he immersed himself in the literature on AIDS and then—without notifying the White House in advance—went public with a *Surgeon General's Report on Acquired Immune Deficiency Syndrome*. It came as a profound shock to all parties.

The Koop report was nothing less than a call to arms. He not only advocated AIDS education at "the earliest grade possible"—his critics translated that as giving condoms to eight-year-olds—but also championed safe sex, denounced mandatory testing, and characterized any suggestion of quarantine as "useless." Yet as the political scientist Cathy J. Cohen has pointed out in *The Boundaries of Blackness*, Koop "seemed to collapse efforts to deal with AIDS among African Americans with policies targeting Haitian communities; this was symptomatic of the institutionalized ignorance of issues relating to race that skewed many of the white reactions to AIDS in minority communities." But the opposition that arose in the White House to Koop's report was hardly based on racial sensitivity. Education Secretary William Bennett and White House adviser Gary Bauer led the assault on Koop, arguing furiously that his report should have been "more morally judgmental." Skillful in influencing the media, Bennett and Bauer fought Koop at every turn. They insisted on "value-based education" that taught teenagers to apply Nancy Reagan's jingle "Just Say No" to sexual activity. Bauer got the president to further emphasize the message in an April 1, 1987, speech in which he stressed that AIDS education in the schools should focus on the importance of sexual abstinence. The Bennett/Bauer position continued to dominate the Reagan administration's policies, though it failed to silence Koop's ongoing call for compassion—and condoms.[7]

Koop's blind spot about the special needs of the African American community was also characteristic of the *New York Times* coverage. Its very first article on the subject of AIDS wasn't published until late in 1985. What followed was a rash of stories linking African swine flu to AIDS, along with coverage of the discomfort felt by the black world in general with the "immorality" of same-gender sex. As Cathy Cohen has pointed out, the *Times* published only three articles between 1981 and 1993 that focused primarily on black gay men with AIDS—but nine about afflicted women of color, portraying them primarily as "innocent victims" of "bisexual" black men.

The AIDS community reacted to the Koop report as a sign of hope—and there had been few of late—that more attention might finally be paid. By the end of 1987, AIDS had appeared in some 113 other countries. Europe reacted with a massive educational program to inform and protect its citizens. The United States reacted with a denunciation from the right-wing antifeminist Phyllis Schlafly declaring that Koop wanted to institute "grammar school sodomy classes."

The swift growth of ACT UP chapters and confrontational direct action reflected the growing anger in the gay world at the lack of progress against AIDS. Back in 1976 the CDC had spent $9 million within months of the outbreak of Legionnaires' disease (which killed thirty-four people); during the first year of the AIDS epidemic, with more than two hundred people already dead, the CDC spent $1 million. By the mideighties, the lack of research had been accompanied by growing calls—and not just from right-wingers—for mandatory AIDS testing, quarantine, and even tattooing (the latter advocated by William Buckley). People with AIDS were being attacked, not succored—evicted from their apartments, fired from their jobs, confronted by masked and gloved nurses in hospitals, denied even the assurance of safe private space thanks to the Supreme Court's 1986 *Bowers v. Hardwick* ruling.[8]

Even as the federal government refused to marshal its resources to combat the mounting AIDS epidemic and in general cut back on social welfare programs that aided the poor, the Reagan administration seemed to have no trouble at all in spending vast sums of money for other kinds of war—including sending marines into Lebanon, invading the tiny island of Grenada, and supporting brutal right-wing elements in El Salvador and Nicaragua. The coffers stayed closed for sissies and perverts, but they spilled forth without prompting for the promotion of macho violence.

Increasingly, the gay community fought back. The growth in direct-action protest culminated in a massive March on Washington in October 1987. The night before the march, Essex and Wayson did a ten p.m. show at d.c. space and another, joined by Michelle, at midnight. At the earlier showing, at Essex's initiative, the two men performed a piece denouncing RENAMO (Resistência Nacional Moçambicana), a right-wing political party in Mozambique that was backed by the South African apartheid regime. As Wayson remembers it, the audience response was lukewarm; that in itself bothered Essex, but he was annoyed, too, that Wayson didn't know as much about RENAMO as he thought he should. The more Essex became a cultural icon in the black gay community, the more, as Wayson saw it, "he was hurt when he felt like he wasn't understood." Another example was the negative reaction some members of the black lesbian community had when Essex and Wayson used the word "bitch" when performing the piece "To Some Supposed Brothers." Essex regarded the piece as "a powerful feminist statement against the verbal abuse and disrespect of black women" shown by many black men, and he felt deeply frustrated that the message had failed to be appreciated. Similarly, when Essex at one point casually dated a white guy, it became, according to Wayson "a bicoastal scandal"—e-mails were exchanged questioning his credibility as an exemplar of black gay male identity and his "blackness credentials" in general.

At the 1987 march, estimates of the size of the crowd, as always, varied. But as a participant—I went with my partner, Eli, the man I'd met the year before and with whom I still live—I felt confident that the outpouring, led by PWAs, some in wheelchairs, was "huge"— hundreds of thousands. The *New York Times* estimated the crowd at two hundred thousand, but we thought *Newsday* was closer to the mark in citing upwards of half a million. "Miles and miles of marchers," I wrote, went by "in interchangeable blue jeans, wool shirts and sneakers, making the strong visual point that 'we are everywhere, and everybody." Watching the TV coverage that night of the simultaneous Columbus Day Parade in New York, with its paramilitary drill units and rifle clubs, I was glad that in *our* march no one brandished a single weapon; nor were any police needed to discipline the crowd. I saw only one bunch of angry, confrontational people—the Jesus freaks, carrying their hate-filled banners, screaming their violent slogans.[9]

It would be a mistake to conflate the heightened number of gay people now committed to direct action against governmental AIDS apathy with the whole of the gay community. Mike's "quintessential image of an urban gay man in the Reagan 1980s" was someone "sick; shunned; frightened and frightening; and largely unprotected by either law or popular opinion." Plenty of gay people remained cowed in silent terror—at the disease, at coming out to family and friends, at employers who applauded the recent Justice Department ruling that in regard to federal contracts, employers were entitled to fire employees simply on the *suspicion* that they were HIV-positive and might "casually transmit" AIDS in the workplace. Still others in the gay community, though not ill or in terror, retreated to an ostrich-like head-in-the-sand attitude.

Just two months before the March on Washington, when Eli and I vacationed on Fire Island, we stopped off one day to visit Larry Mass, Arnie Kantrowitz, and Vito Russo, who'd taken a house together in Cherry Grove. We found Vito in a justifiable rage over the seeming indifference of the island's gay inhabitants toward AIDS; he'd written a fiery letter to the *Fire Island Times* denouncing the smug atmosphere in the community, and it had caused "outrage." When, that same week, we had dinner in the East Village apartment of three of Eli's friends, we found a different sort of inactivity—due to illness, not apathy. One of the three, sick with hepatitis and tuberculosis, could hardly sit at the table. The second had already been hospitalized once and had a T cell count of 0. The third had also been hospitalized but was currently feeling okay. The three men had in varying combinations been lovers for some fifteen years and were deeply supportive of one another; the atmosphere that night was "chatty" and "up." Their untheatrical valor reduced me to near silence, and tears. No protest march for them. All three would soon succumb to the disease.

Richard Dworkin had been urging Mike for some time to get back into his music. He not only believed in Mike's vocal talent, but felt he needed a respite from the tension and acrimony of his life as a PWA activist. Earlier, they'd formed the band Lowlife. It had recorded a few songs and done a two-week tour in Fort Lauderdale and Key West—irrepressible Mike sometimes twirling a baton, yodeling, and playing synthesizer simultaneously—but Lowlife had lasted only until 1986. Sometime in 1987, Richard played the record *Nina Simone and Piano* for Mike—not simply for its own glories but to demonstrate to Mike that recording an album need not involve a huge production, complicated arrangements, or a ton of money—which Mike had long assumed.[10]

Richard's strategy worked. The power of the Simone record convinced Mike that neither a lot of musicians nor a lot of cash was needed to produce something musically and emotionally powerful. Yet some connections *were* needed, and it was Richard's musical background that produced them. Back in the 1970s, when living in San Francisco, Richard had learned to play the drums and had also studied jazz with the saxophonist John Handy. He wanted to play with and for the gay male community—"giving it a voice it never had before"—and ultimately that came to include Blackberri (who both Essex and Joe Beam knew), the group Buena Vista, Casselberry and DuPree, and Steven Grossman, who became Richard's roommate.

With Buena Vista—named after the big gay cruising park—Richard sometimes played at the Stud, the hangout (in Richard's words) of "the hippie fags, the freaks of San Francisco." For the first time, he was able to perform "an out-and-out love song sung by one guy to another guy." He had also played for dancers in performance and was part of a group that organized a loft jazz space called the Blue Dolphin in the garage of a Victorian house at Seventeenth and Sanchez in the Castro District. Through a friend who was the keyboard player for the pro-gay Glide Memorial Church in the Tenderloin, Richard, out of his love for black gospel music, occasionally attended services there— though he was "raised and confirmed an atheist from birth."

The first post-Stonewall gay male record had probably been that of a group called Lavender Country, who Richard saw perform in San Francisco in the early 1970s. Steven Grossman's album *Caravan Tonight* had claim to the first "out" gay record on a major label. (One of the main reasons Richard had left San Francisco for New York was his inability to get Grossman, who was an accountant by day, to stick with music consistently.)

When he'd first come to New York, Richard had seen an ad in the

Village Voice advertising for gay jazz musicians to play five nights a week in a gay bar. The bar turned out to be a New York City branch of the Monster, the well-known Fire Island hangout. Richard thought he'd "died and gone to heaven." It proved something less than that, but it did produce a steady gig for a while. One night the bass player turned excitedly to Richard and said, "Look over there, I don't believe it! It's Fred Hersch"—the jazz pianist who was also on the faculty of the New England Conservatory of Music. Richard recalled the incident three or four years later as he looked through a list of recording studios in Manhattan and saw that Hersch owned one of them. Richard went and talked with him and Hersch couldn't have been more accommodating: he gave Richard and Mike an exceedingly low rate—something like $25 an hour—and even included an engineer in the package. (Hersch was gay and HIV-positive but hadn't come out—but after meeting Mike and being encouraged by him, he openly acknowledged both his sexual orientation and his health status. He was one of the few established figures in the jazz world to do so.)

Richard and Mike conceived of the record, which they named *Purple Heart*, as including several songs earlier recorded by Lowlife, and the rest of the album as pretty much just Mike singing and often playing the piano as well (though others did too, including his lesbian friend Marsha Malamet). Mike had written about 40 percent of the songs and lyrics, including the two that became best known, "Living in Wartime" and "Love Don't Need A Reason (co-written with Malamet and her friend Peter Allen). What could be called Mike's romantic view of love suffuses his lyrics, but no more so than his pervasive political awareness:

> They try to break our spirits
> try to keep us in our place
> They do it to the women
> and the poor of every race
> We face a common enemy:
> bigotry and greed
> But if we fight together
> we can find the strength we need
> we can find the strength we need . . .
>
> (from "Living in Wartime")

Love don't need a reason
Love's never been a crime
And love is all we have for now
What we don't have
what we don't have is time . . .

(from "Love Don't Need a Reason")

The phrase "love don't need a reason" derived, according to Mike, from reporters periodically dragging a reluctant Richard Dworkin into several interviews and invariably asking him something along the lines of, "Why would you get involved with somebody who has AIDS?" Richard's moving reply was that "love's a crazy thing . . . it doesn't need a reason."[11]

The uniqueness and beauty of Mike's voice was immediately recognized by most people who heard it. Its tone bright and pure, it had a special keening, wry quality, a pervasive vulnerability. In terms of intonation, Mike was technically very good—that is, he sang in key, hitting the right notes, never slurring his words. Always the perfectionist, he would fault his rhythmic skill—"I'm just a white boy from the midwest," he liked to say. In his natural voice, he could sing quite high, a characteristic of many popular male singers—such as Kenny Loggins, Michael McDonald, or John Fogerty (of Creedence Clearwater Revival)—and Mike could sing falsetto as well.

Singing publicly, unfortunately, was often "torture" for him. He felt that he'd inherited from his father "this absolutely impossible perfectionist system of judgment," and he constantly judged each note as he sang it: "Was this the best note I could have possibly sung? Did I sing it well enough? Did I hold it long enough? Was it entirely in tune? Did the vibrato come in at exactly the right moment?" Eventually, Mike would be less hard on himself, but when he performed in the late 1980s, he kept "waiting for people to shoot me or start laughing." Only the support of close friends and of Richard kept him going.

When *Purple Heart* was released, Mike was too ill to undertake a tour—which pre-Internet was the only practical way to sell an independent album. Mike would later remember that the album "dropped like a stone." But either his memory was faulty or his modesty was working *way* overtime. The reviews were not only plentiful, but mostly raves. The reviewer in *The Advocate*, Adam Block, called it "the most remarkable gay independent release of the past decade" and he especially loved one of the two sides—the bebop, rock-like one (the second side was mostly cabaret-style ballads, with Mike accompanying himself on the piano). The other critics outdid each other with praise. David Kalmansohn in the *Los Angeles Dispatch* called the album "startlingly sophisticated . . . a mature, original work." Christopher Wittke in *Gay Community News* called *Purple Heart* "a great album," David Lamble hailed it as "a virtually flawless debut" in the *Bay Area Reporter*, and Will Grega, in his *Gay Music Guide*, gave it a flatout rave: "Nothing less than the most stunning gay album recorded to date." Two of the best cuts on the album had been recorded by Lowlife in 1985, and the least favorite among some of the critics was the hypersentimental "Love Don't Need a Reason."

The praise eventually sank in and Mike learned to be proud of the recording—though in a few years his voice would drop down about three semitones and what the deeper sound lost in vulnerability, it gained in maturity. This would be especially apparent on Mike's final album, *Legacy*, which he would come to feel was "the best thing I've ever done."

The release of *Purple Heart* in 1988 came soon after the publication of the 352-page *Surviving and Thriving With AIDS: Collected Wisdom*, volume 2, a collection of essays by many hands (volume 1, *Hints for the Newly Diagnosed*, had been half the size). Along with editing *Surviving and Thriving*, Mike contributed several essays and interviews of his own; Richard served as associate editor and Mike's co-worker Jane Rosett (PWA's virtual in-house photographer) as the art editor. Between them, they saw to it that the volume contained, along with a great deal of advice about sex, families, and treatments, two separate sections that were pathbreaking: "Women With AIDS" and "People of Color and AIDS." Mike asked GMHC for help in distributing volume 2, but it refused after learning that it contained certain criticisms of the organization, and in particular of a GMHC editorial in its publication *Treatment News* that claimed "the preponderance of evidence to date is irrefutable" as to the positive value of AZT.

The book makes for poignant reading today. Many of its contributors have long since died, and most of the debates over treatment issues (such as the efficacy of lipids, AZT or AL-721) have long since been settled. But the bravery, determination, and valor that suffuse its pages can never go out of date, representing as they do the remarkable gallantry so many showed in the face of what Mike called "the ineptitude and murderous lethargy of the federal government." The volume also has historical importance. It documents how, despite suffering that was often acute, many people with AIDS managed to resist, to take charge of their own treatment, and to call public attention to the country's catastrophic disregard (with some honorable exceptions, like Matilde Krim, Elizabeth Taylor, and philanthropist Judy Peabody) of those facing death in the prime of their lives. *Surviving and Thriving*— note the persistent optimism, against all odds, contained in that word "thriving"—demonstrated, in the same way that the fierce defiance of ACT UP and other direct-action groups did, the determination of the despised to battle for survival.[12]

Mike took the battle to the annual convention of the American Academy of Dermatologists, where he gave that august gathering, and the federal government, a blistering rebuke. The slow pace of response to the enormous suffering and mounting deaths—the business-as-usual attitude—represented in essence "passive genocide," Mike told his audience, the "political perception that the value of the lives affected by AIDS doesn't justify a swift, humane or top-notch response." Why, he asked the audience of physicians, had only eleven full-time staff positions for AIDS research been filled when Congress had authorized 127? Why hadn't DHPG, gamma globulin, fluconazole, and foscarnet been approved for varying AIDS conditions when the data on them were at least as impressive as that supporting AZT, which *had* been approved?

To take just the example of foscarnet, Mike said, he'd recently come across an announcement from the National Eye Institute that its pending drug trial would be confined to "patients with non-sight threatening" CMV retinitis. "Excuse me?!" Mike indignantly asked. CMV retinitis *always* affected eyesight (often resulting in blindness), and it was already known that foscarnet was effective in treating 75 to 80 percent of those cases. Similarly, Dr. Arye Rubenstein had had a great deal of success in extending the lives of infants with AIDS by using gamma globulin. Yet the medical establishment still opposed its release without a traditional placebo-controlled trial. In Mike's view that amounted to criminal misconduct; who would not recoil, he asked, at "the thought of sick infants being strapped down in order to receive an IV saline solution as a placebo, when we 'know' from clinical experience that gamma globulin will extend their lives?"

Mike quoted Joe Sonnabend on the inherent conflict between the concerns of a researcher and those of a private doctor. The researcher was willing to withhold prophylaxis—to let people die—in the name of rigidly controlled lengthy trials, even when clinical data had already confirmed a given treatment's efficacy. In other words, researchers would deny the best available patient care and insist on placebo trials because "we haven't developed reliable laboratory markers of disease progression." "Well, I for one," Mike declared, "am not willing to die for the greater good of others because I believe there are other ways of approaching AIDS treatment trials which can produce good data without sacrificing my life." This was precisely why CRI in New York was exploring "dose comparison trials, historical control trials and the development of reliable laboratory markers of disease progression beyond T-cell subsets. . . . We simply do not believe it is ethical to sacrifice individuals in the name of some arbitrary standard of proper science."

The ACT UP activist Jim Eigo came up with the notion of "parallel trials": they would enroll anyone with HIV "who had no available treatment options," which in 1988 meant "an overwhelming number of people with AIDS," who'd been "routinely excluded from trials due to gender, illness, or conflicting medications." Eigo argued that the data collected from parallel trials wouldn't be "clean enough" to secure a drug its final approval," but rigorous Phase 2 clinical trials would be proceeding simultaneously. Eigo and the members of his affinity group in ACT UP sent the proposal to Dr. Anthony Fauci, the head of federal AIDS efforts. Within a few weeks, Eigo detected phrases from their proposal in some of Fauci's speeches, and soon after, Fauci came out publicly in favor of the activists' position—which then became standard.

When the gay/lesbian Whitman-Walker Health clinic in Essex's hometown, Washington, D.C., ran a series of ads urging gay men to "try living without anal sex" entirely—even anal sex with condoms—Mike spoke out angrily against the proposal. Precisely who had the right, Mike asked, to issue value judgments on the varying forms of sexual expression—to say nothing about the difficulties of trying to enforce those judgments. He suspected that behind the suggestion of forgoing anal sex was "squeamishness about the asshole—the subtle self-loathing that buys the libel that sodomy is 'against nature' and that AIDS is some divine retribution for such an 'unnatural' act as taking-it-up-the-tush."

Mike had been mounting the barricades on this issue as far back as 1985, when GMHC had distributed a recommendation, based on guidelines formulated by the New York Physicians for Human Rights, that gay men "try to avoid anal sex." Mike had blasted the suggestion. "Those who enjoy getting fucked," he wrote at the time, "should not be made to feel stupid or irresponsible. Instead, they should be provided with the information necessary to make what they enjoy safe! And that means the aggressive encouragement of condom use!" Yes, he acknowledged, condoms could break, but it should be left to the individual to decide how much risk he was willing to take, to weigh the value of his life against the value of a particular form of sexual expression—especially since "AIDS is the day to day management of uncertainty. . . . We cannot say with absolute certainty how risky a particular sex act with a particular individual might be. . . . Fucking is so important to some of us that we're willing to take some risks that others might not be willing to take."

What the Whitman-Walker clinic *should* be doing, in Mike's opinion, was spreading the word that a scientific study completed in 1985 had proved the general ability of condoms to prevent the spread of AIDS. It should also, in his view, be leading the demand for stricter standards for condom manufacture and inspection (to minimize leakage and tears), educating gay men about the *proper* use of condoms and lubricants, and demanding a national AIDS educational campaign "which speaks bluntly in non-clinical language that people can understand." Given Mike's incensed tone, he got back a surprisingly placid, understanding letter from Jim Graham, administrator of the Whitman-Walker clinic. "I do not think you are 'too harsh' on . . . the Clinic," Graham wrote. "These are difficult times for us all, and there are bound to be strong disagreements. I know we are acting in good faith with the best motivations as I am sure you are as well." He did point out that when the FDA tested 204 batches of latex condoms in 1987, it found that 20 percent had a failure rate (leaking water under pressure). Yet he agreed with Mike that people "don't always use condoms the right way, even when they think they are." Mike had become so used to raising his voice in order to be heard at all that Graham's calm response must have taken him by surprise.

In one of the essays he wrote for *Surviving and Thriving*, Mike revealed that he'd recently been diagnosed with a KS lesion on his leg and as a result was taking naltrexone—which at low levels some believed stimulated the production of endorphins, which in turn might have a beneficial effect on T cells. Mike had also become convinced "that there is a bi-directional mind-body connection" and as a result—despite his scorn for Louise Hay—had taken the "AIDS Mastery" course. He also "religiously" prophylaxed with aerosol pentamidine and, less religiously, experimented with acyclovir and Antabuse. He'd even been plasmapheresed—that is, had "a sort of blood cleansing, where they hook you up to these huge centrifuges and spin pints of your blood" to remove "viral debris."

But he championed none of those treatments. In his experience, as he'd argued earlier, one factor stood out as characteristic of long-term survivors: political involvement—putting up "one hell of a fight"—which he felt could be sustained only "if it comes from a loving place; anger has its place but it burns up quickly and can burn your spirit up with it." He applauded groups like ACT UP, but given what he called his "limited energy"—after all, in 1988, he'd turned out an album and a book, not to mention multiple speeches and appearances—he preferred to concentrate on his work with CRI "on doing drug trials faster, cheaper and better than the feds are doing." Despite his "limited energy," Mike managed to get arrested at a civil disobedience protest on the steps of the Supreme Court in October 1988.[13]

Passing by the bulletin board at the New York City Gay Community Center on Thirteenth Street one day, Richard spotted a tacked-up note soliciting responses for forming a gay a capella group. "Perfect!" he thought. "Perfect for Mike," whose relentless superego was always watching and judging when he performed (or indeed did anything). In an a capella ("without accompaniment") group, the lead often shifts; it's atypical for someone to keep it through an entire song—and that would help dilute Mike's guilt-inducing perfectionism.

And thus it was that the Flirtations (the "Flirts") was born and would over time develop a strong fan base. Jon Arterton and Elliot Pilshaw had originated the idea and put up the note on the bulletin board. When Mike went to talk to them, he was excited to discover that Aurelio Font was also involved; he and Aurelio had been in the New York City Gay Men's Chorus and he much admired the quality of Aurelio's voice. (Though a founding member of the Gay Men's Chorus, Mike later referred to it as "loathsome"—"they're so FULL of themselves; they think they're the best in the world; so pretentious.") T.J. Myers, who in 1990 would die of AIDS, also joined the Flirtations; he was "a gotta-sing, gotta-dance kinda guy" who for a while had been in the dance company of Rachel Squires, the manager for a time of the Flirts. Soon after the group formed, Elliot Pilshaw, whose voice wasn't deep enough to carry the low end, gave way to Cliff Townsend, an African American with a trained bass voice.

A capella singing has its roots in a variety of religious traditions—Gregorian chant being one—and in the early twentieth century doo-wop and barbershop became well-known variants in the United States. The most popular groups by midcentury were probably the Hi-Lo's, the Four Freshmen, and the King's Singers. A new wave of popularity had been inaugurated when Bernice Johnson Reagon founded the all-woman African American ensemble Sweet Honey in the Rock in 1973. By the late eighties a significant number of well-known artists performed a cappella music, including the Persuasions, Bobby McFerrin (whose innovations probably did more than anyone else to produce the a cappella renaissance), and the Nylons, who many thought had a gay sensibility. The number of professional a cappella groups grew in the country from about one hundred in 1985 to more than seven hundred a dozen years later. By the 1990s many contemporary vocal "bands"—but not the Flirtations—would use electronic assistance to produce a range of startling effects with their voices.

Everyone in the Flirtations was on the left politically; the Flirts in fact billed themselves as "the world's only politically correct gay male a capella group." All five were not only involved in the gay movement, but also supported other liberation movements, including feminism and the black struggle; one of the songs they performed was "Biko," as well as the antiapartheid anthem "Something Inside So Strong." The group's first album wouldn't appear until 1990, but they started performing on the streets of Greenwich Village soon after first meeting in 1988.

When Joe Beam died from AIDS on December 27, the printed obituary simply announced that "the exact cause of his death was not immediately clear," though friends said that he'd "been in ill health recently and had been extremely depressed for several months." Essex, of course, knew better and provided a far more ample tribute. "The work Joe did," Essex wrote, "enriched the community in ways that have yet to manifest themselves. His life was a light for many of us." Essex also memorialized his friend in the poem "When My Brother Fell":

> When my brother fell
> I picked up his weapons
> And never once questioned
> Whether I could carry
> The weight and grief,
> The responsibility
> He shouldered
>
> . . . .
>
> When I stand
> On the front lines now,
> Cussing the lack of truth,
> The absence of willful change
> And strategic coalitions,
> I realize sewing quilts
> Will not bring you back
> Nor save us . . .

"Sewing quilts" was a reference to the Names Project AIDS Memorial Quilt, displayed on the Washington Mall for the first time during the 1987 March on Washington for Lesbian and Gay Rights. Seeing the vast patchwork of panels that family members and friends had sewn together was an overwhelming experience for many—a visual counterpart of the desperate toll in lives already lost. But to Essex, the quilt primarily memorialized white lives, and perhaps he also objected (as did others) to the project's lack of politics.

At the time of his death, Joe Beam had begun work on a sequel volume to *In The Life* of black gay male poetry and prose. It had been slow going, and Joe had frequently and gently been trying to cajole people into sending contributions. With Joe's death, his mother, Dorothy, became determined to fulfill her son's contract with Alyson Publications for the second volume. She'd come a long way from the hesitant, uncertain mother who'd first heard her son tell her that he was gay. "There is some kind of fear in the black population," she now felt, "that says they have to hide their gay sons. . . . They say to pray for the gay sons. I don't have to pray for God to change my son because that's how he made him."

Dorothy Beam was a fighter. In her own life, she'd worked during the day and gone to school at night to earn both a college degree and a master's from Temple University. And once she became a teacher, she bucked school administrators and other teachers who treated students with learning or emotional disabilities as "throwaways," making them her special protégés. She was, in other words, distinctly on the side of the underdog, the outsider—and on behalf of gay people, she was tough on the black community. It was guilty, she told an interviewer, "on two counts. First, forgetting that AIDS is taking its toll on the community, and secondly, for not facing the fact that this disease can be prevented by taking proper precautions. Safe sex is a duty, and AIDS can be anyone's disease."

Dorothy Beam was determined to take up her son's projected anthology and make sure that it reached conclusion. Before his death, Joe hadn't gotten very far with the new volume; he'd sent out some notices to the press, had begun to receive a few manuscripts, had chosen a title—*Brother to Brother*—and had left behind a list of possible contributors. Dorothy Beam set tirelessly to work contacting them. She also turned to Essex, Joe's closest friend, for consultation and advice. As more and more manuscripts started to arrive, she photocopied each one and mailed it from Philadelphia to Essex in D.C.

As the material and the need to consult about it began to accumulate, Essex made the decision to move to Philadelphia in order to facilitate working with Dorothy on the project. She and her husband invited him to move into their home, where he could all at once work uninterrupted, save money, and feast on Dorothy Beam's fried chicken. Essex himself sometimes cooked for the Beams—as well as cut the lawn, trimmed the hedges, and shoveled snow. The anthology became something of a family affair.

Sometimes Dorothy Beam would come down into Essex's work space in the basement to "get a hug," and he even arranged a meeting between her and his own mother. Dorothy was "like an older aunt," Essex said. "I don't feel I am a surrogate by any means." For her part, Dorothy told one interviewer that she noted similarities between Essex and her son; even her husband had noted that "Essex is a lot like Joe." Both were "warm, sincere, and humane" personalities; both held "a great deal within"; both "want to do right."[14]

Unlike Essex's own mother, Dorothy Beam became more and more of an activist; she even took a course in counseling relatives of gay people. Some of her friends were scandalized about her having "a gay person living in your house"—to which she characteristically replied, "my son's gay friends are welcome at my house anytime. They hurt the same, they have the same problems. In fact they have more." Several of her friends advised her to take the manuscript material and "throw it in the trash and forget it. . . . It is going to weigh heavy on your heart and you are not going to be able to get yourself together if you keep working with the book." That advice made her angry, and she responded to it with variants of "I thought this gay business was a big problem. It is not a big problem. You made a problem out of it. I want other parents to see that it is no disgrace having a gay child. The disgrace is when you try to put it in the closet."

Essex never hesitated in taking on the anthology, though 1988 hadn't been the best of years for him. Guarded as always about his privacy, he obliquely referred to having had to cancel a performance "due to circumstances related to my health. It is very much my mental health. . . . I am slowly returning to myself. . . . Believing this period of my life to be a test, I can't say I have survived it with the best qualities of my person." No additional details have surfaced about whether Essex's difficult year related to side effects from medication or from AIDS itself. But whatever the case, Essex accepted Dorothy Beam's invitation to take over her son's work without reservation.

Joe Beam had left behind few notes or editorial comments. This left Essex all at once without direction, yet entirely free to follow his own impulses. The black lesbian writer Barbara Smith gave him unstinting encouragement and coaching on everything (as Essex phrased it) "from questions of copyright to questions of copyediting"; ultimately she advised him on the choice of manuscripts and even took on the onerous job of reading page proofs to provide Essex with another set of eyes for catching errors.

By August 1989, some ninety manuscripts had poured in, but in that early batch Essex was "still waiting," as he wrote Barbara Smith, "for some 'exciting' poetry to come over the transom." He was beginning to realize that poetry "is not taken very seriously by many," and for him there was "the additional loneliness that sometimes comes from relating with Black gay men as writers." He found that his "great respect for language and the transformational powers inherent in it" was rarely shared—and especially in regard to effective expression "in poetic form"—by other black men. At the risk of misinterpreting what Essex meant by "respect for language," it seems worth pointing out that he doesn't explicitly acknowledge—either in the letter cited or in the *Brother to Brother* anthology—the lively, inventive African American vernacular that differs markedly from standard English—what James Baldwin meant when in 1979 he wrote, "People evolve a language in order to describe and thus control their circumstances, or in order not to be submerged by a reality that they cannot articulate."

Ultimately Essex gathered a pool of some 140 manuscripts. He knew that he didn't want "a lot of coming out stories"; *In The Life* had already done that. Essex's interest "was making the brothers speak more honestly about their experience—let's get away from the surface froth, and really dig underneath the issues we talk about." He ended up selecting nearly three dozen writers, several of whom appear more than once. The hefty finished volume came to nearly three hundred pages of closely printed text, with Essex including several of his own significant poems and essays. He also appended a long, vibrant, even fierce introduction, dating it "January 1990."

In it, he not only provided a detailed history, dating back to the Harlem Renaissance, of black gay male literature, but also mounted an angry attack on the white gay world in general and one of its celebrities in particular—Robert Mapplethorpe, then known for his series of "erotic" (Essex called them "racist") portraits of black men. He angrily denounced the post-Stonewall white gay community as having been basically unconcerned with the lives of black gay men and lesbians—and Mike Callen would have agreed with him. White gay men, Essex pointed out, become "other" in this country only when and if they choose to come out of the closet. But all blacks "are treated as 'other' regardless of whether we sleep with men or women—our Black skin automatically marks us as 'other.'"

Essex made the further point that unless the racial divide that characterized the gay world was somehow healed, the gay community could never "become a powerful force for creating *real* social changes that reach beyond issues of sexuality." If he was surely accurate in declaring that "there was no gay community for black men to come home to in the 1980s," any prescription for the failure of solidarity had to include, along with white racism, the endemic homophobia that then characterized the straight black community. Some individuals on both sides (gay and black) of the equation were attempting in the 1980s to heal the division, but in Essex's view all that the AIDS crisis had succeeded in doing was to "clearly point out how significant are the cultural and economic differences between us. . . . We are communities engaged in a fragile coexistence if we are anything at all."

Photographer Robert Mapplethorpe was for Essex the iconic representation of the white gay community's lack of serious concern "with the existence of black gay men except as sexual objects." Mapplethorpe died of AIDS in 1989, while Essex was at work on the anthology, but that didn't stay his hand. He excoriated Mapplethorpe's catalogue *Black Males* as well as his 1986 *The Black Book* as centrally supportive of the stereotype of black men as headless, heartless creatures with monstrous phalluses. To Essex and others, Mapplethorpe's famous *Man in a Polyester Suit*, a photo that focused on a large, flaccid black penis dangling out of an unzipped trouser, reiterated the standard sexual fantasy of blaxploitation movies of the 1970s. "What is insulting and endangering to black men," Essex wrote, "is Mapplethorpe's *conscious* determination that the faces, the heads, and by extension, the minds and experiences of some of his black subjects are not as important as close-up shots of their cocks."

Essex wanted to make it clear that his critique of Mapplethorpe wasn't mistaken for prudery. "I don't have any problem with erotic art," he told one interviewer. "In fact, I think much of it, when rendered well, can be very beautiful and very moving. I think that Mapplethorpe was an excellent eye and an excellent talent. But again, that doesn't negate the question of why are the heads of some of his images missing? . . . *The Man in the Polyester Suit* . . . should have been called, *Black Dick in a Polyester Suit*, because that's essentially what it is. . . . Being on the outside and looking at that image, for me it just continues to perpetuate this whole notion that we are beasts." Essex refused explicitly to call for censorship; he had no wish to see Mapplethorpe's work banned from exhibition. What he did call for was an end to silence about calling "racist" representation by its name and exempting artistic work from political analysis. The reactions of some white gay men to his criticism of Mapplethorpe further confirmed his position; they "reacted as if what I had said," Essex wrote, "was sacrilegious. They also acted as if black men had no right to critique Mapplethorpe."

Underscoring Essex's opinion, the British filmmaker Isaac Julien (*Looking for Langston*) and the art history professor Kobena Mercer in the essay "True Confessions," which appeared in *Brother to Brother*, were no less denunciatory about "the exclusion of race from the gay agenda" and the objectification of the black subject in Mapplethorpe's racist "phantasms of desire." They acknowledged that the mythology of "black macho" was further maintained by sexist elements in the black community itself, which made the stereotype a more general site of struggle. A multipronged confrontation was necessary—against white gay racism, against sexism within both black and white male communities, and against the heterosexual black world's homophobia, as heightened by the current agenda of such revolutionary black nationalist leaders as Eldridge Cleaver. "Black nationalist sensibility," Essex wrote, "positions homosexuality as a major threat to the black family and black masculinity." No black gay man, Essex pointed out, "had openly participated in the 1960s Black Arts Movement"—and certainly not James Baldwin, who was never drawn to nationalism of any kind.

Though the nationalist sensibility had considerable support in certain black circles, Essex located his own yearning for "home" in the larger straight black world. "Our mothers and fathers are waiting for us," he wrote. "Our sisters and brothers are waiting. Our communities are waiting for us to come home. They need our love, our talents and skills, and we need theirs. . . . They will remain ignorant, misinformed, and lonely for us, and we for them, for as long as we stay away, hiding in communities that have never really welcomed us or the gifts we bring." In the late eighties, the expectation that the straight black world was "waiting for" its gay children to "come home" partook to some degree of wishful thinking. The Dorothy Beams of that world had opened their doors and put candles in the windows, but the pulpits of many black churches were still issuing thunderbolts against "perverts" and equating AIDS with "God's righteous wrath." For too many black gay people the choice was akin to the devil and the deep blue sea.

As a young man Essex had characterized black literature from the Harlem Renaissance of the 1920s through the protest era of the 1950s and 1960s as a period that "consistently ignored homosexuality except as something comic—or as a tragic example of white corruption of black manhood." After Essex came out, he began to recognize that "some of the finest writers in African-American literature were homo- or bisexual." Still, the Harlem Renaissance was a period where "your sexuality was tolerated at best, or overlooked or considered an aberration." Thus it was that W.E.B. Du Bois had objected to works like Claude McKay's homoerotic *Home to Harlem*, writing that he "distinctly felt he needed to take a bath" after reading the book.

Yet Essex felt that gay men of African descent had played a significant, if at times closeted or coded role in the Harlem Renaissance; such writers as Claude McKay, Alain Locke, Wallace Thurman, Countee Cullen, and Langston Hughes often wrote in sufficiently suggestive ways as to allow for subsequent "de-coding." Only Richard Bruce Nugent, whose short story "Smoke, Lilies and Jade" continues to be admired, was daringly upfront about same-sex desire. Essex was fascinated enough by the Harlem Renaissance writers of the 1920s that he drew up a seminar syllabus, "Evidence for Being," that he taught in the spring of 1991 at the Institute for Policy Studies in Washington, D.C., and he also did a series of readings and performances at the Rodde Center, People Like Us bookstore, and the Randolph Street Gallery. Post-Renaissance, Essex felt there wasn't enough black "gay" literature to allow for any claim to a "tradition."

But as Essex argued in the introduction he wrote to *Brother to Brother*, the 1980s had proved "a critically important decade" for the reemergence of same-gender desire in African American literature. Not only did a significant number of publications and journals appear—*Blacklight*, *Black/Out*, and in L.A. *BLK*, to name but a few—but as well the collective in New York City called "Other Countries" brought together a community of writers for workshops, readings, and eventually a journal. A number of black gay poets self-published their work—including Essex, Donald Woods, and Roy Gonsalves, who also founded a literary journal. This efflorescence of black gay writing produced some novels that "crossed over" to a mainstream audience; this was especially true of Randall Kenan and had already proven true for Samuel Delany.

The new flowering of black gay art was being consciously hailed as "a second black renaissance." The New Yorker David Frechette, the poet and cultural critic (and a founding member of the black gay collective Other Countries), headed one of his articles in 1989 "Renaissance for Black Gay Writers." In it, Frechette, who later became yet another AIDS casualty, singled out Essex as in the forefront of the new movement, giving special prominence to the choral poetry group's recent performance of his poem "Civil Servant" at the Kitchen. The long poem, now well known, describes the infamous Tuskegee experiment in Alabama, where for decades two hundred black men with syphilis were given, without their knowledge, placebos rather than medication so that government scientists could study the long-term effects of the disease when *not* treated.

"Civil Servant" chillingly focuses on the role of Nurse Eunice Rivers, a black woman who worked on the experiment:

> I could perform my job no other way:
> obey instructions or be dismissed,
> which would end my nursing career . . .
> I didn't talk back,
> raise my voice in protest,
> or demand the doctors save the men.
> It wasn't my place to diagnose,
> prescribe, or agitate . . .
> I never thought my duty
> damned the men.
> They were sick with bad blood,
> but I thought they were lucky.
> Most Colored folks in Macon
> > went from cradle to grave without ever visiting a
> > doctor . . .

As the men died, I wept
with their wives and families.
I was there to comfort them,
to offer fifty dollars
if they let the doctors
"operate"—
cut open the deceased
from scrotum sack to skull . . .
I never thought my silence
a symptom of bad blood.
I never considered my care complicity.
I was a Colored nurse, a proud
graduate of Tuskegee Institute,
one of few, honored by my profession.
I had orders, important duties,
a government career.

The performance of "Civil Servant" at the Kitchen was followed with Essex's "poetic manifesto, "To Some Supposed Brothers." Like Mike Callen, Essex was a confirmed feminist who deplored the dominant male sexism of the day:

You judge a woman
by what she can do for you alone
but there's no need
for slaves to have slaves . . .

But we so-called men,
we so-called brothers
wonder why it's so hard
to love *our* women
when we're about loving them
the way America
loves us.

Frechette ended his article by hailing the Hemphill event at the Kitchen as a significant marker of "a new renaissance," but Essex himself gave prime credit for the outburst of black creativity to black lesbians like Cheryl Clarke, Michelle Parkerson, and Jewelle Gomez for "breaking the silence surrounding their experiences." He also singled out two filmmakers for special praise: Isaac Julien (a member of the British film collective Sankofa) for *Looking for Langston* and the greatly gifted Marlon Riggs (who later died of AIDS) for the pivotal 1989 documentary *Tongues Untied*, in which Essex and his poetry would prominently appear.

While Essex was still at work on the anthology, Washington, D.C.'s mayor stopped the Tenant Assistance Program and sought as well a 38 percent cut in the annual AIDS budget—though the number of new AIDS cases in the United States had by then reached nearly 43,000 and the number of deaths 27,680. One of the newly deceased was the first black news anchor on network television, Max Robinson. Public discussion surrounding his death in December 1988 exemplified the attitudes current in the black community and informed much of the commentary in the anthology. How Robinson contracted AIDS remains to this day a subject of speculation, but mainstream African American discussions of the matter largely precluded same-gender sex—or, for that matter, intravenous drug use—as the cause.[15]

Robinson had expressed the hope that his death would become an occasion to educate blacks about AIDS, but neither the obituaries nor the statements that issued from black spokespeople allowed room for discussing the possibilities either of homosexuality or of drug addiction. Jesse Jackson, for one, spoke of Max Robinson as a family friend who'd confided his HIV status to the Jacksons, even while "reassuring" them that he'd been infected *not* from homosexuality but from heterosexual promiscuity. Yet Jackson failed even to suggest how rare it was for a man to contract AIDS from intercourse with a woman— even less likely if the "promiscuity" involved protected sex. Had Jackson—or someone—bothered to make those points, Robinson's dying wish that his passing would be used to educate other blacks about AIDS might have been met. Instead, disinformation was substituted—and AIDS continued to hit the black community hard. By 1989, 25 percent of all persons with AIDS in the United States were African American. Among those newly diagnosed, the figure jumped to 36 percent.

At its completion late in 1990, the manuscript for *Brother to Brother* ran to more than 550 pages; as a result of further cutting, it was reduced to

490 pages—with Essex having to inform five contributors that he'd had to pull their work. By December 1990, the manuscript of *Brother to Brother* was at the typesetters. Audre Lorde and Samuel Delaney both agreed to blurb the book, which was published in 1991. Essex hoped that *Brother to Brother* would both demonstrate and consolidate how much had been achieved in black gay literature, as well as inspire future accomplishments. His dearest wish was to end the emasculation of "not speaking out," of remaining mute in the name of preserving the possibility of "middle-class aspirations." He understood those aspirations as a hoped-for compensation for "the shame and cruelties of slavery and ghettos." But in his opinion it wouldn't work. "Whitewashing" the black experience would neither help the race nor impress "the racists, who don't give a damn."

To help promote the anthology, Essex traveled the country and also did a number of interviews on TV and radio. He felt the effort—a considerable challenge given the ups and downs of his health—was well worth it. Not only did the book sell well (it started out as number nine on national gay bookstore bestseller lists), but by extension, he felt, it could open up dialogue within the general African American community. During many of the engagements he undertook, Essex talked often and openly about what he called "the dysfunction" of the black intelligentsia, and in particular assimilationist black academics who kept their posts, he argued, by toeing the greater society's party line. "To my mind," he said during one interview, "they're no better than Jerry Falwell."

Essex also lambasted "other consciences of the black community," with Spike Lee a particular target: "He's been hostile to the black gay experience, and reinforces the homophobia found in the black community." Essex singled out Lee's film *Jungle Fever* and the scene in which a group of black women complain that black men are either addicts, or in jail, or homosexual. It was a bracketing Essex detested: "I'm just sick of being lumped in with those categories!" "All of what his films have done," Essex added, "is breed more factionalism." Which made Essex all the more grateful, he said, for younger black filmmakers like Michelle Parkerson, Isaac Julien, and Marlon Riggs: "There's a sincere hope there that dialogue from the marginalized and disempowered will be handled by people who don't have a commercial interest but a humanistic one."

But as one reviewer of *Brother to Brother* put it, currently black gay men "have historically occupied the untenable position of being part of two communities and fully acceptable to neither." As if in confirmation of that view, the one "white" review I was able to find—in *Publishers Weekly*—was largely negative, characterizing the anthology as "offerings of dubious literary merit." Black reviewers were mostly more appreciative. The writer Don Belton, for example, proclaimed *Brother to Brother* "every bit as fine a work as its predecessor, and it brings up to date much of the dialogue begun by the earlier collection."[16]

But there were dissents. When the black gay writer Donald Suggs reviewed *Brother to Brother* in the *Village Voice* (October 1, 1991), he offered an unusual criticism of the section on AIDS: "I needed to know less about how these men experienced AIDS in their daily lives and more about the ways in which their own responses to AIDS were shaped by the attitudes of those around them. Even Black PWAs who can afford health care suffer the poverty of the Black community's resources in dealing with AIDS." Suggs did praise Essex's "outstanding selection of poetry" but further objected to his choice of "a cheerleading quote" from Joe Beam as a preface to the anthology, namely, "Black men loving black men is a call to action, an acknowledgement of responsibility." Suggs thought that Charles Harpe, another contributor to the anthology, "better identifies the root of our creativity, both as writers and as black gay men. It is, he [Harpe] says, the 'beginning of [the] feeling that the word *faggot* did not accurately name the man I was or the man I was aspiring to become.'"

In a comparable vein, the *New Republic* review raised the question of "whether we can have a gay literature that is not merely about its own gayness, but is true to the variety of ways in which gays relate to each other and to the world." The reviewer apparently preferred gay writers like Samuel Delany, Michael Nava, and Joe Keenan, who placed gay characters in settings where homosexuality was "simply taken for granted" and the characters were shown "exploring worlds, solving murders, getting laughs" that required their authors to employ "the advantages of indirection" in discussing sexuality. But for many readers of *Brother to Brother*, the subtle virtues of "indirection" paled, became something of a literary luxury, when placed in the context of a community devastated by AIDS and desperate for succor.

The section in *Brother to Brother* devoted entirely to AIDS was given the overall title "Hold Tight Gently." Its searing content consisted of seven poems and seven prose pieces. One of the longer essays, by Walter Rico Burrell, a journalist with a master's degree from UCLA, consisted of excerpts from his AIDS diary. Burrell had submitted the piece by mail and when Essex initially read it he wasn't prepared for the scorching honesty of the diary entries—and burst into tears. He called Burrell on the phone and their shared pain reduced them both to crying. In the excerpts, Burrell revealed that he'd decided to give AZT a try, but when he took the doctor's prescription, along with his Blue Shield medical insurance card, to a pharmacist, it was handed right back to him; "this prescription," he was told, "is going to cost more than two hundred dollars and we aren't allowed to make any third-party transactions on a sum that large."

"Jesus!" Burrell wrote in his diary, "I was going to have to fight to get the very medicine I needed to hold the disease at bay. I immediately thought of all those street people, poor people, people who didn't have the resources I had, the job I had, the insurance I had. Christ! What would happen to them? Were they doomed to death simply because they're not middle-class enough to afford to fight AIDS?" The answer was yes, though some state and federal subsidy programs would subsequently kick in. The answer is still yes for many in the United States and also for the millions afflicted in developing countries.

When the anthology was published, Essex sent a copy of the book to Burrell. It was returned—marked "deceased." Burrell had died of AIDS—as would nearly all of the fourteen authors represented in that part of the book.

The AIDS section of the anthology also included a piece by Assotto Saint—who worked in an office where co-workers would wipe the phones with alcohol after he used them—about the death of his long-term lover. The account began with his lover developing a small spot on his right foot, "purple with the stain of a crushed grape." Soon after, the spot "multiplied like buds on a tree in early spring. It multiplied all over his feet, his legs, up his ass, inside his intestines, all over his face, his neck, down his throat, inside his brains. For nine months of fever and wracking coughs, nine months of sweat and shaking chills, nine months of diarrhea and jerking spasms, it multiplied, and wrenched him skinny like a spider." And all through it, Assotto held him when he "gagged, choked, and vomited," helped him sit up and cough, "changed his diapers, washed him, massaged his back, smoothed the bed sheets, caressed him until he'd fall asleep, then awaken from a nightmare struggling for air." When the doctor said he was near death, Assotto called his lover's mother. She arrived cursing, "huffing and puffing, waving her righteous finger" in Assotto's face, telling him "You done perverted my son, you low-down immoral—" Interrupting, Assotto sat her down hard and told her he didn't give a damn about getting her blessing. He was thoroughly tired of the heterosexual version of caring.

The poem "Hope Against Hope," by Craig G. Harris (who died of AIDS in November 1991 at age thirty-two), in *Brother to Brother* exemplified one gay version of caring:

> he swore no virus would beat him
> armed with rose quartz
> and amethyst, homeopathic remedies,
> Louise Hay tapes
> and the best doctors
> at San Francisco General
> he fought it
> like a copperhead going
> against a mongoose
>
> when he lost
> we all wore purple,
> tucked him in white satin
> with his crystal shields,
> and thought of Icarus
> soaring toward the sun . . .

Though Essex felt that "home" for black gays was far more likely to be found in the black community as a whole than in the white gay one, *Brother to Brother* contained a number of strong pieces that showed his open-eyed awareness that many leading black intellectuals and academicians continued to denounce homosexuality. He printed parts of a 1989 interview that he'd done with Isaac Julien, which detailed how the Langston Hughes estate had "disrupted the original version" of Julien's film *Looking for Langston* by forcing the deletion of several of Hughes' more homoerotic poems. The estate's reaction to Julien's decision to "take a black cultural icon and basically undress him" was, in Essex's view, "based on the black middle class's belief that it's important to project the *right* image." It was part and parcel, he felt, of "the manifest determination of major black publications such as *Jet, Ebony, Ebony Man, Black Scholar, Emerge, Callaloo*, and many other black periodicals and journals" to perpetuate "the lack of visibility and forthright discussion of gays and lesbians."

That line of argument was continued in *Brother to Brother* in Ron Simmons' interview with the black filmmaker Marlon Riggs. (His award-winning *Ethnic Notions* was soon followed by the stunning and controversial *Tongues Untied*.) Simmons, a good friend of Essex's, pointed out in the interview that homosexuality had "been ridiculed and spoken of with absolute scorn by some of our most brilliant writers, scholars, and leaders—Amiri Baraka, Haki Madhubuti, Nathan Hare, Robert Staples, Molefi Asante and Minister Louis Farrakhan—most of whom view homosexuality as one more pathology resulting from white racist oppression." To that list one can easily append additional names: Frantz Fanon, the psychiatrist Alvin Poussaint, and Eldridge Cleaver.[17]

Essex himself would devote an entire essay (in his collection *Ceremonies*) to Dr. Frances Cress Welsing, one of the lesser-known, yet influential, advocates of the "homosexuality as pathology" theory. At a 1987 London conference on AIDS, Welsing had declared that the U.S. government had deliberately created HIV in order to rid the nation of undesirable blacks. She had also written several attention-grabbing articles that in 1990 were collected in her book *The Isis Papers*, which enjoyed considerable prestige among black cultural nationalists. Essex found Welsing's views more dangerous than those of better-known figures because she grounded her homophobia in African American history, explaining it "as evidence of Black Males *adapting* to oppression." But not everything, Essex insisted, can be ascribed to racism. Homosexuality, he declared, was a *natural* variant; nature, not white racism, had created sexual diversity. Anthropological studies would later conclusively show that homosexuality was an indigenous phenomenon in certain African cultures.

In her book, Welsing also advocated the traditional patriarchal family structure—dominant male, submissive female—and this further offended Essex's feminist perspective. Her views, in his opinion, widened "the existing breach between Black gays and lesbians and their heterosexual counterparts, offering no bridges for joining our differences." Instead of fostering an appreciation of diversity, Welsing offered a brand of heterosexism that, in Essex's opinion, would continue to fracture and disable the black community.

In the Simmons interview in *Brother to Brother*, Marlon Riggs struck a note that was soon to become a mantra ("intersectionality") of queer theory and can also be read as moving in a somewhat different direction from Essex in regard to race. "The way to break loose of the schizophrenia in trying to define identity," Riggs said, "is to realize that you are many things within one person. Don't try to arrange a hierarchy of things that are virtuous in your character and say, 'This is more important than that.' Realize that both are equally important; they both inform your character. Both are nurturing and nourishing of your spirit. You can embrace all of that lovingly and equally."

In a powerful essay of his own ("Black Macho Revisited: Reflections of a Snap! Queen") in *Brother to Brother*, Riggs expressed his belief that at the heart of black America's "pervasive cultural homophobia is the desperate need for a convenient Other *within* the community, yet not truly *of* the community, an Other to which blame for the chronic identity crises afflicting the black male psyche can be readily displaced." For black men struggling with discrimination and ostracism, poverty and powerlessness, self-doubt and self-disgust, the "faggot," Riggs suggests, is an *essential* Other, a despised Other not to be helped even during as desperate a trial as AIDS.

"Because of my sexuality," Riggs wrote, "I cannot be Black. A strong, proud, 'Afrocentric' Black man is resolutely heterosexual, not *even* bisexual. Hence I remain a Negro." "Contemporary proponents of Black macho," Riggs added, converge with white supremacists "in their cultural practice, deploying similar devices towards similarly dehumanizing ends." He offered the comedy routines of Eddie Murphy as an example. Murphy unites "Negro Faggotry, 'Herpes Simplex 10'—and AIDS—into an indivisible modern icon of sexual terrorism. Rap artists and music videos resonate with this same perception, fomenting a social psychology that blames the *victim* for his degradation and death." Riggs, like Essex, rejected an essentialist vision of race, including the nationalist version that argued a historical (before the arrival of whites) narrative featuring strong, noble African men. "And women—were women. Nobody was lesbian. Nobody was feminist. Nobody was gay."

Essex wrote Barbara Smith that despite all the hard work and travel on behalf of *Brother to Brother*, his health was "good and stable" and he'd put on eight pounds. He added that in the coming year he'd have to make more money somehow or "find myself returning to the work environment." In a separate letter co-signed by Dorothy Beam, the pair warmly thanked Barbara for her multiple efforts on the book's behalf: "The historical moment will show that concerned individuals such as yourself and others were there in the way communities are supposed to be there for one another."

6

Drugs into Bodies

The situation for black gay men and lesbians wasn't notably differ-ent in New York City than in Washington, D.C. Black and His-panic elected officials offered little leadership on the issue of AIDS, and although three new organizations—the Hispanic AIDS Forum, the Minority Task Force, and the Association for the Prevention and Treatment of Drug Abuse—had been formed in the eighties, none had gotten widespread community support or sufficient funding. The established media were also of little help. On the first page of its Met-ropolitan section, the *New York Times* published an article ("Homo-sexuals Detect New Signs of Friendliness Amid Bias") in the late eighties that failed to make a single reference to the situation of black lesbians and gay men, thereby reinforcing the long-standing invisibility of both. For good measure, the *Times* mentioned that antigay violence had been decreasing (i.e., "New Signs of Friendliness")—a claim the New York Gay and Lesbian Anti-Violence Project directly contra-dicted with figures that proved an *increase* in violence.[1]

Nor did the *Times* bother to mention the numerous antigay com-ments increasingly emanating from the city's white male leadership. In that regard, his eminence Cardinal O'Connor had long led the pack, denouncing homosexuality, as early as 1983, as "sinful and unnatural." He thereafter regularly reaffirmed the Roman Catholic Church's insistence that same-gender love and lust were iniquitous. (Other churches, it should be added—and especially the Unitarians and Episcopalians—were more benevolent.) When for a short time (before reversing itself) the National Conference of Catholic Bishops decided to allow condom use for the limited purpose of avoiding HIV, Cardinal O'Connor thunderously opposed the decision and helped to overturn it, even as he continued to denounce any form of safe-sex education. For him, the solution to the crisis was simple: *abstinence*. Though students in high schools went right on having sex and using drugs, O'Connor, denying reality, insisted on withholding from them the information and tools that might save their lives.[2]

New York City mayor Ed Koch, a great friend of the Cardinal's (they even published a book together, *His Eminence and Hizzoner*), did declare a "state of concern" about AIDS, but the mayor's "concern" wasn't great enough to warrant significant outlays of money to help fund education, treatment, or housing for homeless people with AIDS. When a candlelight vigil and a demonstration of protest both failed to budge the mayor, a group of angry GLAAD members formed the Lavender Hill Mob to stage "zaps" designed to disturb Koch's equanimity. But Koch was nothing if not stubborn. Even after it became clear by the late eighties that drug addicts in the city had high rates of HIV infection due to shared needles, Koch refused—in direct opposition to the recommendations of his health commissioner, David Axelrod—to allow needle exchange.

When I spoke at the unveiling of Stonewall Place in Sheridan Square in June 1989, Koch was the other speaker. Preceding me, he read the official proclamation aloud. Even though I was standing next to him I was unable to hear a word he said—thanks to the large crowd of some five hundred intense young demonstrators shouting their disgust at his complacency and jabbing the sky with their "Koch Is Killing Us!" signs in the shape of tombstones. Hizzoner's smug, fixed grin never left his face, but he was smart enough to leave the platform the moment he finished reading the proclamation. I then extemporized my own opening line—"I take no pleasure in sharing a platform with Ed Koch"—to gratifyingly clamorous applause.[3]

I assumed the crowd—young, intense, engaged—consisted mostly of ACT UP members. Certainly they'd pilloried Koch before, and would again; he, in turn, referred to them publicly as "fascists." Fascists they were not. But they were, by design, tactically neither respectful nor "respectable"—to the disgust of the more conservative members of the gay community. ACT UP was designed to replace normative channels for change (electioneering, lobbying, petitioning) with disruptive, direct-action street demonstrations commensurate with mounting gay desperation at the ever-climbing number of AIDS cases and the deaths of many young people in their prime. As ACT UP's ranks swelled in the late eighties, it carried out a series of public protests that galvanized the media, gave hope to those with AIDS, and roused the retaliatory scorn of the stand-patters. And it did so with theatrical panache. It plastered the city with provocative posters and daringly designed materials from one of the dozen or so ACT UP affinity groups, Gran Fury, a bunch of professional artists who volunteered their services (they even managed to sneak their famous parody of the *New York Times*—which they called *New York Crimes*—into hundreds of newspaper vending machines).[4]

No direct-action event better exemplified ACT UP's growing impact than its 1988 demonstration in front of the Food and Drug Administration (FDA) in suburban Washington, D.C. The demonstrators had prepared well. ACT UP's Treatment and Data Committee had prepared a forty-page pamphlet, *FDA Action Handbook*, and had also held a series of teach-ins to guarantee that the demonstrators were well informed about current research issues. A savvy media campaign also preceded the action, ensuring that it would be well covered. The action itself centered on well-thought-out demands, primarily that the drug-approval process be shortened, that the "unethical" practice of double-blind placebo trials be ended, that people "from all affected populations at all stages of HIV infection" be henceforth included in clinical trials, and that Medicaid and private health insurance companies "be made to pay for experimental drug therapies."[5]

The civil disobedience action at FDA headquarters was determined, prolonged, and raucous. A variety of costumes, props, T-shirts, and posters was employed—"We Die, They Do Nothing"; "The Government Has Blood on Its Hands"; "One AIDS Death Every Half Hour." The D.C. police, wearing masks, rubber gloves, and riot gear, some on horseback, reacted with brutality and arrested nearly two hundred of the activists. But much of the police action was captured on film and aired on the TV news that night, which ensured the message would be heard. In the year following the demonstration, officials at the FDA and the NIH began to include activists in their deliberations, and double-blind placebo trials were replaced by ACT UP's suggestion of parallel tracks, whereby different doses of the same drug were given to all participants.

All that was to the good. But certain stark facts remained true: there was still no reliable treatment for AIDS, let alone a cure; no one was willing to predict when efficacious drugs might emerge from a seemingly empty pipeline; no one was quite sure which sexual activities, if any, were truly "safe." Did kissing, fellatio, and cunnilingus qualify? What about condoms? Were they usually safe or did they tear or leak with some regularity? Were some condoms better than others in providing protection? Was it true that the partner on "top" during anal sex was much safer than the "bottom"—and if so, just how much safer? It's no wonder that in unknown numbers, some gay men were choosing celibacy or monogamy, though often neither suited their temperaments or their sense of what "gay liberation" actually meant.

Consuming worry over such questions seemed to the gay writer Darrell Yates Rist obsessional. To the astonishment of many—since Rist was himself HIV-positive—he published an article in *The Nation* early in 1989 denouncing ACT UP, and by implication all AIDS activism, as "fashionable hysteria" and, further, theorized that such "keening" reflected a "compulsive . . . need to partake in the drama of catastrophe" (apparently akin, in his mind, to the gay male worship of diva tragedians like Judy Garland). Rist's article struck many as a shockingly misguided piece of invective. I was one of those who responded in *The Nation*, writing that "the legions of the young in ACT UP who've stationed themselves on the front lines deserve something better than being characterized [as Rist had] as 'clones' and 'chic street protesters.'" Rist had further denounced the ACT UP demonstrators as "immoral because they are panic-mongering"—which was tantamount to saying that no one need fear dying of AIDS, that profound fear ("panic") was illegitimate. Nor did Rist even once in his article implicate governmental apathy or the straight world's general indifference as causal factors that had *necessitated* the formation of ACT UP and its nervily audacious actions.[6]

Rist and those who thought like him were unable to stop or slow ACT UP/New York's momentum. Its dramatic series of protests continued: demonstrations on Wall Street, at Trinity Church, and in Grand Central Station; an action against the Burroughs Wellcome drug company that led to a reduction in the cost of AZT; a four-day-long picketing of Sloan-Kettering Cancer Center; several angry zaps of Mayor Koch—and a host of others. All were theatrical, imaginative, shocking to many (including conservative gay men), and usually consequential. For sheer drama, as well as subsequent wrath, none exceeded the demonstration (co-sponsored with WHAM!—the feminist Women's Health Action Mobilization)—at St. Patrick's Cathedral in December 1989. That action would mark a critical divide in the organization's history and produce an outraged response from both the general public and a considerable segment of the gay community.

Certainly St. Patrick's, in the person of its representative figure, John Cardinal O'Connor, had, through its poisonous denunciations, more than earned the enmity of gay activists. From a free speech perspective, O'Connor had every right to deplore safe-sex education, clean needles, condom use, and abortion. But his ignorance-is-bliss campaigns of disinformation literally threatened the lives of many New Yorkers, including members of his sexually active parish. O'Connor also vigorously opposed the repeal of antigay discriminatory laws, was vehemently antichoice, and successfully urged the National Conference of Catholic Bishops to oppose all needle exchange programs. "The truth is not in condoms or clean needles," O'Connor claimed. "These are lies—lies perpetuated often for political reasons on the part of public health officials."[7]

O'Connor even outdid his predecessors when he banned the gay Catholic group Dignity from holding meetings in any Catholic church. When members of the group held silent protests against the ban in St. Patrick's, O'Connor got an injunction to clear them out. Further, he actively supported the activities of Operation Rescue in its terrorist campaign against abortion and family planning clinics. His position ran directly counter to ACT UP's prochoice stance, along with its struggle to end the policy of women being routinely excluded from AIDS trials because of their "reproductive capacities"—that is, the potential damage to fetuses. When the Supreme Court in 1989 issued its *Webster v. Reproductive Health Services* opinion, which gave the states more power to restrict access to abortion, WHAM! and ACT UP joined forces in demonstrations to "Stop the Church."

The special venom of O'Connor's invective against gay people made life still more difficult for them, more filled with the guilt and shame that socially induced homophobia had already bred into them. O'Connor's voluble hatred and distortions of the truth ran counter to a true Christian's allegiance to love and to alleviate suffering. He'd hurled down the thunderbolts of "sin" and "sickness" for so long and with such vehemence that it was all but inevitable that the time would come when they'd be hurled back.

On December 10, 1989, a dozen or so members of ACT UP/New York scattered in the pews of St. Patrick's, while about a thousand demonstrated outside the cathedral. When the signal was given in the midst of the cardinal's sermon, various ACT UP members threw their bodies into the aisles in a "die-in" act of civil disobedience and hurled condoms into the air, while others chained themselves to the pews and shouted "Your works are killing us!" at O'Connor. One former altar boy deliberately dropped a consecrated communion wafer on the floor— thereby giving the "pious" press a focal point for howling denunciations of so "sacrilegious" an act. Mayor Koch, Mayor-elect David Dinkins, and New York Governor Mario Cuomo all deplored the scandalous excess of invading "sacred" space. The police dragged the protesters into the street and arrested more than one hundred of them (the few who'd been inside the church, plus many outside). Within gay circles, a number of leading spokespeople, including journalists Randy Shilts and Andrew Sullivan, deplored ACT UP's "adolescent" tactics as "discrediting" the community. "Good gays," apparently, did not engage in militantly confrontational behavior—that was reserved for cardinals and mayors.

There was dissent within ACT UP/New York itself about the St. Patrick's action, and the division involved more material issues than the fate of a communion wafer. In her brilliant book *Moving Politics*, Deborah Gould pinpoints a rift over priorities within the membership ranks of ACT UP that would grow over time. Some members insisted that ACT UP's prime goal of speeding up medical research and getting more "drugs into bodies" should remain its singular focus. Others remained committed to the more expansive social agenda of combating sexism, racism, and classism within ACT UP itself and in the culture at large. The tension between the two positions would lead ACT UP/San Francisco to split into two organizations: ACT UP/

Golden Gate, focused on research, and ACT UP/San Francisco, concentrated on broad social change. Two years later, ACT UP/New York would see a comparable split when its Treatment and Data Committee (all white, all male, except for one woman, Garance Franke-Ruta) would split off into a separate entity, the Treatment Action Group (TAG).[8]

A significant number of those who joined ACT UP/New York had never been politically involved in the gay movement during the seventies—and in some cases (like Larry Kramer) had derided it. ACT UP would throughout its history remain predominantly white and male, but several of the lesbians who joined its ranks—preeminently Jean Carlomusto, Maria Maggenti, Liz Tracy, Sarah Schulman, Heidi Dorow, Ann Northrop, Terry McGovern, and Maxine Wolfe—brought with them considerable experience and savvy from having worked in other progressive movements, including the feminist one. Of the various committees that formed within ACT UP by the late eighties, the Women's Caucus (mostly white at first, but subsequently with some influx of HIV-positive women of color), the Housing Committee, and the Majority Action Committee paid particular attention to issues relating to sexism and racism. The Women's Caucus successfully pushed for a CDC redefinition of AIDS to incorporate the fact that for women full-blown AIDS manifested not as KS but as bacterial pneumonia, pelvic inflammatory disease, and cervical cancer.

Maxine Wolfe was perhaps the most vocal of these women. She challenged, often accurately, the political perspective of many male members of ACT UP. "I had assumed," she argued at one point, that ACT UP "was a lesbian-and gay identified group, but people didn't want to be called lesbian and gay activists; they wanted to be called 'AIDS activists.' And they seemed to believe in the health-care system, even if it had gone awry. They even respected doctors!" But if Wolfe didn't think ACT UP was politically "the be-all and end-all," she remained active in its ranks because she saw "people *develop* a political perspective," saw "men who wanted to hide being gay behind their AIDS activism" do a teach-in on lesbian and gay history, saw more and more members "develop a gay-liberation and not a gay-rights perspective." She believed that over time ACT UP's agenda gradually expanded and more and more young people came "to understand that what we want is the right to exist—not the right to privacy; the right to a life, not to a lifestyle; and a life that is as important as anyone else's, but not more important than anyone else's."

The Housing Committee, the Majority Action Committee, and the Women's Caucus tended to draw ACT UP's most politically radical members, those who believed that issues like universal health care and decent housing were inextricably bound up with the effort to push for faster, more accessible drug research. The divisions within ACT UP weren't always clear-cut; some activists whose focus was primarily treatment issues—Jim Eigo, for one—also worked hard for a more expansive activist agenda.[9]

If you were living at or below the poverty line, couldn't afford to pay rent or see a doctor, or were an IV drug user, the development of more effective treatments was likely to be beyond your means in any case. This lack of resources may help to account for the willingness of some of the poor to believe in the miracle cure of Kemron (which consisted of a small amount of alpha interferon), announced at a press conference held in Nairobi early in 1990. Scientists who'd been experimenting with interferon dismissed the new drug as worthless in countering AIDS, but when the president of Kenya, Daniel arap Moi, praised it at a press conference as the long-awaited cure, interest in the African American press soared. The PWA Health Group, among other buyer clubs, jumped on the bandwagon and began hyping Kemron. The *Amsterdam News* accused white scientists and activists of downplaying the drug's importance because it had originated in Africa. Kemron continued to have a following in the black neighborhoods of New York, L.A., Philadelphia, and Washington, D.C.—that is, until additional studies failed to duplicate the original results, and Health and Human Services Secretary Louis Sullivan, himself an African American doctor, publicly concluded that Kemron was worthless.

Other issues relating to race came to loom large in the tensions that developed within ACT UP. In New York, Allan Robinson, one of several black gay members of ACT UP, was scornful of the dominant white male sense of entitlement: "They were goddamned angry. They were angry because they thought they had everything—trips to Brazil and Fire Island, hanging in the clubs, boyfriends, drugs, money, and living perhaps on Eighty-First Street and Central Park West. They were angry because they were being treated like everybody else." The prominent Latino activist Moisés Agosto ultimately became disillusioned with ACT UP over race and class issues: "The majority of people I looked up to [in the Treatment and Data Committee] . . . were not really that much into doing work related to access to care and treatment for disenfranchised communities." In 1992 Agosto shifted his energy to working with the National Latino Lesbian and Gay Organization.[10]

Members of the Majority Action Committee (MAC) were well aware that people of color were afflicted with AIDS out of all proportion to their numbers, not only in the United States but globally. In April 1989, only 9 percent of the participants in New York City's AIDS program trials were black, though they accounted for 33 percent of the city's AIDS cases; it hardly made sense to speak of blacks as members of a minority, even if that *was* true of their status within ACT UP. Jim Eigo, one of the more influential white members of ACT UP, spoke for the radical contingent in general when he argued that ACT UP should engage in a demand for universal health care. Members of the Housing and Majority Action Committees also put particular emphasis on meeting the needs of people of color and ending minority invisibility. They visited various black churches in order to promote ACT UP's work, to provide information, and to broaden awareness of the widespread suffering that AIDS had wrought in communities of color. MAC members profited from the prior activity of San Francisco's Third World AIDS Advisory Task Force, which as early as 1985 had pushed an agenda that foregrounded the enormity of the needs of people of color afflicted with AIDS, who often lay beyond the outreach of AIDS organizations. The San Francisco group had not only produced a brochure specially designed for people of color, but in 1986 had succeeded in holding the first Western Regional Conference on AIDS and Ethnic Minorities.

New York City's MAC never fully matched that achievement, but it did come to understand and emphasize that a number of blacks and Hispanics had become infected as a result of IV drug use—and understood, too, that strong resistance would greet any attempt to establish a clean needle program; many black as well as white leaders denounced such a notion as sanctioning the spread of drug use. The members of MAC also came to realize that many minority members who'd contracted AIDS through same-gender sex didn't necessarily, or even often, self-identify as gay—it was the difference between behavior and identity: one did not automatically adopt a gay identity simply because one had had sex, occasionally or often, with members of one's own gender. MAC and ACT UP/New York in general made enough strides in sensitizing themselves to the needs of people of color to lead conservative gay writer Randy Shilts, in a January 1991 cover story for *The Advocate*, to make the astounding claim that ACT UP's "growing irrelevance" was primarily due to the fact that it currently seemed more concerned with poor blacks and Hispanics than with gay white men.[11]

That assessment would have stunned many minority members of ACT UP. While it was true that from the beginning ACT UP/New York had formally declared that AIDS "disproportionately affects men and women of color," the acknowledgment had to some extent been pro forma. Mike Callen, for one, felt "there was a huge gap between ACT UP rhetoric and behavior." Those ACT UP members who insisted on focusing their time and energy on pushing for faster research and better drugs tended to be the more privileged members—highly educated, middle-class white men. Those who chose instead to concentrate on issues relating to race and gender populated the organization but did not control its direction. In Mike's view, ACT UP's preferred description of itself as "multicultural, diverse, and democratic to a fault" was overstated. Perhaps unfairly, he felt ACT UP was essentially "a very hierarchical boys group," and the leading "boys" had been raised to have "arrogant certainties." If Mike was guilty of undercrediting the impact of the Housing, MAC, and Women's committees in ACT UP, he never doubted that its direct-action tactics helped to awaken the nation to the plight of those suffering from AIDS.

Fighting the scientific, governmental, and pharmaceutical establishments through confrontational activism did remain ACT UP's number one priority, especially during the first four or so years of its existence. The starkest contrast within ACT UP involved the opposing priorities of the Treatment and Data (T&D) Committee and those of MAC (as well as most of the Women's Caucus). T&D focused on getting "drugs into bodies," MAC on getting minority, female, economically disadvantaged bodies access to health care—and then taking on additional institutional inequalities. For some, the whole business of ranking oppressions was offensive, especially since the mounting conservative tide in the country as a whole lumped them all together as an unsavory collectivity, a distasteful Other.

But thanks to the ACT UP demonstrations, the country's conservatives could no longer ignore the tremendous toll that AIDS was taking, nor continue to assume that gay people were a tiny, cowering minority. Media coverage of ACT UP demonstrations was considerable, and the images many Americans saw on television or in their newspapers contradicted the long-standing stereotypes of frightened sissies and their roughneck sisters. By 1990, there were fifty openly gay elected officials around the country (compared with half a dozen in 1980), and the Human Rights Campaign, a national gay lobbying group, ranked twenty-fifth on the list of the country's most powerful fund-raising organizations. In 1987, only one-third of adults believed that homosexual relations between consenting adults should be legal. By 1989, a Gallup poll revealed that the figure had jumped to 47 percent.

It would be a mistake to draw too rosy a picture. Draconian sodomy laws still remained on the books in twenty-four states, and the legislatures of only two states—Wisconsin and Massachusetts—had passed laws barring discrimination against gay people (and only seven U.S. cities had as yet put "domestic partnership," which granted gay people some of the same rights as married couples, on the books). Additionally, gay people were seven times more likely to become victims of violent assault than other Americans; for trans people, the numbers were still higher. It would only be with the brutal murder of Matthew Shepard in 1998 that the American Psychoanalytic Association would hold its very first forum on homophobia (there had been countless ones through the years on the "causes" and "cures" of homosexuality).

Yet the softening of homophobia was real. In a culture with a profoundly contradictory heritage of conformity and innovation, the way forward would necessarily be gradual (though only if the demands were for full and instant change; you ask for the whole pie in order to get a slice of it) and would periodically be marked by retreats. Yet nowhere else in the world was there a comparably vibrant and effective gay rights movement. In the 1970s, when the first gay civil rights measures were submitted to public referendum, only 29 percent of the voters reacted to them favorably; by the early nineties, the percentage had risen to 39 percent—and would continue to climb.

Had ACT UP been more centrally concerned with feminism, poverty, and racism, both Mike Callen and Essex Hemphill might have been tempted to join. But Essex was probably too disaffected ("The absence of willful change / And strategic coalitions . . . will not . . . save us") to participate in any white-dominated organization. And Mike, as editor of *Newsline* and president of CRI, already had his hands full, even as he tried to somehow fit in music making and the maintenance of his own health. He admired ACT UP's many achievements but had his doubts about its attitude of "damn the FDA and full speed ahead: drugs into bodies." He wasn't interested in CRI "undertaking ANY trial which, from the outset, it believes will not contribute to FDA approval and therefore the wider availability of promising therapies." CRI, like ACT UP, was centrally concerned with trying to find effective drug therapies but felt that could best be achieved through community-based trials, not confrontational street actions. In this regard, the radical-minded Mike was tactically to the right of ACT UP—but not consistently so, since he'd been involved in any number of demonstrations and had several times been arrested. He was also a more committed feminist and more racially conscious than many of the white men in ACT UP.[12]

By 1989, CRI was having internal troubles of its own. Critics charged the organization, and Sonnabend especially, with failing to write up the results of some of its trials, and in particular those involving Antabuse, lentinan, and the egg lipid, AL-721. Some of the criticism of CRI was more broadly gauged—and more hurtful. At the start of the year, Lou Grant, a quiet, unassuming African American board member, unexpectedly issued an "open letter" that produced a shock wave in the organization. Prior to the letter, Mike had made several efforts by phone and in person to allay Grant's apprehensions about CRI's direction. In response, Grant had told Mike that his work had been "extraordinarily important . . . in many ways I owe you my life." Yet in his open letter Grant now called Mike "a self-appointed leader/ hero . . . an AIDS pimp . . . [who didn't] respect the members of the board" and had misappropriated funds that NIAID had awarded for minority outreach.

Grant's accusations were unfounded, but that didn't prevent them from deeply wounding Mike. If Grant had been his only critic, he might have sloughed off the charges as the drivel they were. But he'd been in an on-again, off-again struggle with some of the individuals and policies of GMHC and ACT UP as well. Mike fully acknowledged that both organizations "did very good, important work," but he felt that GMHC particularly was based on hierarchical, patriarchal organizational models of which he disapproved. It was different with ACT UP. Many of its members would have self-described as anarchists— that is, anti-authority, and especially the authority of church and state— but Mike felt that everybody in ACT UP "knew that there was an elite—that nothing could get passed without [the approval of] the T&D (Treatment and Data), the Mark Harringtons and the Peter Staleys" (probably the T&D's two best-known members).

Considerable deference toward members of T&D did exist within ACT UP, though some excused it as the result of the hard work its members had invested in mastering the science relating to AIDS, and the respect that mastery had earned among professional researchers. At the same time, the occasional arrogance and condescension with which some T&D members treated other members of ACT UP with less knowledge and less access to the powers that be also played a role in creating resentment against them. But at no time, contrary to Mike's indictment, did the T&D Committee fully control ACT UP's agenda or dictate its policies.

Mike's overemphatic criticism of T&D had long been fueled by its periodic patronization of both Sonnabend the individual and CRI the organization. In Mike's view, "ANY serious critique of the problems of basic AIDS science inevitably spring from Joe's views and his writings"—for example, his 1988 article "Fact and Speculation." Mike felt that Sonnabend's work had been cannibalized without proper attribution—that he was often condescended to as a mere clinician, as someone not involved in basic research.

Mike also felt that ACT UP played a central role in trying to destroy CRI's credibility. It had, for example, criticized CRI as "racially and sexually biased," whereas in fact by 1989–90 it had enrolled more women and people of color than all AIDS Clinical Trials Group (government testing) sites in Manhattan combined. When advised, moreover, that CRI would do well to have a prominent member of ACT

UP serve on its board, Mike "sniffed around and found out who the most famous, most respected ACT UP member was" and "manipulated" to get him—Mike never publicly named him—on the CRI board. So what happened? According to Mike the new member "came late to every meeting and left early. He abstained from every vote." What he *did* do was arrive at one meeting "with a 10-page letter from ACT UP reaming CRI for this failure and that failure." When he started to read the letter aloud at a board meeting, Mike stood up and stopped him cold: "No, I will not have this. Not after three years of blood and guts. Not after what I did to get you on this board!"

As Mike himself said, "AIDS activism can be a brutal business. . . . We have not learned how to disagree without being disagreeable to each other. . . . Anger cannot sustain activism over time." He decided that for at least the time being, he'd had enough of the accumulated accusations and stepped down as CRI's president. He freely acknowledged that "very real failings," and in particular his own energetic perfectionism, warranted criticism—but not Lou Grant's "venomous, mean-spirited" ones, nor what he saw as ACT UP's spurious ones. It might have helped Mike to know that internecine conflict, sometimes bordering on warfare, has characterized almost all movements and organizations designed to produce social change. At one low point, as founder and director of the Center for Lesbian and Gay Studies (CLAGS), I remember sharing my hurt feelings with Tim Sweeney, who's headed several major LGBT organizations. Tim had come by to talk about the "leadership project" he'd taken on for the Rapoport Foundation. We bounced war stories off of each other, sharing the puzzlement and pain that (so Tim reported) every director of every LGBT organization feels—where mistakes become cosmic crimes and no good deed goes unpunished.

Mike was "weary of crisis management"—his own and CRI's. He seems to have been hurt most by Lou Grant's charge that he'd used funds earmarked for minorities for some other purpose entirely—the implication being that Mike was a racist and even a thief. Yet there isn't a scintilla of evidence to support such a claim. Of the people then enrolled in CRI trials, 25 percent were people of color—much higher than was typical, though still only halfway toward Mike's stated goal of "making the demographics of CRI trials reflect the demographics of AIDS in NYC." As he wrote to the board, "I for one will not rest until people of color are equitably represented in CRI trials."

At one point in Grant's correspondence with Mike, he emphasized that CRI's "fiduciary responsibility" should not be compromised by any person's desire "to restructure this capitalist system or destroy it." He added that it was important to separate "utopian dreams [i.e., Mike's] from the needs of an organization that has to thrive and survive in the real world." In other words, Mike's left-wing views were being held responsible, at least in part, for CRI's financial problems. The indictment had little merit overall, but Grant's specific complaints did have some: the recent choice of an administrative director was to prove unwise and the amount of long-range financial planning being done at CRI was insufficient.

The turmoil within CRI continued for the better part of a year. Grant soon turned his fire on the fact that the board over time had had "three chairpersons (all white men—the usual unconscious and costly, but nonetheless vicious and stupid racism/sexism), none of whom took hold of the meeting and provided needed direction." On top of that, Grant accused Drs. Sonnabend and Bihari of using up board time to share technical medical information better exchanged elsewhere. As well, he continued to criticize Mike as sometimes being "very willful"—which he could be—of showing "great strength" as a leader but not leaving enough room for others "to express their own leadership," and of acting the victim, "the wounded butterfly." Grant attributed the latter to Mike's need as a performer for constant "affirmation and approval." From there, the charges degenerated further. By the end of the year Grant was calling Mike and his supporters "sick egos" who "don't know what the fuck you're doing."

There was also considerable grumbling about CRI's response to supplying Compound Q, the latest in a long series of purported miracle cures. The board of directors voted unanimously to collect data on the substance, though several members expressed concern that CRI might be liable for damages if the organization appeared to be encouraging the compound's use. Mike was very clear that CRI could not even indirectly encourage people to take a substance of "unknown risks and unknown benefits." If community physicians were willing to monitor those individuals who decided to run the risk and take Compound Q, then it would be proper for CRI to collect and analyze data about the substance. Mike sided with board member Dr. Bernie Bihari, who warned that there was good reason to believe that Compound Q "makes infected macrophages burst," which could lead to swelling of the brain, pancreatitis, and intestinal bleeding. But given the desperation that many in the gay community felt, still more antagonism toward CRI followed for its "cowardice" in refusing to take on Compound Q.[13]

Late in 1989, Sonnabend privately wrote, "I now worry that the idea of CRI is more romantic than practical. Self-empowerment without professionalism cannot work, at least on technical matters such as designing and constructing clinical trials." CRI would rebound in 1990 and also experience an uptake in revenues. But the following year, it would merge into the AIDS Community Research Initiative of America, a group that would continue to emphasize the importance of empowering PWAs.

CRI's parent organization, PWAC, was itself having financial trouble. PWAC had expanded its programs to include support groups for mothers of PWAs, Spanish-speaking PWAs, women, and people of color. It had also established a drop-in center ("the Living Room"), which served meals three days a week, ran a hotline, held public forums, and published *Newsline* monthly (with a Spanish-language edition in the works). Unfortunately, as PWAC's good works expanded, its income receded. One of its main benefactors had been amfAR, co-chaired by Mathilde Krim; the independent organization dispensed money for research to a number of both university- and community-based projects. Krim had herself been arguing for some time that the standard double-blind placebo trial was "an insult to morality," and she had also defended community-based trials against those critics who'd questioned whether local physicians had sufficient knowledge of sophisticated lab techniques.

She and Mike not only shared views on such matters but had become somewhat friendly. AmfAR had funded several of CRI's trials, but in 1989 it rejected the organization's proposals five consecutive times—even though Mike had been led to believe that they stood a good chance of being funded. Mike thought the reasons given for the rejections were "insulting" and he complained about it to Krim. She expressed her embarrassment and vowed to make changes at amfAR. Yet when CRI submitted an *emergency* request to amfAR for $50,000 to partially fund the salary of a medical director, months passed without word, and when it did come the award was reduced, without explanation, to $30,000 and CRI was told that the money could *not* be used for the requested purpose.[14]

An angry Mike wrote Mathilde a long, blistering letter in which he spelled out his "contempt" for amfAR, even as he tried to exonerate her personally for what he considered its failings ("Mathilde, I have never been able to express the depth of my admiration for you. That someone not immediately, personally threatened by AIDS should be so tireless on our behalf makes me weep sometimes"). But he felt he had to tell her that amfAR had become a "den of thieves." The problem, as he saw it, was that she'd set out to create a foundation to fund AIDS research that the federal government had failed to do but, "in an attempt to legitimize" amfAR, had invited in "the very scientists and establishment types responsible for the deadly delays at the federal level."

The result, according to Mike, was that "amfAR has lost whatever fire in its belly it ever had." He claimed that the staff at amfAR had pretty much circumvented her, that the organization had become "a sewer of self-interested scoundrels for whom AIDS is low on the agenda," that a West Coast/East Coast competition for funds had developed without her knowledge, and that each successive director of amfAR—and Mike named them, calling each either a "disaster" or an "asshole"—had made matters worse.

I can't pretend fully to assess the accuracy of Mike's claims: no detailed history of amfAR exists, and no response to his letter from Mathilde Krim has turned up in my research. But Abby Tallmer, then an employee of amfAR, confirms most of Mike's indictment and adds as well that at that point in time, there was "low employee morale." Two additional things can be said with reasonable certainty: Mike *was* a truth teller and, judging from his record as a whole, he wasn't one of those activist-warriors who sometimes confuse advancing an agenda with building up their own reputations.

When *Time* magazine, for example, featured a photo of Mike along with its article "Longer Life for AIDS Patients," instead of glorying in his prominence, he wrote a furious letter to the editor denouncing the contents of the piece. It had contained a number of odious comments, including "New drugs are giving hope but also raising difficult questions"—namely, that the "staggering" bill for medical care would only "postpone by a few years the eventual calamity of early death," and—the most offensive single remark to Mike—"many of the lives being lengthened are either dangerous to others or sexually isolated and childless." Dangerous to others? The implication was that predatory gay sociopaths with AIDS were stalking unsuspecting and innocent people. As for the article's closing phrase, Mike was succinct: "being dead is a worse fate than being 'isolated and childless.'"

The angry tone Mike took with Krim may have partly been a function of the periodic physical exhaustion that accompanies serious illness, and Mike's growing sense "that AIDS is closing in on me." He was now getting KS lesions at the rate of one a month and could "literally feel my body rotting. Political games I might have been willing to play a year ago are simply no longer tolerable." Simultaneously, he was beset by a crisis at PWAC. He'd stepped down as president of PWAC in order to concentrate on editing *Newsline* and attending to the rest of his activities and commitments and by the summer of 1989 had pretty much "stopped trying to figure out what is *really* going on" with the organization as a whole.

But his editing of *Newsline* soon became an issue in itself. Mike received a hand-delivered letter from PWAC's current executive director announcing that henceforth he'd be expected to submit each issue of *Newsline* to a board committee for approval. The reason given was that Mike was no longer a "full time, fully committed Coalition staff member." That was a cruel, deeply hurtful description of the fact that Mike, due to health issues, had of necessity been spending more time than usual out of the *Newsline* office, and failed to give even a token nod to the central role he'd played in PWAC up to that point. Besides, the notion of a committee passing on the contents of every issue of *Newsline* in Mike's mind would "hopelessly delay timely publication and would lead to censorship." In the face of such a blinding lack of appreciation, let alone understanding, of his multiple activities on behalf of AIDS education and research, Mike simply threw up his hands and—after four and a half years of presiding over PWAC's publications—submitted his resignation.

He pointed out—"just for the record"—that he'd never considered himself an "employee" of PWAC, had never been notified of staff meetings, and had neither a desk nor a telephone in the office. Though he'd "hate to see the *Newsline* become a house organ like GMHC's shamelessly self-promoting *Volunteer* newsletter," he expected that it would. In regard to his own future, he thought he'd devote himself to outreach to hemophiliacs, IV drug users, women, and people of color— all of whom, he felt, had failed to be sufficiently included in AIDS programs. He'd hoped for a more graceful departure from PWAC, but in his travels he'd long noted the prevalence of what he called the "eat the founders phenomenon. . . . I long for the days when we trusted each other and simply went about the business of accomplishing agreed-upon goals."

Mike's lover, Richard, was furious—as were Mike's close friends—at the way he'd been treated after all his hard work for PWAC. Richard became so angry that he once tried to compute on an hourly basis how much money Mike might have earned at a minimum-wage job—which he didn't have—and on top of that factored in the prodigious phone bills they incurred when calls came in from around the world asking for Mike's advice. In the early years of the epidemic, moreover, when Mike had spoken widely on safe-sex practices, he'd rarely been offered either plane fare or an honorarium. And besides, as Richard kept reiterating, Mike wasn't devoting nearly the amount of time to making music that his talent warranted. The Flirtations stood ready and eager to rehearse more and to turn out a first CD before the end of 1990. To that end, Mike now rededicated his energy.

Though the lead vocal on any given song in the Flirts' repertoire constantly shifted, Mike's unique voice was central to the group's success and he was its recognized star. Part of the reason was his ability to sing falsetto effortlessly. Before 1990, Mike rarely used that ability professionally; in fact he was somewhat embarrassed by it, apparently feeling that his effeminacy was pronounced enough without adding further embellishment. But one day, when he absentmindedly started singing falsetto, Richard dashed in from the other room. "What was *that*?!" he asked in astonishment. "It's beautiful!" The falsetto took much less work for Mike than singing in his natural voice, and with Richard's encouragement, he thereafter added it. A happy side effect was that singing in general became less of a torment and much more fun.[15]

A capella singing lends itself to "messing" with lyrics and adding twists—particularly gay political ones—to tunes like "He's a Rebel," "Something Inside So Strong," "Surfin' U.S.A.," and "Mr. Sandman." (The latter served as the brief background music for the party scene in Jonathan Demme's 1993 AIDS film *Philadelphia*—though Demme rejected the campy lyric "Give him two legs like Greg Louganis / But make him public about his gayness," and also excluded the Flirts from the soundtrack album.) "Messing with lyrics" was especially true for doo-wop songs of the 1950s, which audiences in 1990 were still conversant with.

The group did a considerable amount of touring even before its first album appeared in 1990. In 1988 alone, the Flirts did more than thirty concerts, including a wide variety of events and benefits—events like the AIDS Candlelight Vigil, the AIDS Walk, the National Lesbian and Gay Health Conference, and the Gay Pride Day Rally; and benefits for organizations including ACT UP, GMHC, Identity House, the Names Project (AIDS Memorial Quilt), the National Gay and Lesbian Task Force, and GLAAD. In 1989, they performed at least as many concerts, this time including one at the high-toned Alice Tully Hall.

Given the built-in tedium of touring, Mike's wit became an invaluable asset, especially at mealtimes. Cliff Townsend, the group's bass, recalls one evening at a restaurant when Mike asked the waitress if the turkey on the menu was fresh or the compressed, processed kind often served; when she assured him that it was fresh, Michael responded, "So you're saying that if I went back in your kitchen, I'd find a carcass in there?" Another time, when staying at a hotel that included a "continental breakfast" and being served a single piece of dry toast and some coffee, Michael asked the waiter, "This is your continental breakfast? From what continent, Biafra?!" Mike also had a tendency to ad lib when the Flirts performed, and Townsend remembers the time Mike told the audience that "as a group we tend to defy some stereotypes about gay men. But then, of course, we also confirm a few. You've all heard of the Four Tops? Well, here you have the Four Bottoms."

Richard produced their first album, simply entitled *The Flirtations*, recorded direct to digital two-track in New York City at Classic Sound and Manhattan Recording Company in November 1989 and February 1990. The critical reception was overwhelmingly positive. The gay music critic Will Grega, for example, wrote that "between the brilliant harmonies, general silliness, and giddy repertoire, a splendid time is guaranteed for all." Gene Price, music critic for the *San Francisco Bay Times*, hailed the Flirts as "the most entertaining, vocally enchanting, all-male singing ensemble I have ever heard." And the group often got standing ovations. Their tour in 1990 extended as far as Vancouver, where they ran into some momentary trouble: they made the mistake of revealing to a customs official that the records they had with them were intended for sale—which led to their prompt detention. Feigning haughtiness, Michael told the official, "*That* will teach us to tell the truth!" To which the officer sternly replied, "No Canadian would say that"—and proceeded to go meticulously through every one of their bags before finally giving them the nod to cross the border.

The group's concerts, as one of them put it, had arrived "at that annoying point where it's half way between part-time and full-time . . . I think within a year, we'll get enough bookings to keep us at it full time." Michael had a wittier take: "I'd say 90 per cent of my time is spent on activism, five per cent on music and five per cent on being a housewife. I'm trying to divide up that 90 per cent—like sleep for a change."

Once back in New York City, the group returned to rehearsals with the goal and expectation that their next record would appear in fairly short order. But in August 1990, group member T.J. Myers succumbed to AIDS. His place in the Flirts was taken by Jimmy Rutland, who was gradually integrated into the group. Their second album, *Out on the Road*, was recorded live on December 3–7, 1991, and would appear in 1992.

Marlon Riggs was an "army brat" born in 1957 in Texas, but he grew up, starting at age eleven, in Georgia and then West Germany. He returned to the United States in 1974, got a BA from Harvard in American history, and returned to Texas to work at a television station. The endemic racism he encountered made him decide to leave the state and take a master's degree at UC Berkeley. He made a number of short documentaries on a variety of themes, then turned his professional attention to the subject of racism. It took him five years to raise the $230,000 budget for his first feature-length film, *Ethnic*

Notions, a documentary on the historical depiction of black Americans in the popular media, which won him an Emmy nomination in 1989.[16]

Riggs next turned his attention to making *Tongues Untied,* which would become by far the most controversial of the eight works he produced between 1987 and 1994. He wanted to attempt to do for black gay men what a number of filmmakers and writers—Michelle Parkerson, Audre Lorde, Barbara Smith, Cheryl Clark, and Jewelle Gomez—had begun earlier for black lesbians. To reach his goal of exploring black gay male identity, Riggs wove together a wide variety of elements and crossed a variety of genre boundaries. He utilized lyric poetry (mostly work by Essex), vogue dancing, music by Billie Holiday and Nina Simone, "vérité" footage, autobiography, montage, and "Snap!-thology" (finger snapping). The latter was of special importance to Riggs. For him, "snap is a form of resistance, a form of saying, 'Yes, I'm different and I'm also proud of it.'" For similar reasons, he utilized the "so-called effeminate gestures in vogueing"; it was a way to "deliberately distinguish yourself . . . to affirm those gestures which the dominant culture looks down upon. . . . It becomes a virtue rather than a vice or flaw." He used Essex's poem "A Homocide," about the murder of a black drag queen, in a comparable way, moving the poem beyond an expression of grief to a longing search for community and love.

With himself, Essex, Wayson Jones, Craig Harris, and Larry Duckett as the film's chief performers, Riggs created a vibrant tapestry that combined defiance and anger, flamboyance and wit, pain and frankness. Addressing black homophobia and antigay violence, in one sequence he showed black "ministers" fiercely denouncing homosexuality, and in another a young black man being mugged by a foul-mouthed ("Fag! Punk! Queer!") gang of black toughs. As Kobena Mercer has pointed out, Riggs (as well as Isaac Julien in *Looking for Langston*), rejecting silence and exclusion, addressed his audience directly on the subject of black homosexuality, confronting it with the lived experiences of black gay men. As Riggs told an interviewer, "*Tongues,* for me, was a catharsis. It was a release of a lot of decades-old, pent-up emotion, rage, guilt, feelings of impotence in the face of some of my experiences as a youth. . . . [It] allowed me to move past all of those things that were bottled up inside me, that were acting as barriers to my own internal growth. . . . I could also finally express my rage about being treated as a pariah by the black community when I was younger, as my differences became more and more marked."

Riggs had a highly sophisticated attitude toward the standard issue of whether black gays primarily identified with and owed their allegiance to being black or being gay. "Neither," was Riggs' response: "I try to invalidate that argument. Part of the message of the video is that the way to break loose of the schizophrenia in trying to define identity is to realize that you are many things within one person. Don't try to [arrange] a hierarchy of things that are virtuous in your character and say, 'This is more important than that.'" No single voice or attitude dominates *Tongues Untied*; there is no unifying "typical" narrative of what it is like to be a black gay man. Riggs' views on "identity"—much debated in these years within intellectual circles—incorporated the current innovative investigations of "queer theory" and contributed to their expansion as well.

Unwilling to compromise his vision, Riggs was well aware that the provocative *Tongues Untied*, unlike his earlier film *Ethnic Notions*, would have trouble finding an audience. *Ethnic Notions* had been shown on many PBS stations, but *Tongues Untied* could hardly count on a national venue and had to mostly rely instead on film festivals and college audiences—despite receiving a number of favorable reviews and even awards (eventually including Best Documentary at the Berlin International Film Festival, and Best Video at the New York Documentary Film Festival). The very first showing of *Tongues Untied* was at the American Film Institute Video Festival before an invited audience of some 150 to 200 "largely white" fellow filmmakers and artists. Preceding it, Riggs had been isolated in the editing room day and night and had had no advance work-in-progress screenings to give him some sense of what to expect. At the festival, people reacted so enthusiastically that Riggs was profoundly shocked. The second showing of the film—at the Film Arts Festival at the Roxie Theater in San Francisco—was before a sold-out crowd filled with Riggs' primary intended audience of gay black men. At the film's close, the audience rose as one to give Riggs a standing ovation.[17]

Given the difficulty of finding outlets for screening *Tongues Untied*, Riggs was pleased when an invitation arrived to show the film at the Washington, D.C., Filmfest at the Kennedy Center. But he was far less pleased with the way the screening turned out—and Essex was downright apoplectic, calling the event a "disgraceful embarrass-ment." He wrote a long, scorching letter to the directors of the festival in which he itemized the assorted insults of "this shabbily handled affair." Six weeks in advance of the screening, Essex had himself sub-mitted a list of the technical needs—microphones, music stands, and so forth—that the artists planning a performance along with the screening would require. Arriving at the theater an hour ahead of time, Essex discovered that none of the equipment had been assem-bled and that the directors denied ever having received such a request. Essex and Larry Duckett had to chase the theater manager around for some forty-five minutes in an effort to obtain the needed equipment, but that produced only four microphones—two of them dead—and music stands so wobbly that one actually fell apart when handled. Essex found the situation "galling," since the Kennedy Center was a national performing arts space with first-rate equipment of every kind.

To top off the shoddy business, people who'd reserved tickets in advance were told after arriving that their names weren't on the box office list. Angry "chaos" followed in the lobby. Once the performance finally got started, it turned out that the two microphones that did function were too loud for the room (the artists' request to do a sound check had been denied) and no technical personnel, they were told, were available to make the needed adjustments. On top of all that, once the screening began, the images that appeared jumped shakily up and down. After five minutes, Riggs, Essex, and Ron Simmons raced to the screening booth—only to find that the projectionist was occupied with something else entirely and paying no attention to what was happening on the screen. He was finally persuaded to stop the film and rethread it. The only partial consolation for the botched event was that it had sold out.

The following year, the PBS documentary series *POV* (Point of View) scheduled *Tongues Untied* for a ten p.m. showing. A national viewing audience at last seemed possible. The Reverend Donald E. Wildmon, president of the American Family Association, a conservative media watchdog group, expressed his wish for as many people as possible to view *Tongues Untied*, secure in the belief that its "offensive" nature would swell conservative ranks. But Wildmon failed to get his wish. Affiliated stations aren't required to broadcast PBS programs and a number of them immediately announced that they wouldn't show the film during prime time; eighteen of the top fifty markets refused to show it at all. In total, 174 out of 284 stations—more than 60 percent—that ordinarily carried the *POV* series refused to show *Tongues*. Perhaps most hurtful of all, a number of local black leaders spoke out against the film. One bank vice president sounded a common note: "I had a strong concern that it was sort of degrading to African-American men, and just represented a small segment of the population," too small to be allotted that amount of time.

Another kind of controversy opened up within the black gay community itself. It centered on the bold lettering that closed the film: "Black men loving Black men is *the* revolutionary act" (the phrase originated with Joe Beam). When it became known that Riggs' lover was in fact a white man, one well-known figure in the black gay community, Cary Alan Johnson, published a review in the left-wing *Gay Community News* in which he wrote: "that Riggs has a white lover struck me as ironic and may leave some feeling cheated. I do not fault Riggs for his choice of a partner, only for what I see as a deception. . . . If Black men loving Black men is truly '*the* revolutionary act' . . . then why isn't he acting?" Since the British filmmaker Isaac Julien also had a white partner, the issue for a time became heated.[18]

And Essex jumped right into the middle of it. He characterized Cary Alan Johnson's remarks as "blatantly intrusive," even while acknowledging that many black gay people were suspicious, if not downright hostile, about those who took white partners. Did that mean, Essex asked, that "we burn the writings of James Baldwin and Lorraine Hansberry (they had white lovers)? Should we not acknowledge civil rights activist Bayard Rustin, chief organizer of the 1963 March on Washington (he had a white lover, too)? Should we not honor the significance of poet Pat Parker's work (she had a white lover)?"

Essex directly entered the debate over "identity" that Riggs himself had earlier outlined. "What is this 'blackness' that is being addressed?" Essex asked. "Is one still being black if one is out attacking innocent citizens? Is it black to be buried denying one was ever homosexual? Is it black to be fucking without a condom? Is it black to be shooting each other dead in the streets? Is it black to be selling cocaine or crack to black people?" Was it "revolutionary" to love *any* black man regardless, say, of his behavior—like betraying friends, employing violence, preferring lies to truth, terrifying children?

Besides, Essex went on, the phrase "Black men loving Black men is *the* revolutionary act" was never meant to refer to strictly sexual or romantic matters: it was meant to "speak of a responsibility we must each have and maintain as it relates to home, community, self and each other"—in other words, Essex argued, Riggs was envisioning something more encompassing than physical intimacy, something like the generalized support and comfort black men should try to offer one another. Isaac Jackson, another black gay writer, joined the debate to ask, "Is this a movement for all black gay men—or only those with black lovers? . . . Relationships in general between gay men are so hard to maintain, why must we chastise the black man who found what satisfies him, regardless of the color of his lover? . . . Why do we always come out of one limiting situation right into another?"

In Essex's view, the implication of Cary Alan Johnson's comment was that the black gay journey Riggs depicted in *Tongues Untied* was fraudulent, not credible, simply because his lover was white—a remarkably thin criterion, in Essex's view, for evaluating cultural documents. Or, for that matter, lives. A few years later, in his unpublished novel, "Standing in the Gap," Essex has one black gay man say to another,

> Just because you've decided that there's no place in your life for white men doesn't mean the brothers who are dating white men aren't being fulfilled in their relationships. And it doesn't mean they are less black than you. . . . As far as I'm concerned your thinking isn't any different than the thinking of black nationalists who believe our homosexuality is caused by white people, and that we aren't really black because we're homosexuals. You can't tell how black a person is based on who he's sleeping with or loving or his sexuality. What you really sound like is a bigot and a hypocrite when you suggest such a thing.

It reminded Essex of the reverse snobbism of those who located black "authenticity" in those who grew up in ghettos. In his view, "a ghetto childhood in and of itself does not make one 'black' nor define 'black culture.'" Nor, obversely, should it be assumed that interracial lust and love were functions of self-hatred. To see such pairings as somehow aberrational was, Essex argued, to suggest "that the natural roles of white and black people are to be, for all time, adversarial and corrupt with cruelties and indignities."

Riggs had his own reaction to the attack on his interracial relationship: "I didn't want people to believe that black men loving black men," he told an interviewer, "was a total kind of love that excluded any other, that it was a monolithic love. And I didn't want people to think of that love solely in sexual-romantic terms. I still think that for African-American men, our learning to love ourselves and each other would be a paramount act of revolutionary sentiment and behavior, because the opposite so much prevails now. But by acknowledging the importance and place of interracial love, one also says that there are other kinds of loves that are part of our universe."

Essex had found working on *Tongues Untied*—despite the Kennedy Center debacle—a "wonderful experience," and he felt sure that his collaboration with Riggs would continue (he felt the same about working again with Isaac Julien). Within a year, *Tongues Untied* traveled to the Soviet Union, Scandinavia, New Zealand, Canada, and Germany and was also bought by the BBC. What that taught him, Riggs said, was that "when you speak from the heart, people understand, even when you speak in ways that are troublesome." Within a short time of the release of *Tongues Untied*, he produced a new eight-minute work, *Anthem*, based on the Langston Hughes poem "I Too Sing America" but also including the words of black gay poets like Essex, Donald Woods, and Colin Robinson—to accompany the fast-paced screen images ranging from cock rings to ACT UP's "Silence = Death" logo to a pink triangle superimposed on a map of Africa in African National Congress colors. About Essex's poetry, Riggs said, it "moves me extremely just reading it, and it did so before I ever met or heard him."

A few years later, Essex and Isaac Julien, in a conversation intended for publication, extended the issues relating to "identity" into a different sphere. Sympathetic as the two friends were, they strongly disagreed about whether black gay men should participate in Louis Farrakhan's pending Million Man March. Julien considered the suggestion unthinkable. The Nation of Islam's political base consisted primarily of lower- and working-class heterosexual black men, and the reigning discourse among them centered on "black macho." Julien felt being excluded from that kind of "oppressive masculinity" was "a part of what it means to be queer. That's what our work has been about."

Essex agreed with Julien's point but felt "the power of the possibility of black men coming together" overwhelmed it in importance. Despite his aversion to Farrakhan and black nationalism, he felt drawn to gay participation in the march—"my blackness is the priority." He didn't believe that current macho notions of masculinity worked for anyone—and certainly not for black women. But whether many of Farrakhan's followers saw patriarchy as a liability was of course the point of contention. The evidence suggests they did not. The March's organizers and many of its participants took as a given that the male-dominated family was the essential building block of black unity—and that meant the exclusion of faggots.

Essex held out the hope that the organizers of the March might be pressed to include gay men as speakers, and even if not, that black gay participation in the March might help to end gay and lesbian invisibility. For the same reason, the National Black Gay and Lesbian Leadership Forum, while declining formally to endorse the March, encouraged black gays to participate. Keith Boykin, executive director of the Forum, led a contingent of some two hundred black gay and bisexual men in the March and subsequently wrote of it with sonorous awe: "We stood on the mall in the nation's capital in all of our beautiful diversity. . . . There was hardly a whisper of criticism as we marched along that day. The crowd of men on the mall split like the parting of the Red Sea as we marched and chanted, and most of those who had any reaction at all simply clapped. . . . Almost all of us left with a sense of awe and wonder in the possibilities for the future." Boykin neglected to mention in his account that Ben Chavis, national director of the March (and until recently executive director of the NAACP), had rejected the suggestion of a black gay speaker.[19]

Earl Ofari Hutchinson, the distinguished African American academic, writing in 1999, expressed the view that up to at least that point Afrocentric attitudes toward black gay men hadn't changed one iota as a result of their participation in the Million Man March. They were treated civilly at the march because, in Hutchinson's opinion, their participation marked "a tacit signification that all Black men, regardless of sexuality, face many of the same problems." If true, that recognition alone might be considered sufficient to justify the views of Essex, Keith Boykin, and others that participation had been worthwhile. Yet Hutchinson felt certain that there had been no "sea of change" in black nationalist attitudes toward gays. He cited a 1997 TV interview with

Rowland Evans and Robert Novak during which Farrakhan explicitly stated that he continued to regard homosexuality as an "unnatural act" and would do his utmost to discourage it.

While discussing the March with Julien, Essex stressed the overriding importance of black gay men *participating* in the larger black community's life. As an example of the need to intervene on a daily basis, he told Julien about a recent episode when he came upon three or four "young brothers . . . bigger than me" writing all over the storefront windows in his neighborhood with magic markers. "Something in me just snapped," Essex said. "I'm sick of there being no intervention. I told them, 'Don't do that. That's a black business. You're destroying property.' I was scared to death, but I wasn't going to my apartment and locking my door. . . . Even a simple intervention could cost our lives."

In the end Essex would be too ill to attend the Million Man March, but his wish to do so speaks volumes about his priorities: "returning home" to the black world had always been his chief concern, but he stubbornly knocked on the door as an openly gay man insistent on being accepted for who he was, tenacious in that insistence. In his speech at the annual OutWrite conference in 1990, he advised black gay men and lesbians that "we are a wandering tribe that needs to go home before home is gone."

With calculated optimism Essex went on to say that "our communities are waiting for us to come home. They need our love, our talents and skills, and we need theirs." Essex knew perfectly well that he was exaggerating; his own father, after all, had never accepted his homosexuality and had never been much of a presence in his life. And he personally knew any number of black gay men desperately ill with AIDS who more than anything had wanted to return to their families of origin to be taken care of and to die, but whose families had been unable or unwilling to take them in. Learning, often for the first time, of their son's sexuality and illness, some of these families expressed their shock and grief as "shame and anger" and had disowned "their own flesh and blood, denying dying men the love and support that friends often provided as extended family." Yet Essex put his hope in those many other families he'd known and seen who had understood and had "bravely stood by their brethren through his final days."

Those examples gave Essex the evidence to speak of the *potential* of a united black community and, at least as important, to draw a contrast with what in his view was the more entrenched hostility of the white gay world. Essex felt that initially he'd been "naïve" in approaching the gay community. Alluding to the common practice during the 1970s and 1980s of blacks being "carded"—kept waiting and waiting on line, and then being asked for *three* photo IDs before even being *considered* for admission to certain white gay bars and discos—Essex advised his audience in 1990 "not [to] continue standing in line to be admitted into spaces that don't want us there."

His earlier assumption that "here [in the white gay world] you have a group of people under persecution, denigrated, working from spaces of disempowerment, if you will, working from spaces of invisibility, et cetera. One would suspect, at least on the surface, that those conditions would sensitize individuals to the struggles of others." But that had been "hardly the case" in his experience. A chief concern of his about the white gay community was "its failure to make connections with other oppressions, with other spaces of disempowerment that need to be looked at and joined." The "bonds of brotherhood . . . so loftily proclaimed to be *the vision* of the best minds of my generation" had revealed itself, in his opinion, as empty rhetoric. The "disparity between words and action was as wide as the Atlantic Ocean and deeper than Dante's hell." There was no "gay" community for black men to come home to in the 1980s. "At the baths, certain bars, in bookstores and cruising zones, black men were welcome . . . the black man only needed to whip out a penis of almost any size to obtain the rapt attention withheld from him in other social/political structures of the gay community." Nor had Essex noticed any recent shift of opinion: the white gay world still operated, in his opinion, from "a one-eyed, one-color *community* that is most likely to recognize blond before black, but seldom the two together."[20]

Nor, Essex felt, had the scourge of AIDS bound black and white together into anything more than

a fragile coexistence, if we are anything at all. . . . What AIDS really manages to do is clearly point out how significant are the cultural and economic differences between us, differences so extreme that black men suffer a disproportionate number of AIDS deaths in communities with very sophisticated gay health care services. . . . Our most significant coalitions have been created in the realm of sex. What is most clear for black gay men is this: we have to do for ourselves *now*, and for each other *now*, what no one has ever done for us—we have to be there for one another and trust less in the adhesions of semen and kisses to bind us. The only sure guarantee we have of survival is that which we construct from our own self-determination.

In justifiably pointing up the racism that disfigured the white gay world, Essex, for dramatic emphasis, was teetering on some half-truths. There were many reasons, besides white gay indifference, for the disproportionate number of black AIDS deaths, including lack of access to affordable health care, the initial insistence of both black churches and black leaders that AIDS was a gay white disease to be contracted only by sleeping with whites, or a plot by the government to destroy black people—as well as the reluctance of many black gay men to admit to same-gender sex or to acknowledge that they were infected.

By the time Essex gave his OutWrite speech in 1990, traditional attitudes and organizations had begun to change; even the black church had started to show heightened concern. This shift had a lot to do with the work of black AIDS activists like Gil Gerald. And the extent of the shift can be exaggerated; one case in point is the fierce controversy, with many black and Hispanic leaders spearheading the opposition, that surrounded New York City's efforts to provide clean needles to addicts; one of David Dinkins' first acts after becoming mayor of New York City was to dismantle the city health department's small-scale needle exchange program.[21]

Essex was well aware that the black world—the "home" he aspired to—was rampant with crime, drug trafficking, and "self-destructing" youths ending up in prison. And he freely acknowledged that such a world frightened him. One evening in the summer of 1989, wearing shorts, sneakers, and an old gray T-shirt, he left his apartment to buy cigarettes, juice, and cat food. As he approached Sixteenth and Irving Streets, three teenage figures jumped out from behind the bushes, slammed him up against a parked van, and put a cocked gun to his head. "Shoot him! Shoot him!" the smallest of the three shouted. "For the hell of it," Essex later wrote, "he wanted to blow me away." One of the other two had his arm against Essex's throat and kept slamming him into the van. He had enough presence of mind to remain "calm and passive." After they took the $13 he was carrying in his shorts, they released him and casually walked away. Essex claimed that if a gun had materialized in his hand, he "would have used it without mercy." Later, he indignantly blasted "black people [who] have only one political reflex—the assumption that racism is the root of every issue in the black community."

A second incident further unsettled him. A group of young blacks marched around a store near his apartment, taunting the Asian shopkeeper, Yong Chang, with racial slurs and verbal intimidation, in retaliation for Chang's son having shot and killed a black male who'd reached for a knife when attempting to rob the store. The police had ruled the killing a justifiable act, and Essex was in agreement with the ruling: "I, too, would have shot the robber. . . . Tell me why is it racist to defend your property and your life?" It isn't, but Essex's further gloss on the incident—the dead black man "chose to be a criminal no matter what socio-economic conditions may have motivated or can explain his actions"—could be contested. Others would prefer to argue that it was the "socio-economic conditions" that did the choosing.

Nor did Essex have any patience with blacks who insisted that the recent downfall of Mayor Marion Barry—he'd been caught on camera smoking crack with a prostitute—was the result of a concerted white plot to destroy a powerful black male. Essex would have none of it: "To suggest that the federal government went out of its way to catch Barry was an attempt to obscure the issues of Barry's conduct, his character, and the legality of his actions . . . particularly regarding his drug use in a city where his leadership was supposed to bring the community out of the throes of a savage drug crisis." Black leaders, in Essex's view, were just as accountable for their actions as anybody else, and if Marion Barry was a victim at all, "it was as a result of his own wrong-doing." Nor did Essex have any sympathy for the argument that such tragedies could basically be traced back to white racism. Racism was real and had profound consequences, Essex felt, but it couldn't legitimately be used to "transform flawed men into martyrs," nor convince us that "criminals are victims. . . . Barry is responsible for his transgressions and his downfall. Not the government. Not white people."

Essex admitted that he himself had politically "steered clear of any heavy group involvement," except for membership in the National

Coalition of Black Lesbians and Gays. His group experiences had always been in the cultural context of performance art—Station to Station or Painted Bride, for example. He told one interviewer that he didn't "expect ACT UP and Queer Nation to march in the neighborhoods that I know against the drugs that are in those communities." But he did feel "as a black gay man . . . [that] something needs to be done in those communities. . . . It's not as if they [ACT UP and Queer Nation] don't have my support as a gay man and that we can't work together when our goals are parallel, but I have to take care of home. . . . I just can't sit back. That's what I mean about coming home. My sexuality isn't so big a thing that it's going to overwhelm my desire to see us [black people] live and survive."[22]

Essex did participate in fund-raisers for AIDS in the D.C. area and also gathered together artists regardless of sexual identity to benefit a homeless shelter (they raised $500 and ten cases of canned food). As well, he often wove material relating to AIDS into his performances—even if, in 1989, the reviewer for the *Los Angeles Times* disparaged the AIDS material as "melodramatic excesses." "There's been a certain knowledge of giving back," Essex said at one point, "that's been instilled in me by family." He also felt that support groups for black gay males, like those pioneered in the women's movement, "would be a great undertaking in terms of consciousness." By the end of the eighties, there was evidence that such groups were spreading around the country: GMAD (Gay Men of African Descent) in New York City, Black Gay Men United in Oakland, Unity and ADODI in Philadelphia, Black Men's Network in Delaware.

But if Essex didn't expect majority white organizations like ACT UP to devote resources to combating drugs and crime in black neighborhoods, he could grow exceedingly angry at the opposite suggestion that black gays relied heavily on white-dominated groups for shared political or medical needs. He pointed to people like Gil Gerald, Craig Harris, Chuck Hicks, and Colevia Carter as prominent examples of how black gays and lesbians were performing "the back-breaking and poorly rewarded work" of black organizing. In regard to AIDS, he believed it was absurd to argue, as some did, that the cultural differences between the black and white communities were *so* huge—though they were real—that the black community needed to establish entirely separate institutions, right down to different flyers, in order to reach their own constituencies. That argument, Essex believed, was one more offshoot of a racist paradigm. In fact, the caregiving services and educational materials that the white-dominated Whitman-Walker clinic were offering, he felt, were being fully utilized and were fully "understood" and appreciated by black gays.

When the publication *Network*, out of Newark, Delaware, interviewed Essex in 1990, its reporter Chuck Tarver remarked that "a number of creative folks have succumbed to AIDS." Essex picked up on the remark and elaborated it further: "I think there was a fundamental mistake made in the early 1980s. Because the initial deaths were largely White gay men, Black people didn't think they had anything to worry about. That was like sitting on the train tracks with the train bearing down on you and saying, 'I will not get hit by this train.' And that was crazy. . . . I partly think that some of the issues of racism were played out in that as well. Because for some Black people, it was almost glee for them that it was White people who were dying and not Black people. It set into motion a certain inactivity that has proven itself to be very fatal."

Stalemate

At the June 1989 International AIDS Conference in Montreal, a good deal of optimism was expressed about AIDS soon becoming a manageable disease. The optimism hinged on the number of "promising" drugs—like the nucleoside analogues ddI and ddC—currently in the pipeline. A variety of federally sponsored AIDS clinical trials began (with blacks, Latinos, women, and IV drug users woefully underrepresented), and within a year it had become disappointingly clear that the new drugs, taken either singly or in combination, lacked efficacy.[1]

Some activists felt that the drugs still held promise and that the pharmaceutical companies should provide the funding for additional, larger trials. But many others, activists and otherwise, fell into a kind of blunt despair. The bubble had burst. Nothing of promise was on the horizon. Nothing stood between a person with AIDS and inevitable death. By early 1990, more than fifty thousand people had died of AIDS in the United States, with twice that number known to be infected with the HIV virus. Drug after drug had been run up the flagpole with a surge in hope, then just as quickly lowered. There was no magic bullet. By 1991, ACT UP/New York, the country's largest chapter, would begin to splinter into factions, each claiming to represent the "right" priorities.

In a climate of growing desperation, Mike Callen unblinkingly stared the facts in the eye and issued a lengthy, lucid, cool-headed assessment of the current situation—all the more remarkable given the state of his own health. He'd recently been diagnosed with KS of the lungs, was often "literally breathless," and had been given a maximum of one to two years to live. He was nonetheless determined to prevent "this latest moral panic" from crushing the liberatory spirit of the gay sexual revolution. In 1990, statutes declaring homosexuality illegal were still on the books in twenty-six states, and many Americans still believed that any sex that was not connected to marriage, procreational in nature, and confined to the missionary position was vaguely shameful and unacceptable.

"What breaks my heart," Mike wrote, "is my sense that the vast majority of gay men and lesbians appear to be in essential agreement with their oppressors—at least about the married and missionary part of 'appropriate' forms of sexual expression"—which made them "virtually indistinguishable, sociologically, from their conservative suburban heterosexual counterparts." Many gay men, Mike felt, were "just like our parents in the sense of wanting a marriage, house in the suburbs, career, and the right to dip into the gay sexual revolution now and then." By contrast, Mike wanted them to spend whatever political capital they had "defending the right of gay men or lesbians to explore radical forms of sexuality—that is, sex which isn't 'married' nor essentially missionary, the kind that used to occur in bathhouses, backrooms and private sex parties, specifically non-monogamous, group sexual expression." Mike credited feminist sex radicals—in particular, Gayle Rubin's groundbreaking essay "Thinking Sex: Notes for a Radical Theory of the Politics of Sexuality"—for having turned him into a serious student of sexual politics.[2]

Mike believed that in the seventies gay men had effected "an unprecedented revolution in sexual practices," and he felt strenuously that the revolution—even in the face of AIDS—needed safeguarding. In his view, that could happen only if what he called "the many grey zones" around safe-sex practices could be rationally debated, which in his opinion they weren't being: "At countless 'Eroticizing Safer Sex' workshops, the 'right,' 'politically correct' answers are parroted by agonized, confused and conflicted gay men fearful of being drummed out of the fraternity of cool, AIDS-adjusted, post-AIDS babies. A vast ocean of silence surrounds what gay men are actually doing—or actually wanting to be doing."

As the granddaddy of safe-sex guidelines, Mike had reached firm conclusions about certain sex acts that most discussions of safe sex either avoided or distorted. One such act was oral sex. There had been much hemming and hawing on the subject; as of 1990 the official position of GHMC and other gay "mainstream" organizations (in contrast to those in Canada and Australia) was that any cock sucking taking place without a condom fell into the category of "unsafe sex." Nonsense! Mike roared. There simply wasn't enough evidence to warrant such a conclusion—that is, so long as ejaculate wasn't swallowed. Besides, in the actual acts he witnessed in his travels (when he felt "obligated" to visit local sex emporiums and "observe" behavior—like the serious-minded investigative reporter he actually was), he'd "never, ever seen anyone suck a dick with a condom on it," and, to the extent he could tell, rarely saw anyone swallowing cum. He felt that gay men intuited what was or wasn't safe sex better than the honchos of the AIDS establishment.

Mike felt the same about rimming and fisting and called for their removal from the list of high-risk activities; both carried health risks, of course, but AIDS wasn't one of them. He knew from painful past experience that "the safe sex circles will shout from the rocks that I'm a 'murderer,' that I'm complicit in the deaths of anyone who is 'confused' by my raising 'irresponsible' doubts about safe sex. Well, I mince, but I don't mince words: fuck them. I had a hand in the *invention* of safe sex! I've paid my fucking dues! In the Spring of 1983 . . . Joe Sonnabend, Richard Berkowitz and I first officially proposed that cumbersome concept of 'avoiding exchange of potentially infectious bodily fluids.' Let's just say that the AIDS establishment didn't immediately embrace safe sex. In fact, we were initially attacked for 'promoting promiscuity,' which in fact we were happy to do, provided everyone rigorously avoided the exchange of bodily fluids. The best advice the AIDS establishment had been able to come up with was pathetically, perhaps murderously, useless: 'try to reduce your number of sexual partners and try to limit your sex to people you 'know.' "

Mike didn't pretend to have definitive answers about the potential danger of oral sex; what he was railing against was the refusal of the "authorities" to present convincing data that it *was* risky. He was pleased that private sex clubs had begun to open again: the Glory Hole Church in San Francisco; the basement of the Christopher Street bookstore; the Meatrack in L.A. The fog was lifting, "life-affirming sex-positive sunlight" was reappearing. He himself had never been a fan of cock sucking; he was part of the first gay sexual revolution based on anal sex—"which, after all, is both an art and a skill."

The second, post-AIDS revolution, he felt, was "based almost entirely on oral sex." Why? Because the authorities had irresponsibly equated getting fucked with getting cum up your butt. It was the latter, not the former, that dangerously exposed one to AIDS—which the inserter's use of a condom mitigated (though condoms *did* sometimes break). And thus it was that they'd thrown out "the baths with the bathwater." Whenever Mike told someone that he still liked to get fucked—with condoms, of course—"they often literally gasp or take a step back" as if he was a "diseased pariah . . . an apparition from the past. 'You still do *that?*' they ask, their voices quivering with barely contained disgust. Yes," he'd say, "getting fucked and sugar are my reasons to live."

And unlike many others, Mike had no problem getting fucked with a condom—"after a few seconds, it heats up." But he acknowledged that "physiologically there has to be a difference between skin on skin and skin on latex." Still, he added philosophically, "This is the time in which we live. I'm OK with that. I can eroticize that. . . . I'm an adult. Life is precious." He thought that gay men on the whole had done a remarkable, even unprecedented job in achieving behavioral modification—a much better job than, say, smokers or dieters had ever been able to do. He pointed to the recent 50 percent increase in heterosexual syphilis and compared it approvingly to the lack of any increase among gay men.

Mike liked to joke that he was becoming known as "a safe-sex bag lady"—the reason being that when he went out on one of his investigative sex tours, he'd fill every available pocket with condoms and water-based lube. "Whenever I see two men about to fuck, I shamelessly approach to look for evidence of a condom. I'm not averse to reaching my hand down and feeling for the rubber-band-like end of the condom near the base of the top's penis. If I don't see or feel a condom, I wordlessly reach into my pocket, produce one, rip open the packet, shake out the condom, produce some lube, tap the top on the shoulder, smile, and offer him the condom." Nine times out of ten, Mike claimed, the top took it and thanked him. "If I'm feeling bold," Mike added, "I whisper: 'it matters to me whether you both live or die'; I smile, and move on."

Mike tried to interview various government epidemiologists and AIDS educators with the goal of pinning down the actual rate of rectal gonorrhea among gay men—which was astonishing, given the declining state of his health and his limited energy. His assumption was that rectal gonorrhea would prove the best surrogate marker to evaluate the current level of unprotected anal sex among gay men (though it was possible, as he recognized, that it might be easier to contract AIDS than gonorrhea). "Well, kids," he reported—his wit intact, even if his stamina wasn't—"you'd think I was asking for classified state secrets." The few AIDS educators who'd agree to take his call were "arrogant and supercilious," declining to provide any information. A few government officials were more forthcoming, though cautious. A staff person at the New York Department of Public Health sniffily told him that no such data were being kept, and to do so would be offensive. A second New York official revealed that such data *did* exist and promised to phone Mike back. "Surprise, surprise; no one has," Mike wrote.

But he struck pay dirt with his calls to the San Francisco and Seattle Health Departments, both of which confirmed his hunch that very little unprotected anal intercourse among gay men was occurring. In both places, according to a 1990 census, the annual rate for rectal gonorrhea in gay men had gone down steadily, year by year. For Mike that was cause not only for celebration but also for pride: gay men had done an unprecedented amount of self-policing, of behavioral modification, and had done so in "a virulently homophobic, violently sex-negative atmosphere in which it was difficult, if not impossible, to get federal funding for explicit, no-nonsense safer sex education." The gay male community had real cause, Mike felt, for self-congratulation—"if never complacency."[3]

Having produced the Flirtations' first record, Richard Dworkin did little with the group subsequently. He and Mike in fact came from different worlds, musically: Mike from piano/vocal cabaret—his heroes were Barbra Streisand and Bette Midler—and Richard, though he enjoyed some of the female singers that many gay men of his generation liked—Joni Mitchell, say, or Laura Nyro—had gotten into music through the very different route of rhythm and blues, of Motown. After he'd moved to San Francisco in the 1970s and started playing music professionally, Richard had also been drawn to free jazz groups and was part of a collective that had organized a loft-jazz space. But if Richard's basic taste in music differed from Mike's, he continued to encourage Mike's involvement with the Flirts. In the years 1990–92, Mike started to edge away from PWA activism, thus freeing him up to tour more with the Flirts and to rehearse for their second record, which would appear in 1992.

His gradual withdrawal from activist work after a decade of intense involvement was a carefully considered move; he summed up his attitude toward activism as "bitter, burnt-out and soul-weary." He recognized that he'd lost the fight against the "free-for-all philosophy" implied by the ACT UP rally cry of "drugs into bodies"—which he sardonically reduced to "any drug into any body." As someone who had AIDS, he well understood the kind of desperation that led many to clutch at any straw. But he continued to regard the practice as ill-advised, as likely further to compromise already weakened immune systems.

ACT UP's Treatment and Data (T&D) Committee, that small circle of activists composed primarily of middle- and upper-class educated white men, had by 1990 gained considerable access to AIDS scientists and researchers—even to the point of designing clinical trials together. This "old/new boys network" provoked considerable resentment, especially among women and people-of-color activists within ACT UP, who felt their special needs continued to be insufficiently addressed. The charges of sexism and racism brought against T&D were, arguably, overstated, but there was growing resentment over what some considered a merely pro forma acknowledgment on T&D's part of issues relating to women, poor people, and people of color. (Mike had never joined ACT UP, but his primary sympathies were with its detractors.)[4]

By 1990 the division had grown into a serious internal conflict between those whose concentration was centered on treatment issues and those who were deeply concerned as well with other aspects of the AIDS epidemic, like health care insurance and housing, that most members of T&D never had to worry about. But if their locus of desperation was different, it was no less intense; most T&D members were HIV-positive and feared that delving too far into "side" issues might somehow cause delays in the scientific research on which so many lives depended. Ultimately, T&D would break away entirely from ACT UP and would set up independently as the Treatment Action Group.

The mounting toll of deaths and the continuing failure to produce effective drug therapies deepened the level of fear and desolation throughout the AIDS community, as did the attitude of the federal government. Reagan's Supreme Court twice refused to entertain constitutional challenges to allow openly gay people to serve in the military. Draconian sodomy laws still remained on the books in twenty-four states, with only two states (as of 1990) passing laws that barred discrimination against gay people and only seven cities adopting "domestic partnership" legislation. At the same time the amount of violence against gay people soared, a shadow companion to the ever-rising toll of AIDS deaths.

No gay person had to look very far to find cause for despair. Though I was of an older generation, I saw the growing desperation firsthand, initially as a volunteer phone operator at PWAC, then as increasing numbers of younger friends and acquaintances died. The person I most admired and felt closest to at PWAC abruptly came down with advanced lymphoma. He was (as I wrote in my diary) "the most vibrant and energetic of all the people at PWAC. . . . I thought of him as an encouraging example of how one can be HIV-positive and yet uncompromised in health. He turns out instead to be an example of how suddenly and unexpectedly the virus can impinge." When I visited him in the hospital, he was full of confidence about the prospects of recovery.

The health of other friends and acquaintances—like the writers Allen Barnett, Paul Monette, and George Whitmore, the organizer Greg Kolovakos, or Damien Martin, co-founder of the Harvey Milk School—was beginning to slide precipitously. Closer to me personally were Vito Russo, Ken Dawson, and Tom Stoddard. Though I wasn't an intimate friend of Vito's, when his health began rapidly to deteriorate in 1990 I became part of his caretaker team—of which Arnie Kantrowitz and Larry Mass were the mainstays. In June Vito was still (as I wrote in my diary) "a bundle of positive energy," yet within weeks he became "fiercely sealed off," as if putting himself in "an ice-cold deep freeze" to survive the grinding hell he was going through.

By late July he was in the hospital getting chemo, then in and out for more of the same, though the treatments seemed to make him weaker, not stronger. If anything, the chemo seemed to be heightening his suffering, and by mid-September he was noticeably fragile and thin. But Vito wasn't the self-pitying type. A tough Italian American born and raised in New Jersey, he had a strong, resilient will and "faced every crisis in a resolutely positive way." Still, when I was helping him pack up for yet another trip to St. Vincent's Hospital, he seemed to me for the first time "obviously frightened . . . he kept gulping the fear down, concentrating on the tasks at hand: 'Do you think I should pack a sweater?' etc. He bravely managed a smile when he asked me if I thought "he could sneak out of the hospital one day to see the film 'Postcards From the Edge.'" Vito died on the morning of November 7, 1990.

Ken Dawson was the executive director of Senior Action in a Gay Environment (SAGE), the gay seniors organization, building it from a small-scale operation into a leader in the field of geriatrics. He was a remarkably handsome man, and, what was much more rare, a warm and genial one as well. He and I had briefly dated in the early eighties, and we'd become friendly. Socially I saw Ken and his lover, Todd, fairly often, and the slippage in his health became steadily more apparent. At dinner one night, Ken (as I wrote in my diary) "looked drawn and ill, and spoke in a low, energy-less voice light years from his vibrant self—though he bravely stayed the full evening."

We celebrated his forty-fifth birthday in his hospital room in 1991. The literary agent Jed Mattes (who later also died of AIDS) brought a cake, Eli and I party favors, and seven or eight people lifted their seltzer water to toast him. As Ken was about to blow out the candles on the cake, Jed said, "We're all wishing just what you are." Ken told us that all his tests had improved, and he seemed to actually enjoy the party. "This is more than WASP training," I wrote in my diary, more even than a saintly disposition; it's genuine optimism." It didn't last. A collapsed lung had him in and out of the hospital, and his stoic spirit began to sag. Ken died in April 1992. "Why," I scribbled in my diary, "does it seem to be mostly the decent ones."

Tom Stoddard served for six years as the executive director of

Lambda Legal Defense, the well-funded legal arm of the gay movement, and during his tenure the staff grew from six to twenty-two. He
authored the gay rights bill that had (finally) passed the New York
City Council in 1986, and, handsome, telegenic, and articulate, he
became one of the country's best-known advocates for gay civil liberties. Tom had an enormous zest for life—sex, food, travel, you name
it—and eagerly pursued all of it, which made his slow decline all the
more painful to watch. He held on until the "miracle" protease inhibitors became available but was one of those unlucky people who
didn't respond to them, and he died in 1997.

On and on the list goes. Every gay man alive in those years, and
every lesbian or straight woman with gay male friends, has a similar,
and often longer, list of beloved friends lost to the deadly disease.
Everyone knows somebody—more often, many; for some, the "many"
is in the hundreds—who was dead or dying. Most of them weren't
"artists" and didn't leave behind any tangible product other than the
friends they'd made, the love they'd generated.

In May 1989, Eli and I decided to get tested. My diary picks up the
story:

> May 27: Hard news yesterday . . . Eli is positive . . . my angel who has
> learned to expect no, has gotten an ultimate no. We cried and cried
> yesterday, comforting each other, assuring each other that since his
> T-cell count is normal & there are no other signs of active illness that
> only years down the road is he likely to get into trouble—and by then,
> *surely*, good drugs will be available. There's truth to that, and it's a
> truth we have to hold onto in the days ahead, but right now I can't
> hold the tears back . . . I can't stop touching him, have trouble taking
> my eyes off him for fear he'll be snatched away before I can *fix* him
> inside my soul . . . I feel no relief over my own negative, as if instead
> we had both gotten positives . . . Maybe, just maybe, we'll get lucky . . .
>
> May 29: The nobility of sweetie's spirit makes me feel achingly
> close to him. He is sad and quiet, but entirely uncomplaining. He
> never expected life to go right for him, and then, just as it seemed it
> might, he's been brought back to what he all along assumed would be
> a suffering fate. Perhaps he never felt entitled enough to a good life to
> get angry over the prospect of its being withheld or withdrawn. I

worry that that could lead to resignation, and last night talked to him about how good his odds were, how much I love him, how good our life together will continue to be . . .

June 7: Volunteering at PWAC has taken on a different meaning. I used to read the materials, field the phone calls and proof the *Newsline* with grateful distance. Now I read the memorials and the personal accounts of how HIV-positive turned to ARC turned to AIDS with a churning stomach, a gloomy sense of immediacy.

July 4: I have to fight off the fear (I tell myself I'm being literary— the 19th-century sentimental novel) that goodness such as Eli's can only be a visitation.

Oct. 9: Dr. "Bigelow" says that Eli might stay free of major infection for years, and by then Bigelow expects a combination of drugs will have reduced AIDS to a chronic, but no longer life-threatening disease. I had been sunk in gloom before the results came back, convinced Eli looked thinner & pale, certain the news was going to be bad.

A year later, Eli's T cells had dropped by half, yet Bigelow's prediction would ultimately prove accurate. No one knew, of course, that in 1995 the protease inhibitors would arrive and dramatically change the AIDS prognosis, so when Eli's numbers continued to drop, Bigelow for the first time suggested that he enroll in an experimental GP120 trial at the Deaconness Hospital in Boston. It would entail fifteen trips over eleven months, and Bigelow (who we trusted completely) assured us that there was no downside to participating—no side effects, no immunity created to future drugs, no negative effect on T8 cells. My friends at PWAC told me that a comparable study had shown a T4 cell decline of 6 percent in those getting the drug versus a 23 percent decline in those not getting it.

Eli decided to go ahead. For the first few trips to Boston I went with him, thinking we could minimize the trauma by "making a kind of weekend vacation" of it, dropping in casually for a few minutes to get an injection while "cavorting" from one touristy good time to another. It didn't work. Eli decided that the best strategy for denial was to fly back and forth to Boston as rapidly as possible—without me. He continued to make the trips, and his T cells (and weight) continued to fall. After his count went down to 240, Bigelow put him on AZT, but he couldn't tolerate it—nausea, exhaustion, anemia—and Bigelow stopped the drug after two months. I administered daily shots of Epogen for the anemia. Then came night sweats and fevers, and Bigelow added Bactrim as a prophylactic against PCP. But Eli's T8 number rose, and one new theory was that for some lucky people T8 cells replaced T4 cells, and were the new marker of stability . . . and on it went . . .

June 18, 1994: My poor sweet boy is so amazing, he carries this awful burden every minute, yet moves bravely through his day, even extracts some joy. In his place, I would whine away my life, and probably be dysfunctional. But now & then his underlying grief bursts through, and he sobs and sobs . . .

Aug. 3, 1994: The decision has been made to drop everyone from the Boston protocol with fewer than 200 T-cells, and Eli's are now— 70 . . . Bigelow will tell Eli *casually* that the study is over and that there will now be a pause to analyze results . . . it turns out Eli was the one out of six who was on a placebo . . . Bigelow thinks my own level of anxiety needs some attention; he gave me the name of a psychopharmacologist . . . If I don't keep myself in decent shape, I won't be there for Eli when he most needs me . . .

June 30, 1995: Eli's again running a low fever. It's happening with more frequency. I loudly ascribe it to an "ongoing Bactrim allergy," but inwardly quake.

And then, when Eli's T-cell count fell below 10, came the unbelievable release of the protease inhibitors . . . and he's reacted well to them down to the present day. In the end, we were among the lucky ones.

Despite Mike Callen's remarkable resilience, by 1990 he was having more difficult health problems, and they were accompanied by greater mood swings and deeper periods of despondency than he'd known before. "I only hope," he wrote, "that those who claim to represent the best interests of those like me who *have* AIDS understand the tremendous responsibility they have taken on. . . . I strongly suspect that the current rush towards virtually total deregulation of drug testing in this country is a disaster of immense proportions."

Though Martin Delaney of Project Inform had done seminal work informing AIDS patients about treatment options, Mike again singled him out to blame for championing the latest "hot" drug being hyped. The official study of Compound Q (trichosanthin), which derived from a Chinese cucumber, had been a small one, and Delaney initiated his own study but without (in Mike's opinion) sufficient safeguards to secure it against contamination. Sonnabend agreed with Mike; he accused Delaney of swallowing anything the authorities told him, though in Sonnabend's view they often held racist and homophobic views. When two people in Delaney's study went into comas, Sonnabend was horrified and declared that Delaney should be arrested. Sonnabend was nearly as hard on the activists of ACT UP, feeling that in their rush to expedite the approval process ("drugs into bodies") they were dangerously diluting needed safety procedures. Alas, when people are dying, out of options and nearly out of hope, taking risks on untested treatments becomes the least of their worries.

Mike was more understanding. He realized that in the absence of properly conducted treatment research on a variety of promising therapies, people would become instantly excited over rumors that an effective new drug had surfaced. When the FDA refused to stop Delaney's "illegal" Compound Q trial, Mike felt it signaled the end of any effort to apply testing standards.

The history of Bactrim suggested to many that to wait for trustworthy trials was literally to court death. A double-blind study as far back as 1977—four years before the outbreak of the epidemic—had conclusively proven that two double-strength Bactrim tablets a day could essentially prevent PCP. Yet after AIDS emerged, the federal government made no effort to urge doctors to use the drug as a prophylactic against PCP. The result? By the beginning of 1989, 30,534 Americans had died of AIDS-related PCP. By the time Compound Q came along, some people with AIDS weren't willing to enter federally sponsored trials unless there was demonstrable evidence that the drug being tested offered more hope than those already widely available, though of unproven efficacy. Mike—and Joe Sonnabend—put some of the blame on (in Mike's words) "the plethora of treatment newsletters and the relentless PR of groups such as Delaney's Project Inform urging what is referred to as 'early intervention.'" The result was that some PWAs, given the lack of alternatives, were still "injecting, ingesting and imbibing" any new substance that came down the pike.

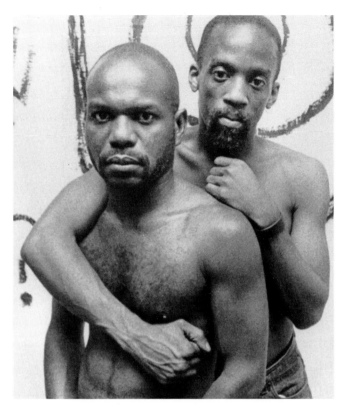

Marlon Briggs and Essex Hemphill in *Tongues Untied*, 1989 (photo courtesy of Signifyin' Works)

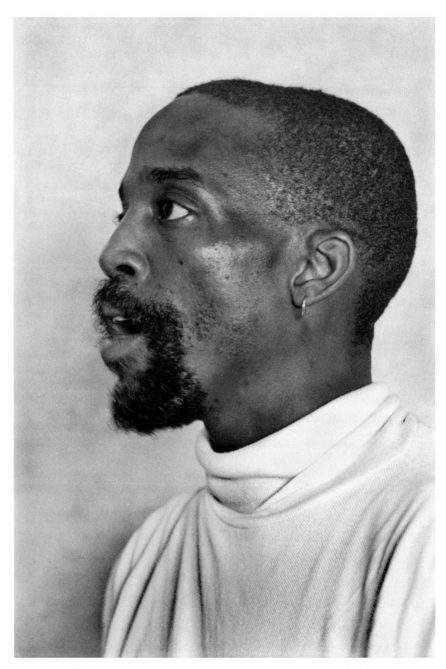

Essex Hemphill at the San Francisco Out Write Conference, 1990 (photo courtesy of Lynda Koolish)

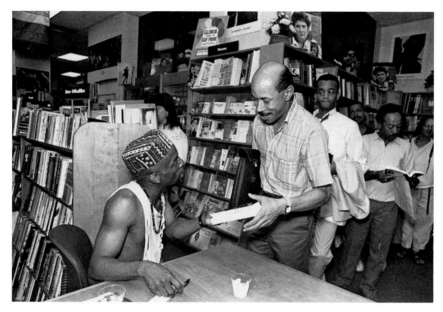

Essex signing *Brother to Brother* following his reading at the Lambda Rising bookstore, 1991 (photo © Sharon Farmer/sfphotoworks)

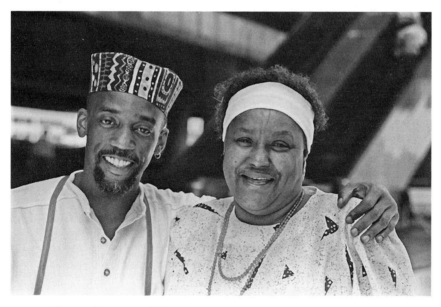

Essex and Dorothy Beam, Philadelphia, 1991 (photo © Sharon Farmer/sfphotoworks)

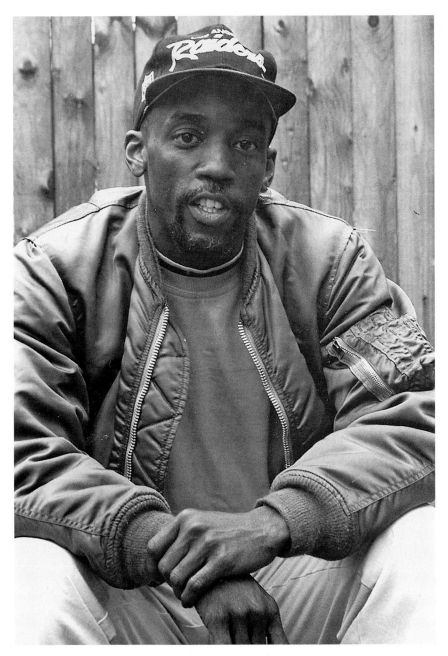

Essex, 1991 (photo courtesy of Richard Marks)

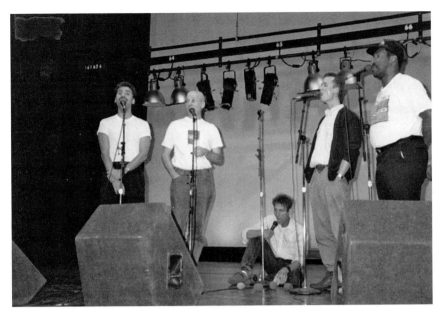

An exhausted Mike soldiering through a Flirtations sound check, 1992—left to right: Aurelio Font, Jon Arterton, Michael Callen, Jimmy Rutland, and Cliff Townsend (photo courtesy of Richard Dworkin)

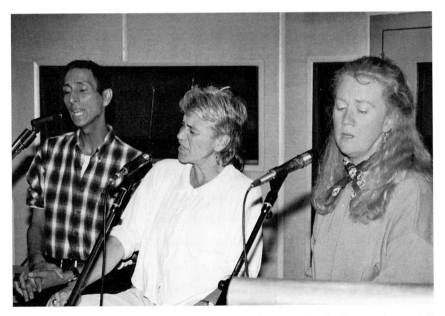

Hyde Street Studios, San Francisco, June 1993, rehearsing for the *Legacy* album—left to right: Michael Callen, Chris Williamson, and Holly Near (photo by Patrick Kelly)

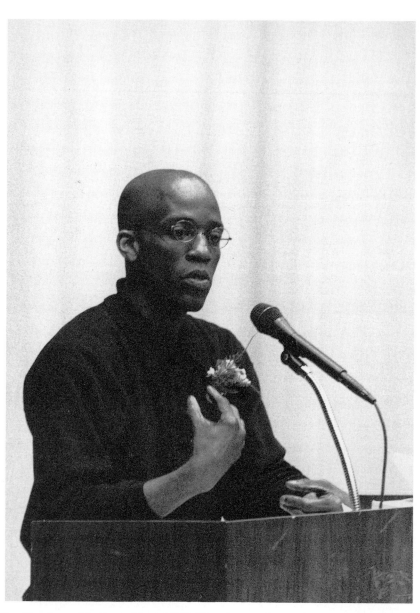

"An Evening with Essex Hemphill," The Center for Lesbian and Gay Studies (CLAGS), CUNY Graduate Center, New York, 1993 (photo courtesy of CUNY)

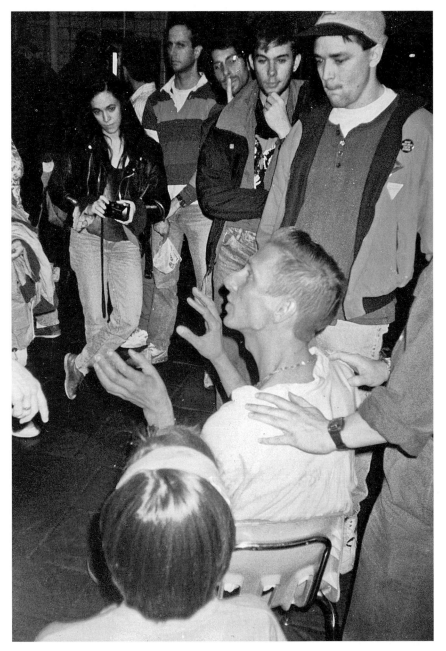

Michael in a theater lobby surrounded by well-wishers, 1993 (photo courtesy of Richard Dworkin)

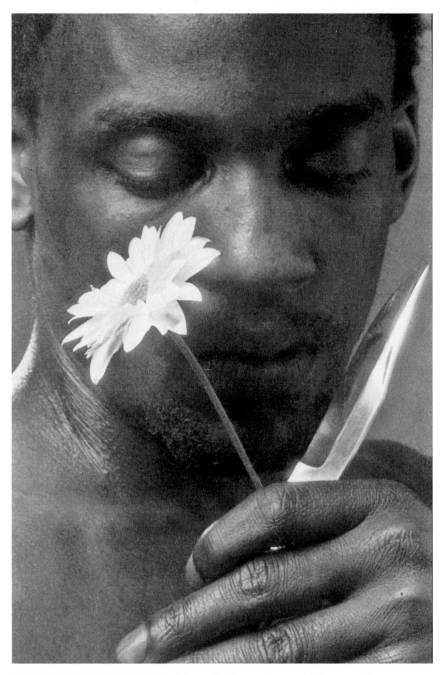

Essex the poet, 1985 (photo © Sharon Farmer/sfphotoworks)

As a result, it had become nearly impossible for the government to fill its clinical trials. Besides, it had become widely known that federal studies were being sabotaged by various forms of "cheating"—patients, for example, would have their pills tested by a lab to see if they were getting a placebo or the drug. At CRI Mike had found out just how "damned difficult" it was to run good clinical trials, but he continued to feel that, properly designed and regulated, they still held out the best hope for finding treatments that worked. He believed most people with AIDS would be more likely "to cooperate honestly and altruistically" with community-based trials than with federal ones.[5]

Mike felt that he, too, bore some responsibility for the current lack of effective drug oversight; he had, after all, helped (in his own words) "to foster the atmosphere of rabid anti-expertism" that fueled the drive to put "any drug into any body." What he'd intended was to open up the definition of "expert" to include the lived experiences of people with AIDS. That had gotten twisted, he felt, "into the absurd notion that all opinions are of equal value—that when, for example, one must evaluate some highly complex pharmacological and toxicological question, the opinion of a PWA who may or may not have finished high school is just as valid as someone who has studied these issues for 20 years."

Despite all the buyers clubs and the ingestion of a wild assortment of untested drugs, the progress against AIDS had been agonizingly slight. By 1990 there had been modest increases in median survival—that is, for middle-class white men, 18 percent of whom were now living on average eighteen months after a diagnosis of full-blown AIDS—as opposed to one year for IV drug users and a mere six months for African Americans and Hispanics. Mike believed that the improved statistics for white men were primarily due to Bactrim and aerosol pentamidine as preventatives against PCP, as well as to a general improvement in patient management—but the prospects for effective treatment were no more promising than when he'd been diagnosed a decade earlier. He agreed with the activists of ACT UP that the failure could be assigned largely to the federal government's slowness and lack of urgency in its response to the disease. But he didn't think that the best antidote was widespread deregulation.

His reasons were multiple. Reliable "surrogate markers"—like CD4 counts—had not yet been established; in fact, a high-powered meeting convened by the National Academy of Sciences had, in late 1989, failed to reach consensus on precisely that matter. It had been Mike's personal experience, and that of many others he knew about, that T cells "bounce all over the place, varying from lab to lab and day to day." He also disputed the common notion that an HIV-positive diagnosis was inevitably a death sentence, and pointed to his own decade-long survival as a case in point. He attributed his survival to having followed Sonnabend's advice *not* to experiment with whatever drug was currently being touted. In this regard, Mike rejected the widespread assumption that a drug either worked or it didn't work. He insisted on a third alternative: taking a given drug could actually *harm* you, could hasten your death. Mike believed that he and other long-term survivors had rightly taken "a wait-and-see attitude about experimental drugs."

That conclusion was difficult for someone like Mike to reach, since his politics were libertarian (that is, he was against blindly obeying authority instead of relying on individual choice). But he'd come to the painful decision that "there are in fact experts better able to assess the risks and benefits of a particular course of action than I." He might have reached a different conclusion if Joe Sonnabend—whom he'd long credited with keeping him alive—hadn't been his doctor, and if all PWAs had access to disparate data and to physicians and scientists willing to take the time to explain the complex implications of any potential drug therapy.

Instead, a "carnival atmosphere," in Mike's opinion, currently prevailed, the result of the pharmaceutical companies' outrageous promotion of their products for the sake of making money, and the unearned certainty of some doctors and scientists bent on promoting their own careers. "The order of the day," Mike wrote, "is anarchy. . . . The stage is thus set for anybody to test any drug, regardless of its toxicity, based on any fucocta theory. . . . The AIDS activist movement has joined with the drug deregulation movement to score a knock-out victory. . . . Federally designed AIDS research has become irrelevant . . . thanks to a plethora of treatment newsletters and the relentless PR of groups such as Project Inform urging what is referred to as 'early intervention,'" which in Mike's view encouraged desperate PWAs to medicate themselves with useless drugs.

Even if all PWAs had full access to the research literature, they would have found it rife with contradictory conclusions and advice. This was true both for recommended drug therapies and for definitions of "safe sex." Mike may have been the founding father (he preferred "Queen Mother") of the latter subject, but not even Mike could evaluate with certainty recent all-over-the-map studies about cock sucking. One such study found that oral sex without a condom carried "significant risk" of contracting AIDS, while another concluded that any top in anal sex who failed to use a condom was at greater risk of getting AIDS than someone who sucked unsheathed cocks. It had reached the point where, depending on your preferred sexual activity, you could probably find a study that confirmed your favorite option as the safest one. Questionnaires about sexual behavior, moreover, were notoriously unreliable. Asking someone whether they played the top or bottom role in anal sex, for example, not only encouraged an either/or answer but failed to control for ambiguity, role reversals, memory lapses, fear of discovery, and distorted self-images.

The unreliability of self-report data had been clearly revealed at least as far back as Masters and Johnson's 1979 study *Homosexuality in Perspective*. The two researchers had studied the sexual fantasies of four groups: homosexual men and women, and heterosexual men and women. The heterosexual men during face-to-face discussions and interviews had described same-gender sex as "revolting" and "unthinkable." They reported no incidence at all in their histories of homosexual experience. As a result, Masters and Johnson had understandably designated them Kinsey O's—that is, exclusively heterosexual. Yet when the two researchers studied their subjects' fantasies they discovered that the men had "a significant curiosity and anticipation about same-gender sex"—and even worried about how effectively they'd perform. (The men's fantasies also revealed, incidentally, that they envisioned themselves more frequently as rapees than rapists—as victims of "groups of unidentified women.") The moral, I suppose, is something like "you can't believe people are who they say they are"— they may well be reporting a vision of their ideal selves rather than their actual ones.[6]

Essex wasn't naturally belligerent—that is, someone who invented slights in order to stir up trouble. But he was a person of intense feeling, and when he believed a genuine injury had been done to him, he could be fierce in defending himself. Twice in the summer of 1991, on quite different fronts, he became militantly contentious. The merits of the first dispute seem clear; those of the second, somewhat less so.

Essex had a gift for meticulously detailed work and proved his own best publicist on *Brother to Brother*. Diligently, he sent press materials to some sixty review outlets and then made follow-up calls to make sure that the books and assorted press releases had arrived in the proper hands. When he contacted an assistant editor at *Book World*, the review section of the *Washington Post*, and was told no such material had arrived, Essex sent a second round to the same editor. When Essex again followed up, the editor again told him that no material had arrived. But Essex wasn't easily put off. He had the UPS shipping bill pulled to verify that the book had been sent (twice), and he had first-hand testimony from another employee at *Book World* who'd overheard the editor telling someone that he wasn't interested "in reviewing gay and lesbian literature."[7]

That did it for Essex. He accused the editor of homophobia, and the editor in turn insisted that "to suggest that we exclude books based solely on an author's sexuality is not only absurd but personally insulting." The lie heightened Essex's anger. He sent the editor a blistering four-page letter in which he first made it clear that he'd never accused *Book World* itself of being homophobic—but rather the editor. Essex reiterated what he'd said from the first: he had a high regard for both the *Washington Post* and *Book World* and was not accusing either of being antigay. He had, moreover, checked again with his firsthand witness and she'd reconfirmed the editor's homophobic words.

Secure in his position, Essex opened up with both barrels: "You should be accountable for your statements and your actions," he wrote the editor. "That's what I respect. Accountability . . . just because you don't agree with a given sexuality it does not mean you have to trade in your integrity and credibility for lies and shabby denials in order to maintain a heterosexist hegemony that can easily find you expendable at any moment, and dismiss you as excess baggage or yesterday's news." Essex closed with this zinger: "I leave you with my best wishes that *you* will be able to manage in a changing world." And he did his bit to ensure that the editor would *not* be able to manage: he sent a copy of his letter to the head of *Book World*. The bottom line? In general, Essex was a sweetheart, but on some issues you didn't want to cross him.

At almost exactly the same point in time, August 1991, Essex took on Phill Wilson, the African American AIDS coordinator for the city of Los Angeles, and in 2014 still a prominent, well-regarded AIDS activist. Wilson invited Essex to come to L.A. under the auspices of the Black Gay and Lesbian Leadership Forum (BGLLF). The visit did not go well. Essex had been invited to offer three public programs under BGLLF's sponsorship. On arriving in L.A. he read, with his usual attention to detail, a number of the free newspapers available to the gay community—and found not a single mention of his upcoming appearances. When he stopped off at the gay bookstore A Different Light, in West Hollywood, the clerks on duty expressed surprise that he was in town.

When Essex confronted Wilson with the absence of publicity, he replied that notices had been sent out to the black press. Not good enough, Essex felt. Since the appearance of *Brother to Brother* (and *Tongues Untied* as well), he'd been drawing "very diverse audiences" to his public offerings. His primary commitment *was* to black audiences, but "when it comes to moving products and building coalitions," Essex expected his sponsors to make "general outreach efforts" to draw in audiences.

He also expected a reasonably accessible site. But Phill Wilson and BGLLF had selected a facility that had no running water or working bathroom (should nature call, patrons had to go across the street to use the bathroom in a restaurant—and deposit a coin to get access to a stall). Essex himself had to piss outside against the wall of the building minutes before he was to go onstage. In his protest to Wilson, Essex drew a devastating comparison between his receptions in San Francisco and in L.A. In San Francisco he spoke to nearly seven hundred people and sold more than 250 books. In L.A. he spoke to thirty-six people and sold "maybe thirty books." Though the San Francisco/Oakland programs were organized by individuals, without "the luxury of an organization or a board of directors to help in the planning," they succeeded in drawing large crowds because they sent notices to the newspapers and generally circulated the flyers, photographs, and bios that Essex had sent them in advance.

As far as Essex was concerned, his one bad experience with BGLLF was enough to warrant an overall condemnation of the organization. He held Phill Wilson, fairly or not, directly responsible: "You are quite accountable for this travesty and unfortunately your board has to suffer my loss of faith through an unknowing complicity, though they are not totally to blame." (Essex copied each member of the board and told Barbara Smith that two of the members had called to thank him "for raising the issues that they have been trying to raise with Phill regarding the structure and running of the organization.") To Phill Wilson himself, Essex wrote how tired he was "of seeing us fail to do the simple things that convey our respect for one another." Then he acidly added: "I don't want my name or my image associated with any of your future activities. NONE." Nor would he attend the group's upcoming retreat—not, that is, "unless I was coming wearing a hockey mask and carrying a chain saw."

A year later, Essex was still reporting to Barbara Smith that his health was "good." It was typical of him to provide no further details: he wasn't a complainer and would rarely if ever elaborate about whatever symptoms he may have been suffering. He did tell Barbara that during the year he'd been hospitalized while in Chicago, but rather than explaining why, he wrote instead about his battle with Medicaid for denying him any financial assistance because he was a visitor from out of state. Essex's lifelong motto—and the way in which he closed nearly every letter he wrote—was to "take care of your blessings." Obversely, one did not itemize or dwell on disabilities and distress.

On November 7, 1991, Earvin ("Magic") Johnson announced his retirement from the Los Angeles Lakers basketball team because he'd tested HIV-positive. To forestall any speculation that he'd contracted the disease through drug use or homosexual contact, Johnson appeared the following night on the *Arsenio Hall Show* and declared "I'm far from being homosexual. You know that. Everybody else who's close to me understands that." The reassurance produced wild cheering from the studio audience. Just in case "far from" left room for interpretation, Johnson removed the ambiguity a week later in *Sports Illustrated*: "I have never had a homosexual encounter. Never." In all likelihood, he speculated, he'd contracted the virus before his marriage when, as a freewheeling star/stud, he'd "truly lived the bachelor's life," doing his best "to accommodate as many women as I could—most of them through unprotected sex."[8]

"Accommodate" made it sound as if Johnson had had no say in the matter, that he was the passive plaything of female lust. It *had* been brave of him to acknowledge explicitly his HIV status, but the gay community was less than enamored with his commentary about it. As Randy Boyd, a young African American writer, put it in the publication *Frontiers*: "To the world, Magic Johnson is one of the innocent victims, like babies. . . . From Rome, George Bush called him a hero. . . . Remember—he [Magic] didn't get it the wrong way; it was some dirty woman's fault, just like Eve."

In a letter to *Frontiers* praising Boyd's piece, Mike Callen reminded everyone that although the government lists "some 4,000 American men . . . as having gotten AIDS from sex with an HIV-infected woman," the facts were a bit more complicated. Two thousand of the four thousand were Haitian men who'd simply been dumped into the heterosexual category. And who were the remaining two thousand? One widespread assumption was that they'd gotten the disease from prostitutes. But in New York City, the epicenter of the epidemic, where many female prostitutes work to support their drug habits, the city's AIDS surveillance unit listed exactly *six* men as having gotten AIDS from commercial sex with a woman (the figure had been eight, but two were discovered to have lied). The point was that the sexual transmission of HIV to men from women was rare.

Mike praised Magic Johnson for his courage, and had little doubt that his revelation "will have a major, positive impact on America's response to AIDS, particularly in the black and teenage communities." There was indeed a flood of media coverage following Magic's announcement, though his recommendation of abstinence probably had little effect on horny teenagers, and though the media coverage of Magic continued largely to ignore the disproportionate number of cases among black gay men. The limited media coverage of AIDS in black or Latin communities continued to focus on its "innocent victims"—women and children—while repeatedly publishing stories about the threat of AIDS spreading to the general population.

Marlon Riggs was more generous toward Johnson than Essex, calling his efforts to educate about AIDS "heroic." But the following year, Marlon Riggs and Essex did see eye to eye about the reluctant disclosure by the tennis star Arthur Ashe of his own HIV-positive status—the result, he claimed, of a tainted blood transfusion when he'd had heart surgery. Ashe had kept quiet about his status until *USA Today* published a story about his gaunt appearance and rumored health, which forced Ashe's hand. Unlike Johnson, Ashe deteriorated quickly—he died in early February 1993—but in the year left to him he did do much to call attention to the disease. Still, as Riggs put it, "many people remain indifferent to, or even contemptuous of, black gay men with AIDS. . . . To the degree that one feels sympathy at all, [it] is extended only to people like Magic or Arthur Ashe who got it 'innocently.' That is, not through homosexual sex or IV drug use."[9]

Marlon and Essex also shared the same judgment on the kind of black representation that mainstream TV featured (when it treated the subject at all). Marlon's new film, *Color Adjustment*, which aired in June 1992 as one of the *POV* series, contained a sharp critique of the hugely popular miniseries about African American history, *Roots*. He jolted "liberal" whites with the accusation that *Roots* actually minimized the evils of slavery while promulgating the myth that "traditional values were all it took . . . to triumph in America"—though Marlon did acknowledge that *Roots* was "a powerful breakthrough against the historic denial of slavery in American popular culture."

Essex also agreed with Marlon's negative judgment of the wildly successful *The Cosby Show*. Yes, Marlon argued, Bill Cosby's show was preferable to previous sitcoms about black people, just as, in the evolutionary hierarchy, *Good Times* was better than its predecessor *Julia*, which in turn was preferable to *Amos 'n' Andy*. *The Cosby Show did* (mostly) avoid "slapstick, buffoonish, eye-rolling, insulting humor," but at the same time it was wholly apolitical. It insultingly avoided most of the issues that afflicted most black families, opting instead for a format that "would be acceptable to the myths of the majority . . . this family could be looked at as, in many ways, no different from any other ethnic immigrant group that had finally reached the pinnacle of success in American society through hard work, family values, integrity, discipline, education." In other words, *The Cosby Show* advanced the pernicious myth that no racial barriers existed to black advancement that wouldn't yield to the traditional virtue of putting one's nose to the grindstone.

Marlon and Essex continued to work together on projects that revealed rather than erased additional dimensions of black life—and especially black gay male life. The first Riggs film to follow immediately on *Color Adjustment* was *Non, Je Ne Regrette Rien*, a thirty-eight-minute profile of five HIV-positive black men, which premiered in 1992 at the New Festival, New York City's annual showcase of gay film and video. Riggs then turned to work on *Black Is, Black Ain't* a feature-length documentary about competing versions of what was considered within the black world itself an acceptably "authentic" identity.

Essex worked along steadily with Marlon, but most of his attention was centered on gathering together a collection of his own writing. It appeared, under the title *Ceremonies*, in 1992. To handle its publication, Essex turned to the agent Frances Goldin, who was a housing activist and also represented a considerable number of authors with left-wing politics (I'd been one of them for a long time and in fact recommended her to Essex). Frances did her usual devoted, obstinate job for him, writing him long letters commenting on his work and sending it out to those publishing houses most likely to be receptive. She and Essex grew fond of each other and forged a bond of genuine trust.

Ceremonies was a selected collection of Essex's poetry to date, including a number from his early chapbooks *Earth Life* (1985) and *Conditions* (1986), and containing as well some half dozen of his short essays. Thematically the collection centered on his life as a black gay man, belittled or condemned by the straight black world (even as he shared its racial indignities) and ignored or patronized by the white gay world. His voice throughout was anguished and angry in equal parts, intensely proud and independent while forlornly in search of sustained connection. He pulled no punches in either his essays or his poetry, bluntly describing his lust and voicing his deep-seated contempt toward those who would censor him.[10]

In his long, blistering poem "Heavy Breathing," he asks an unnamed antagonist:

> And you want me to sing
> "We Shall Overcome"?
> Do you daddy daddy
> do you want me to coo
> for your approval?
> Do you want me
> to squeeze my lips together
> and suck you in?
> Will I be a "brother" then?

Rejected by black men who only want to fuck blondes, he masturbates:

> Occasionally I long
> to fuck a dead man
> I never slept with.
> I pump up my temperature
> imagining his touch
> as I stroke my wishbone,
> wanting to raise him up alive,
> wanting my fallen seed
> to produce him full-grown
> and breathing heavy
> when it shoots
> across my chest;
> wanting him upon me,
> alive and aggressive,
> intent on his sweet buggery
> even if my eyes do
> lack a trace of blue.

He finds the human landscape bleak and ominous; disenchantment haunts his imagination:

> I plunder every bit of love
> in my possession.
> I am looking for an answer
> to drugs and corruption.
> I enter the diminishing
> circumstance of prayer.
> Inside a homemade Baptist church
> perched on the edge
> of the voodoo ghetto,
> the murmurs of believers
> rise and fall, exhaled
> from a single spotted lung.
> The congregation sings
> to an out-of-tune piano

> while death is rioting,
> splashing blood about
> like gasoline.

Most of the essays in *Ceremonies* had appeared elsewhere. In them, Essex spoke as a man caught and torn between the homophobia of the black world and the racism of the white gay one. In "Does Your Mama Know About Me?" he summarized the post-Stonewall white gay community of the 1980s as "not seriously concerned with the existence of Black gay men except as sexual objects. In media and art the Black male was given little representation except as a big, Black dick"—as revealed most strikingly, as he'd earlier argued, in the photographs of Robert Mapplethorpe.

"Coming out of the closet to confront sexual oppression," Essex wrote, "has not necessarily given white males the motivation or insight to transcend their racist conditioning. This failure (or reluctance) to transcend," he continued, "is costing the gay and lesbian community the opportunity to become a powerful force for creating real social changes that reach beyond issues of sexuality." In 1992, this last comment was prescient. Essex's analysis and complaint falls on still more fertile ground in 2014, particularly among younger gays who join older left-wingers in deploring the mainstream assimilationism of the contemporary gay movement.

Though *more* comfortable in the black world than in the gay one, Essex continued to disparage "the middle-class aspirations of a people trying hard to forget the shame and cruelties of slavery and ghettos." His poem "American Wedding" seems designed to mock the traditional rituals of marriage:

> In America,
> I place my ring
> On your cock
> Where it belongs . . .

And in his brief essay "Loyalty," he deplores, "through denials and abbreviated histories riddled with omissions"—he had Langston Hughes, among others, in mind—"the middle class sets about white-washing and fixing up the race to impress each other *and* the racists who don't give a damn . . . I can't become a whole man simply on what is fed to me: watered-down versions of Black life in America. I need the ass-splitting truth to be told, so I will have something pure to emulate, a reason to remain loyal." This was the same indictment Essex had leveled at the white gay community: *don't* distort your own culture in the attempt to win acceptance and appease through assimilation.

Ceremonies reached the gay bestseller lists—and won the National Library Association's New Authors in Poetry Award—but was largely ignored by both white and black mainstream media outlets. The reviews and interviews carried in the gay press were always appreciative, sometimes glowing. Despite Essex's warranted distrust of the white gay movement, it *did* have a left-wing cohort, and one of its reviewers characterized *Ceremonies* as "harsh, stark, and unyieldingly honest." Another smartly caught the book's tone: it's "marked by an acuity of insight and an ironic, often sarcastic, exposing of the bigotry, hypocrisy and ignorance that plague black gays." Alternatively, the collection was characterized as "replete with battle cries, wounded warriors, and soldiers who will not die. The inner struggle with self-identity and acceptance is turned outward and made public." The only complaint I found was in a review that preferred Essex's poetry to his prose, finding "too much venom" in the latter and complaining that "his dogmatism does not invite intellectual elasticity." The reviewer used Essex's attack on Mapplethorpe as a case in point, claiming that it failed to consider the possibility—remote, in my view—that his photographs can be read as *critical* of the distorted view of black men that they simultaneously display.[11]

In one of the interviews Essex did after *Ceremonies* came out, he responded to the question "How is your health?" with the circumspect "It's pretty good. I've had mild disturbances, but I've been fortunate so far, and that is the qualifier: so far." He proved as much by accepting most of the invitations that now came his way, traveling widely to read and speak. Over the next eighteen months, he appeared at Harvard, the University of Pennsylvania, MIT, UCLA, the Folger Library, and the National Black Arts Festival (the first openly gay writer invited to read from his work). He also began to get a number of awards. *Brother to Brother* had already received the Lambda Literary Award for the best gay men's anthology, and now additional prizes began to arrive for *Ceremonies*, including the American Library Association's Gay and Lesbian Literary Award and a Pew Charitable Trust Fellowship in the Arts.

With so much encouragement, Essex decided to try his hand at writing a novel. His agent, Frances Goldin, "adored" him, and when Essex was in New York she'd put him up in her own apartment and cook for him. On one such visit he told her an anecdote about his mother: During a sermon in her fundamentalist church, the minister had railed on and on against homosexuality. Finally Mantalene Hemphill stood up in the middle of the congregation and angrily said, " 'You're talking about my son! And if you don't stop, I'm never coming back to this church!' " And with that, she'd stormed out.

The episode is confirmed and amplified in the manuscript of Essex's novel in progress, "Standing in the Gap," which I recently discovered in the Frances Goldin Agency's files. The section is long but, because it tells us a great deal about the relationship of mother and son, is, in condensed form, worth quoting:

> For a long time she had kept her silence in the face of often blatant condescension, but one Sunday, nearly two years ago, her minister began preaching a sermon about how AIDS is "the just punishment" of homosexuals. Right in the middle of his sermon she stood up, mad enough to start cussing in the church and shouted, "Excuse me Reverend Jenkins! Excuse me! If AIDS is the punishment of homosexuals then it must be the punishment of adulterers, murderers, and thieves, too, and all other manner of criminals and deviates you could want to name! Now, I don't mean to challenge your cloth this morning, but you know my son is a homosexual. He's one of those 'gay' people you trying to condemn to hell, but in my eyes he has committed no crime. Some of these people sitting up in here have sons who would rape them if they were pretty enough. Some of them can barely leave their homes and come here to hear you preach because they fear that when they return home those same sons will have sold everything that isn't nailed down to get some of that crack, and whatever other drugs they got out there. . . .
>
> "Up to this point," she continued, "I've been praying for a wisdom to visit you that would cause you to see we are *all* God's children and no mere man can stand in judgment of another. That's God's privilege,

not man's. I've been praying for you to preach love, but you keep preaching hate from your pulpit. And you ain't nothing but a man yourself, strutting around here with the pennies *I* put in your collection plate jingling in your pockets. But let me tell you, Reverend, as surely as the candle of *my* Lord does not blow out in any wind, I'm not going to sit here and listen to you preach my son into damnation. . . .

"Before I listen to you blasphemy my son, my love, and the dear Lord I trust, I'll leave this church this very day, Reverend. I don't know why our young men and women are dying like they are, and you don't know why, either, but I know in my heart that the God *I* worship does not carelessly take life in order to terrorize us into righteousness! *My* God doesn't punish love! Men do! And you ain't nothing but a man! But my pennies won't be jingling in your pockets no more. I work too hard to be giving my money to a fool. I believe in God too sincerely to trust you to handle my prayers. If you don't know tolerance, Reverend, then how can you possibly recognize a prayer?"

And with that, Mantalene ("Mary" in the novel) gathers up her things, walks out "with her head held high, and she never looked back." Her son—called "Eddie" in the novel—tells her that he's "proud of you for leaving there and joining a church that isn't homophobic and woman hating." But Mary, like Essex's mother, Mantalene, continues to feel "her loyalties torn between her religious beliefs and her son. In this howling gap, her fears for Eddie proliferate. They seep into her dreams long before they're articulated in her prayers. . . . 'I'm angry and sad, and my fears for you have increased tremendously. . . . I want you to survive America. I don't want you fighting to stay alive with handicaps. Homosexuality is a handicap, Eddie. That's how society sees it, son . . .'

"But when she finally came to terms with Eddie's dilemma, and she did see it as that—*his* dilemma, but *hers* as well—she established a delicate balance between suspending all judgment and maintaining all loyalty." She tells her son, "I may never fully understand your sexuality, Eddie, but I don't want to judge you or condemn you for it. I'd love you then. That has always been real clear to me, even as I've struggled to understand. The thought of losing you frightened me into acceptance." Eddie, in turn, "knew he would always have her God-fearing love and she would have his, that was their mutual commitment, but accepting every part of him was not guaranteed, and he knew this, too, as clearly as he knew he was homosexual."

In portraying his mother's conflicted loyalty, Essex had also found a title for his novel: "Standing in the Gap." He spelled out its meaning: "Are you willing to stand in the gap for your loved ones? Can you go prepared for anything and be afraid of nothing? Are you willing to stand in the gap for your community? Are you willing to stand in the gap for the pregnant juvenile black girls? Are you willing to stand in the gap for the black males dying faster than eagles? Are you willing to stand in the gap for the crack addicts, the rape victims, the emotionally and physically abused, the criminally insane, the disenchanted, those stricken with AIDS?"

After Essex completed the first draft of the novel, he sent it to Frances Goldin for her opinion. She read it carefully and sent him back a frank assessment: "As it stands at this moment, it suffers both from structural problems and rhetorical overkill. . . . There is far too much unconvincing dialog and too much lecturing. . . . The book needs more story-telling." Frances knew her comments would come as a blow to Essex and she urged him not to be "dashed" by the criticism, adding that she wouldn't have spent so much time reading and writing about the draft if she "didn't think you were up to great end products."[12]

Proving her commitment, Frances managed to secure a two-book contract for Essex from the conglomerate publishing house of NAL/Dutton/Penguin—which included an advance that allowed him to move into a somewhat nicer apartment. One contract was for a projected anthology of short fiction by black gay men, which Essex tentatively entitled "Bedside Companions," describing it as aiming "to acknowledge and affirm the ways Black gay men support, sustain, and love one another through these critical times." He wanted the collection to "chart territory beyond the coming-out stories and the political treatises on racism. . . . [It] intends to more closely examine home, friendship, family—immediate and extended—lovers, 'brothers,' and the impact life's joys and sorrows have upon these relationships." He appended to the announcement the warning that "No *gratuitous* sex, violence, misogyny, or sexism will be considered."

The second book in the two-book contract was for the tentatively titled novel in progress, "Standing in the Gap." The acquisitions editor at Penguin was Peter Borland, and after he read Essex's first draft of the novel, he sent him a long critique that essentially confirmed Goldin's opinion. Borland reiterated her view that "Standing in the Gap" had the potential to become "a wonderful, literary, important novel," but to reach that goal, he felt a considerable revision was essential. Most radically, he wanted Essex to change the novel's point of view, shifting away from its current "floating third-person semi-omniscient P.O.V.," which he didn't find "particularly engaging." Another large problem, Borland felt, was Essex's "tendency to let the narrator or your characters editorialize or preach."[13]

My own reading of "Standing in the Gap" coincides pretty closely with the Goldin and Borland critiques, especially in regard to the novel's tendency to engage in hectoring lectures that too often substitute for plot and character development. As well, lengthy and repetitive descriptions impede the narrative, and such dialogue as exists in the novel is often pitched at such an artificially inflated level that it's difficult to associate it with the way people actually talk. There are occasional pleasures to be had in the novel's inventive use of language, but they tend to be buried under a defective structure. The book basically alternates between scenes in a dying "Eddie's" hospital room and those describing earlier experiences with his mother and his friends. But a subplot in the novel—the story of Eddie's closest friend, "Tyrone"— gradually takes over the narrative, and it's no longer clear who or what the novel is centrally about. The confusion is heightened by a final scene centered on Tyrone's murder at the hands of a closeted hustler, an anachronistic close that diffuses still further a narrative that thematically had initially focused on the plight of a gay man with AIDS. "Standing in the Gap" has some deliciously sassy moments and more than one skillful scene of erotic encounter. Overall, however, it cannot be judged a success. Alas, Essex was never allowed the luxury of time to revise and work through the novel's shortcomings.

Essex took Goldin's and Borland's criticisms well, and even wrote Goldin that he was "actually looking forward to the work required to create an excellent novel." He'd recently been accepted as a visiting scholar at the Getty Center for the History of Art and the Humanities in California, and hoped to work on the novel during his residency, which began in January 1993. In the meantime he sent Goldin a batch of new poems which he hoped she could get published, under the title "Critical Care."

Unfortunately, her reaction was again negative, though she couched her bottom-line verdict that "we do not see this as right for a trade publisher" in soothing praise for how "moving and lovely" she found some of the poems. She expressed her willingness to submit the poems to Alyson, the gay publishing house, but thought—apparently picking up on Essex's mention of his own early self-publishing outlet, Be Bop Books—a better solution might be for Essex to let Be Bop issue the poems: "There is no advantage to you," Goldin wrote, "to have us handle it as the little money it can earn should not be further diminished by our agency commission."

If Essex felt sadness or anger at these assorted rebuffs, he responded graciously. He did let Goldin know that his presentation at the Getty of "an overview" of his projects had been "very well attended by scholars and staff. The rumor is that they have not had so many guests for what are essentially private talks." But he'd also detected that among the "traditionalists" at the Center, "there is some skepticism . . . concerning the presence of someone like me"—perhaps in part a reference to his lack of scholarly credentials, but more likely an allusion to feelings of discomfort at having a black person, openly gay, in their midst—a reading Michelle Parkerson confirms. She was in L.A. shooting a film at the American Film Institute when Essex was at the Getty, and they got together twice in Santa Monica, where Essex introduced her to the Reel Inn, a wonderful seafood restaurant. He complained to Michelle that "some of the housekeeping staff at the Getty Center had very homophobic attitudes." In any case, Essex did his best to ignore the "skepticism"; instead he spoke glowingly about the wonderful apartment he'd been given and the "dependable and thorough" assistant he'd been assigned. He also made the firm decision to start saying no to invitations to speak, and in general to slow down.

At the midpoint of his yearlong residency, Essex's health worsened. The doctors he consulted diagnosed "intractable sinusitis" and "massive stress burnout," but when Essex discovered that his T cells had fallen to 23, he knew perfectly well that the underlying culprit was AIDS. "I am not too frightened," he wrote Frances Goldin, "but simply stated . . . all is a mess right now." He signed the letter with his standard "Take care of your blessings." For once, an interviewer asked Essex what he meant by that recurring phrase. In response he wrote, "Some of us bake wonderfully, write, paint, do any number of things, have facilities with numbers that others don't have. Those are your blessings. Some of us are very strong and candid and some of us are nurturers or combinations of all of those things. Just be aware of what your particular things are and nurture them and use them toward a positive way of living. That's simply what I mean."

In truth, Essex's own determination to maintain "a positive way of living" was beginning to fray. He had little energy toward the end of his stay at the Getty, and his spirits were only "fair." As a result, the pending anthology and novel were necessarily put on hold. When he did feel like working, he turned to what had always mattered to him most as a writer—poetry. And before leaving the West Coast, he did manage to complete a new series of poems, which he called "Vital Signs"—focused on the actuality of his advancing condition.

8

Breaking Down

Richard Dworkin was trying to figure out what to do about Mike's "disinterest in having sex." The love between them was never in doubt, but Mike, according to Richard, always had some reason for avoiding sex on a regular basis. Though he'd often and proudly proclaim that during the 1970s he'd been a "slut" who'd had three thousand men up his butt, of late he'd been feeling little or no interest in sex—with Richard or anyone else—though Richard would always be game. Mike (as Richard puts it), "was too busy, he was out of town; he was too tired; he was too sick; it was all these things. And there was just a point where I had to do something." Mike told his close friends a different story. He tearfully confided to one of them that his anal fissures made it necessary to "go slow," which put a damper on Richard's enjoyment and made him reluctant to have sex. Whatever the case, Mike, according to one of those friends, "felt like a failure as a partner and as a person."[1]

In any case, a point came in 1988, at the annual Garden Party benefit for the New York City Gay Center, when Richard met a young schoolteacher named Carl Valentino. They hit it off and went home together that same night, even though Carl was due to leave the very next day for summer vacation. When he returned to the city in the fall, he and Richard again got together, and that was the beginning of an affair that went on for about a year and a half. Carl had grown up in Brooklyn, the son of a grocer, and was somewhat active in gay politics, preferring to work behind the scenes. Carl was the kind of person who volunteered to be in charge of the table at an event, or to arrange with a deli to provide food for a committee meeting. He wasn't interested in getting the credit or becoming well known.

Richard made no effort to conceal his relationship with Carl from Mike, since they'd always been aboveboard with each other about everything, and in any case had never sworn fidelity on the altar of monogamy. Still, Richard sensed that on some level the news *had* upset Mike (a sense confirmed by Mike's close friends, to whom he confided his pain about Richard's affair). Perhaps feeling some guilt at not meeting Richard's sexual needs, Mike publicly professed himself happy that Richard was getting laid regularly—it took the pressure off him, he said, and their own relationship seemed more relaxed.

Richard was even happier. He had a devoted domestic life with Mike, and a good sex life with Carl. Everything seemed to be working out so well that Richard decided to introduce Mike and Carl to each other. That could have ended in disaster, but in fact the two liked each other. Both were outspoken, honest, and straightforward, and they became friendly; Carl started volunteering at CRI, and then at Mike's behest joined its board. But as with all Gardens of Eden, the snake in this particular grassy mound soon broke through: Carl fell deeply in love with Richard, who began to return the feelings.

Carl was the first to verbalize discontent: "I want somebody of my own," he'd tell Richard, "this arrangement is crazy." At the time, Richard and Mike had been renting a loft at Duane and Church Streets. After protracted problems with the landlord, and unable to afford litigation, they decided to accept the relocation payment he offered and find another apartment. The real estate market was booming in the late 1980s, and when they finally found a place on Eighth Avenue between Twelfth and Jane Streets, the rent was $1,800 for twelve hundred square feet. They took it, but knew they'd have to find a third roommate to help with expenses. Both of them thought of Carl, but he wanted no part of the arrangement, telling them they were out of their minds! Soon after, Carl broke off the affair with Richard. (Carl would soon become the "gay husband" of the famed avant-garde vocalist and composer Diamanda Galás, herself an AIDS activist and member of ACT UP.)

Two weeks later, Richard—though in no sense a superficial person—met Patrick J. Kelly ("PJ"), one of the head psychiatric nurses at St. Vincent's Hospital. Earlier, Patrick had been a member of the all-male drag troupe "Les Ballets Trockadero de Monte Carlo"—a gay male cultural institution still going strong in 2014. At the time they met, Patrick, who was HIV-positive, was, despite sixteen-hour shifts at St. Vincent's, somehow managing to finish up a master's degree at NYU and, as well, wrote occasional dance criticism for *Dance* magazine and for *New York Native*. He was (in Richard's words) "extremely intuitive, nonverbal; very smart that way, a whole different kind of intelligence. He was like the anti-Mike. Mike was extremely verbal, logical, rational, linear; and Patrick was the complete opposite. The two of them together were everything I could ever have imagined."

And so it began again, with Patrick and Richard sexually compatible and Mike sexually out of the picture and not having sex with anyone else. Patrick lived in an apartment building on Cornelia Street that was going co-op; he had the choice either of buying his place at the insider's price or of getting out. By today's standards, the down payment on the apartment was low, but it was still too high for Patrick to afford by himself. Early in 1991 Mike had gotten a $10,000 advance for the paperback edition of *Surviving AIDS*, so he and Patrick bought the place together—and then quickly resold it at a profit. That left Patrick still needing a place to live. What followed was an intricate set of readjustments.

As Richard knew, Mike had long wanted to leave New York, especially after he was diagnosed with KS. Part of his wish was to put the tensions of AIDS activism behind him, along with his inability to say no to people. His phone rang constantly with assorted requests: "Look, I know how over-committed you are, but it would be really helpful if you could come to just this one meeting"; or "my friend has just been diagnosed and is terribly depressed, could you spare a half hour to talk with him?"; or "we need you to be part of a delegation here, or to appear as part of a panel there—and could you let us know by Thursday?" Mike was too soft-hearted and conscientious to say no, which meant that he was constantly stressed-out about falling behind on his

commitments—since he also sat on the boards of several AIDS organizations and was periodically on tour with the Flirtations. When he
got the KS diagnosis, he felt for the first time that he wasn't going to
survive AIDS, which underscored his wish to get away from his multiple obligations.

For several years, he'd let Richard know that he wanted to move to
Los Angeles. Richard had been reluctant. He liked New York more
than the West Coast and relied on his involvement as a drummer with
various bands for both an income and a creative outlet. And then there
was his involvement with Patrick. Mike agreed to let Patrick move in
with them, but only on the condition that if Mike felt uncomfortable
or unhappy with the arrangement, Patrick would have to move out.
Richard feels, in retrospect, that, on an unconscious level, Mike agreed
to the move as a way of making it easier for himself to leave for L.A. It
had been intensely important to Mike from the beginning of their
relationship that Richard promise never to leave him, and Richard had
reassured him in that regard many times over. Neither of them had
dreamed that Mike would be the one to leave.

He made the decision to move to L.A. within a month of Patrick
moving in. It greatly upset Richard and he offered to ask Patrick to
move out. But Mike showed no sign of wanting to work things out. He
was determined to move. If Richard wanted to join him, Mike said,
that would be fine, but whether together or alone, he was definitely
moving to L.A. Richard (in his words) "felt trapped, and was really
angry about it." Mike had never before been unwilling to talk over a
problematic situation and seek a solution for it; now he "just clammed
up." For his part, Richard felt torn: "I felt that I had brought Patrick
into this situation, and was responsible for him in some way, so I
couldn't just say to him, 'Okay, bye, I'm moving to Los Angeles.' And
I didn't want to move to Los Angeles, anyway."

And so at the end of August 1991—while Richard was playing a gig
in Lugano, Switzerland—Mike told everyone that he was "taking a
hiatus from the fray." He packed his things and left. In L.A. he stayed
briefly with Richard's brother, who helped Mike get settled. Among
the few people on the West Coast he knew even slightly were the writer
and therapist Doug Sadownick and the performance artist Tim Miller,
co-founder of the prestigious theater space PS 122 in New York City

whose innovative solo pieces *Sex/Love/Stories* (1990) and *My Queer Body* (1992) were highly influential.

Once back in New York from Europe, Richard felt "really angry and really unhappy—it was one of the most unhappy times in my life." Mike tried to normalize the situation, but Richard, by his own admission, "was being stubborn and gruff, having none of it." He wrote Mike an angry letter, then quickly followed it with another saying that "what's so extraordinarily sad to me now about that angry letter . . . is that you may not be sure that I know what a sacrificing, good-hearted, caring, generous, loving person you have always been . . . But I *do* know, Michael."

For Richard, the relationship with Patrick, without Mike, somehow "didn't work as well." Patrick as "the anti-Mike, was fantastic." With the three of them together, Richard had felt he had it all. But when he and Patrick were left alone together, the space where Mike used to be felt empty and "huge." As Richard was well aware, the situation wasn't fair to Patrick: "He wanted to be with me, and I wasn't totally there." To make ends meet, they had to take in a roommate, and when Richard went off again on tour, Patrick found a guy who was not only into voodoo, but was also a scam artist. He ran up phone bills, bounced checks, stole their stuff—and then abruptly disappeared, owing them a considerable sum of back rent. And then Patrick himself started to fall ill and soon developed KS.[2]

Meanwhile in L.A., Mike was using every last ounce of his extraordinary willpower to try things that almost anyone else might have considered out of their—and his—reach. Like joining the O Boys (as in "Oh boy!" or "Orgy Boy"), a group of gay men who had started to organize safe-sex orgies; one of the party notices mailed out to the "Orgy Boy Network" captures the group's flavor:

> Some of you have said that the O Boys as a group should not be political. Wake up and smell the hot, ripe cum! This group's very existence is a political statement, and every time you attend a party, you are telling those sex- and self-hating idiots that we will do what we want with our bodies and they can never legislate our morality. Before getting started at a party, or between orgasms, talk to each other! Introduce the new guys around, exchange phone numbers, become friends!

Social politics can be as powerful as electoral politics—and it's always more fun. NOW, grab a dick and pop it in your mouth. Congratulations, you are now a sexual revolutionary!

The O Boys seized on Mike as (to quote Richard) "a sort of good-luck charm, a talisman, a fairy godmother, a patron saint of post-AIDS panic, post sex-negative, post-fear-driven gay male promiscuous behavior." They enjoyed having Mike around, and Mike enjoyed at least some return of his once expansive sex drive.

Mike felt that the O Boys, after a decade of sexual shell shock in the gay male world, represented "the exciting emergence of a new up-in-your-face radical, creative, friendly, hot, group-based sexuality" reminiscent of the pre-AIDS period but also dissimilar from it. This second sexual revolution, in his view, was more realistic about the body's physical limitations, and much more aware that the body wasn't an indestructible pleasure machine "requiring little more than a monthly shot of penicillin to keep it in good running repair." The O Boys were well aware that unsafe sex could kill you and were comfortable in enforcing safe-sex guidelines—of being their brother's keeper, if need be—thereby rejecting the view of the 1970s that it was basically every man abiding by his own guidelines.

They rejected, too, the 1970s tendency to view sex as a serious business, substituting the notion of sex as play; the central image Mike had of the O Boys was that of "week-old puppies in a cardboard box, playfully wrestling with each other for the sheer exhilaration of it." As Mike saw it, the O Boys emphasized friendliness over macho competition, throwing over the 1970s taboo of having sex with friends. In the 1970s the pattern was "to fuck first and then become friends," which inversely meant that once friendship was established sex was no longer an option. As Mike saw it, in the early 1990s, "the new sex radicals move with extraordinary ease from friendship to hot sex and back again." At one orgy he attended, he saw a group of five close friends "go from giggling to sucking and be-condomed fucking . . . [and] when the tidal wave of hot sex had passed, they adjourned upstairs to giggle some more over beers."

The O Boy emphasis on group-based sex gave actual life, in Mike's view, to that oft-cited but infrequently practiced axiom of the 1970s—the "brotherhood of lust." He knew that jack-off clubs had been founded in some urban areas at least as early as the late 1970s and acknowl-edged that "an important goal of the original sexual revolution was to explore creative alternatives to the heterosexual, monogamous dyad." With the second revolution, he felt that sex and sentiment—even love—were reunited. He also understood that outside of the larger cit-ies, most gay men were scandalized by what they viewed as the "ex-cesses" of the urban gay male ghetto. Yet the cutting-edge minority in the metropolises did set the tone—both for the generation of the 1970s and for that of the 1990s. Mike also acknowledged that the O Boys of L.A. were not alone: PRISM and the Jacks of Color, among other groups, were elsewhere roaming down the same paths.

None of this led Mike, despite all his fey effeminacy, to become a follower of Harry Hay's "third gender" theory or to join the group of Radical Fairies that exemplified it. He could flaunt his gender noncon-formity, and his campy wit embodied gay "differentness," but he didn't believe in gay *separateness*. Rather he felt that gay people had the re-sponsibility to share their unique subcultural values with the emo-tionally staid and ritually starved mainstream—gay *and* straight. Nor was he sympathetic to Hay's view that gay men and lesbians had little in common. At the least they shared a common enemy—homophobia. And ideally, in Mike's view, they could all benefit from the egalitarian values of the feminist vanguard.

One of the reasons Mike had given for moving to L.A. had been the need finally to concentrate on his music—both as part of the Flirta-tions and on his own. He said he wanted to write new songs and work on a new record, but for the first six months in L.A. he did little be-yond settling into substandard subsidized housing. For four and a half years he hadn't missed a single Flirts gig, but for now he was slow to pick up again with the group. Its four other members, Mike felt, were being "extremely generous and accommodating"—they even kept him on salary. They also suggested that he skip minor engagements and save his strength for the major ones. During the summer and fall of 1992, he was particularly active with the Flirts. And the gay critics continued to adore them, especially their gay-positive message—never delivered polemically but rather through witty asides and updated verses, such as "Give him two lips like Pagliacci / But not as closeted as Liberace."[3]

Periodically, though, his health would take a dive, and he'd have to retreat from the Flirts and return to the hospital for additional tests or treatments. He scribbled notes under the title "Dinosaur's Diary" (a few months later, under the same title, he'd publish a brief series in *QW*, which had become New York City's leading gay weekly). His first such column, handwritten while still in the hospital, is dated 1991:[4]

5:40 a.m.: ". . . the news that "Danny" [Sotomayor?] had died this morning—died primarily of KS of the lungs and its treatment—that same disease that everyone bustling about me here in the hospital appears to think I have but wouldn't say out loud . . . I kept saying to myself as I went in and out of my sleeping pill haze, this should depress me, this should be an ominous sign. But the cynic in me just couldn't convince the optimist that Danny's final freedom could possibly be bad for anyone, including me . . .

"A Hispanic, bearded man comes to wheel me down to OR [Operating Room] . . . I am a slab of meat which must somehow be defrosted and delivered to another floor . . . he's a man and . . . doesn't carry the burden of the expectation of *caring* . . . He's not mean or cold. I'm just a job, not an adventure. I don't take it personally and . . . when he delivers me into the hands of OR receiving, he makes one surprising, noble attempt to connect, mano a mano. He doesn't touch me—God forbid—but he says, 'Take care, man' . . . I very much want to acknowledge his attempt to connect—even if it's on a gendered bridge I do not like to cross. 'Thanks,' I whitely muster, and he's gone . . .

"My chest X-rays are missing. I'm made to feel vaguely responsible. Didn't I *know* that the procedure could not proceed without those X-rays? The head nurse phones up to my other nurse and firmly demands that my X-rays be brought down . . . The other two women have fallen on my chart and are devouring it . . . they cluck and sigh as they sort thru it. *Ah ha!* Papers are missing. They turn to me—on me?—'where are your CBC results? Did you give a urine sample?' . . . My bad diagnostic Karma continues . . . . My pulmonary specialist casually informs me that I've been 'bumped' to 1:00. 'Sorry,' he says, not being . . . I'd . . . more or less made a grumpy peace with the 4 hour delay when my main nurse mentions casually that she'd be back at 3 to prep me for my transport . . . I know with a sinking certainty that I've been unceremoniously bumped to 3:30 without so much as a thought. Courtesy, that's it. That's what gets lost in the shuffle of American health care delivery. Strangers come and go from your room, without knocking; you're handed pills to take without explanation; buzzers go off just as you're finally dozing off. It's a factory—a conveyor belt. It's not good will that's missing. Most of the people mean well . . . but you're expected to be sick by shift—on their rhythms . . .

"The women lost interest in me . . . One by one they exited until I was ominously alone—abandoned—and without my X-rays . . . Just as my anxiety was beginning to mix with my stomach acids, two black women entered chatting breezily . . . the older black woman noticed me. She stopped instantly . . .'Honey, you all alone here?' she asked. In an instant she was by my side. 'What's your name, sweetheart?' She was so soothing. She actually took my hand and started gently rubbing my right forearm, the one without the IV needle in it. She stage whispered to her companion that they'd have to stay . . .'It's not right to leave patients alone,' she said, with profound dignity and authority. We continued to make meaningless but meaningful chatter till the nurses returned . . .

"Entry of my doctor. Completely casual . . . I'm wheeled in and put happily out. I wake up one hour later in recovery. Groggy and hung over, throat sore, but ravenous."

Mike's hospital stay confirmed the diagnosis of extensive KS of the lungs. Essentially that meant, in his words, "I am, literally, breathless. I am drowning in my own blood. 'They' say a year, maybe two at best, which jibes with my own experience: I've never known a PWA who survived KS of the lungs much longer than that . . . Of course, the [Robert, the prominent NIH scientist] Gallo—or should I say [Martin] Delaney—miracle KS drug might yet save my life. Yeah, I'll hold what's left of my breath!" Mike's skepticism was understandable; Gallo's claim that the retrovirus HTLV-III caused AIDS had been disproven, and Delaney's Chinese cucumber (Compound Q) had also bitten the dust. (A reporter confided to Mike that when he contacted Delaney's Project Inform for Mike's number, he was told not to bother interviewing him—he was "an AIDS fraud.")

Mike of course regretted the failure of the assorted drugs and nostrums that for a decade had been periodically hailed as likely cures. Yet he didn't sink into the despairing state that so many others did in the early 1990s. Even some of the ACT UP vanguard began to lose confidence that the tactics of angry confrontation would yield medical dividends. Ironically, the plight of the dead and the dying had led to a greater acceptance of gay people than previously, but fear of jeopardizing that increased sympathy led the more conservative members of the gay community, and even some members of ACT UP, to urge an end to "excessive" direct-action tactics. The feeling spread that confrontational politics was played out, had outlived its usefulness.

The well-known gay conservative Andrew Sullivan wrote in the *New Republic* that the radicals of ACT UP did not represent the vast majority of gay people, who had assimilationist goals. And Randy Shilts, in an *Advocate* cover story, insisted that militant activism was no longer relevant. Of course, it never had been relevant to either Shilts or Sullivan. As well-positioned white men they could afford to champion "civility," confident that folks like *them* were well on the way to becoming full partners in the inner circles of American life. After all, hadn't Bill Clinton promised in his 1992 campaign for the presidency to overturn the ban against lesbians and gay men serving openly in the military, to make them equal-opportunity killers?[5]

Yes, he had. And though Clinton failed to follow through after winning the election—settling instead for the bizarre "Don't Ask, Don't Tell" policy, which wasn't rescinded until 2011—surely, many argued, his nod in the right direction was far preferable to the exclusionary disdain of the Republicans, to the harsh homophobia of the Reagan-Bush years. In the minds of many gay people, mainstream acceptance was gaining "obvious" traction, and ACT UP's bristling rage seemed to them largely irrelevant, if not downright counterproductive. Yet what that view failed to take into account was the fact that the search for effective treatments for AIDS had *still* come up empty-handed, and that the toll from the epidemic was *still* rising. In 1992 alone, the figures were staggering: 78,000 new cases, and some 41,000 people dead; worldwide the death toll had exceeded 200,000, with the World Health Organization estimating more than 13 million affected. The only treatments thus far had been the so-called nucleoside analogues— AZT, ddC, ddI—with a fourth, d4T, expected soon. But the 1993 Concorde study would soon conclude that these did little if anything to prolong life.

Where was the evidence that traditional forms of political action like electioneering and lobbying—or relying on mainstream sympathy and morality—were more likely than direct-action tactics to produce greater research energy and results? If Americans knew more history, they might have realized that if it hadn't been for thirty years of confrontational pressure from the abolitionist movement—to give but one example—slavery might well have expanded across the continent and become permanently entrenched.

The growing breadth of the AIDS crisis and the growing despair over its failure to produce efficacious treatments, in combination with internal divisions, led to ACT UP's slow decline and ultimate disintegration. In 1992, its Treatment and Data Committee, deeply knowledgeable about the science of AIDS and well connected to the world of establishment research, broke off from the parent group and refocused on *treatment* activism, leaving behind the social activism of the original ACT UP agenda—racism, classism, and sexism—to those primarily interested in them. Sentiments of solidarity weakened and then disappeared. Mike had pursued his AIDS activism outside the ranks of ACT UP, but his feelings of being overwhelmed by years of conflict, and his decision to leave New York, paralleled the decision of many in ACT UP to retreat from the fray and pursue individual salvation. What they shared was the sense that the struggle to save lives had come up empty.

Unlike many others, Mike didn't feel suicidal; what he felt was more like sadness and weariness, which he was entitled to, given how long he'd been pushing himself to the brink. His reduced lung capacity now had him huffing and puffing, further sapping his energy. He'd seen countless friends reach the late stage where he now was of KS of the lungs. Sometimes he even thought that "having some sense of WHEN one is going to die can be a blessing, if you work it right. It allows one to pace and prioritize and make peace." He'd long preached that PWAs should "listen to the wisdom of their own bodies," but he'd always been too steadily on the go to heed his own advice as much as he might have. As he put it, "I was too busy living at a furious pace to pay much attention to the aches and pains, fevers, rashes and diarrhea that constituted what I called my 'AIDS normal.'" It wasn't until he started to cough up blood and been diagnosed with KS of the lungs that he finally decided to "pamper" himself.

He started to shop, go to the movies, take a class to learn how to make puff pastry—he was already a wonderful cook whose repertoire included baking his own bread and making fresh strawberry sorbet. Then there was the "ecstasy" of ordering "a quintessential minestrone" at Café Benvenuto; of delighting in his collection of Betty Crocker fifties kitchen utensils; and of visiting his "favorite spot on earth"—the Huntington Gardens—the estate that contained seven different botanical gardens. Plus he read, and read, and "read some more." "I'm in HOG HEAVEN!" he wrote a close friend. He still felt "raw and bloody from selling my soul to the movement" but now he let sixty-five phone messages that "should" have been returned go unanswered and didn't go near—well, not for a while—the stack of correspondence and bills that had piled up. In retrospect, he couldn't imagine how he'd done all that he'd done for so long. He hoped he'd one day be able to return to the hectic life, and even developed a very clear image, should he get lucky, of what he'd look like as an old man—"cantankerous, opinionated, frisky."[6]

Despite his lack of energy, those first few months in L.A. seem to have been something like a genuine honeymoon for Mike. But his doctors made it clear that it would soon end, that he would have to start chemotherapy if he was to last even the year or two that they'd predicted. His first treatment, in the spring of 1992, was largely uneventful. He had some "vague, flu-like symptoms which were completely manageable with aspirin and anti-nausea medication." That made him totally unprepared for the trauma of the second treatment. It took only fifteen minutes and he left whistling, went to the gym and did yoga, soaked in the Jacuzzi while watching "all the naked gods walk by," came home and fixed himself a feast of fresh fruit and vegetables, went to a movie, read, and went to sleep thinking it had all been a "piece of cake."

Then—wham! He woke, at two a.m., with a high fever, teeth chattering, disoriented, and "with joints and muscles so aching that I literally couldn't lie down or sit up. It was sheer torture." Eventually he fell back to sleep, had a series of frightening dreams, and woke up *thirteen* hours later drenched in sweat and again disoriented. He called Joe Sonnabend in New York, who warned him that the effects from chemotherapy were cumulative and that from here on in he'd probably feel still worse. That shook Mike up. He didn't know if he could face "the geometric progression of traumatic side effects." Since the treatments were spaced two to three weeks apart, he decided to hang in for the time being. He did let his mother know about the chemo, and although she was terrified of flying, she told him that should he need her she'd be on the next plane.

Yet he realized that—to his own surprise—he still *did* want to record another album, or maybe even two. *If*, that is, he could manage it physically and financially. He had a friend in Chicago who swore he'd be able to find the money somewhere, somehow, to produce at least one of the albums. Mike thought of declaring bankruptcy in order to avoid paying some of his bills, and he missed Richard's practical-minded advice on such matters. He missed Richard, period. But he was also deeply angry at him, for what he saw as Richard's rejection. When Richard failed to return a phone call, Mike called again and accused him of having turned his back on the news that he had KS of the lungs, of not wanting to deal with it. According to the account Mike sent to a friend, he yelled at Richard that "the point is, if you'd wanted to speak to me, you'd have called back or written or found some way, and you didn't. I can no longer suffer such abuse, especially at this point in my life. I have my hands full. . . . *You* must sort out whether or not you're up to being involved in my dying process. If you decide not, I'll be sad, but I'll be fine."

Mike wasn't "exactly bitter." He was "still able to remember the good times," was still grateful to Richard "and his willingness, at the lowest possible moment of my life, to [quoting Archibald MacLeish] 'blow on the coals of my heart.' " But Mike did feel abandoned by him and even wrote about Richard in his occasional column, "Dinosaur's Diary," for *QW* magazine: "I miss my ex. To the extent that I ever thought about my death from AIDS, I always assumed he'd be there to help send me gently into . . . whatever. And his gruff forcefulness would be so *useful* to me now. *He'd* know what to do, my mind races. He'd sit me down and tell me what my priorities *ought* to be, and then he'd help me accomplish them. But the divorce has been unusually bitter and protracted. Now I'm very much alone."[7]

Richard read those lines in *QW* and felt deeply, deeply hurt by them. He knew—and so did Mike in his calmer moments—that they still loved each other, and he also knew that their relationship wasn't over. But at the moment he was dealing with Patrick's failing health, as well as having to travel with various bands in order to provide for some sort of income. Their story wasn't over, though what lay ahead would be equal parts comfort and desolation.

Nor had Mike ceased to be political, even—when his stamina allowed—actively so. He feared that the conservative segment of the gay community was in danger of capturing the dialogue about sex, that a *majority* of gay men and lesbians had arrived at essential agreement with their oppressors about what were or weren't "appropriate" forms of sexual behavior. Though Mike no longer patronized bathhouses and back-room bars, he continued to defend them—to defend any kind of sexual expression that wasn't mainstream or hetero-imitative—and he came to openly regret his role in helping the state to close the bathhouses and sex clubs in New York. Mike rejected any safe-sex guidelines that insisted on monogamy as the definition of "maturity"—let alone morality. He believed that gay men in the 1970s had "effected an unprecedented revolution in sexual practices" and the last thing he wanted was to see that legacy destroyed.

Mike was convinced that radical feminism continued to provide the best guide for safeguarding the sexual revolution. He agreed with its disavowal of the widespread notion that sex had been unchanging through time and across cultures, and he rejected the ingrained view that some forms of sex are "better"—healthier, more moral—than others. He felt it important to resist the notion that the particular sex acts *we* preferred "should" be the ones everyone preferred, and he deplored those countless "Eroticizing Safer Sex" workshops that parroted "politically correct" guidelines for all those "agonized, confused and conflicted gay men fearful of being drummed out of the fraternity of cool, AIDS-adjusted, post-AIDS babies." "A vast ocean of silence," he felt, "surrounds what gay men are actually doing—or actually want to be doing. There currently is no permission to discuss, calmly and rationally, the many gray zones of safe sex." The relative risks of some sexual acts were still surrounded, Mike felt, with confusing, contradictory, guilt-inducing guidelines. He rejected the view that every lesbian who refused to use a dental dam when engaging in oral sex, or every gay man who sucked dick without a condom, had a death wish. Mike's attitudes about current safe-sex guidelines prefigured a debate within gay male circles that was about to erupt. The gap between public HIV prevention messages (the "condom code") and the refusal in some gay male circles to abide by it was widening.[8]

More and more gay men were feeling that the condom code was inhuman; they chafed against the tight strictures that circumscribed sexual pleasure. They'd significantly reduced their levels of risky sexual behavior but were unwilling never again to experience the satisfaction of skin-to-skin contact or the intimacy of exchanging semen. They'd accomplished a remarkable degree of self-policing, and doubted that many heterosexual men, with their attitude of entitlement, could ever have achieved a comparable level of behavioral change—hell, most of them couldn't even sustain a diet or an exercise regime.

What's most remarkable about Mike's carefully composed arguments about issues relating to safe sex is that he still cared enough to make them. Here he was, undergoing the torments of chemo treatments, told that his life span would likely be about a year, living alone in a studio apartment in subsidized housing where the toilets still had pull chains and some of his possessions had been stolen from a storage room in the basement—and he was still employing what he called his "sick sense of obligation to others." Had he not been essentially modest, he might have substituted "noble" for "sick."

Essex, too, continued to engage with public issues, though his health was no less compromised than Mike's. He joined with Audre Lorde to do a joint reading, "Gay Art Against Apartheid," and when the prestigious *Journal of the History of Sexuality*—which at the time leaned heavily in the direction of LGBT content—published an essay by a black gay man that Essex found "ridiculous, pedestrian," he used the occasion as a means to make a larger point: namely, that the journal did not have a single black gay male on either its editorial or advisory boards. In his letter of protest to the editor, Essex forestalled one familiar response by writing, "please don't tell me there are no Black gay and lesbian scholars or scholars of color available to work with you all." He offered his help in recommending "a number of very capable and brilliant scholars to you."[9]

Like Mike Callen, Essex roused himself to protest despite increasingly precarious health. His T cell count—the prime indicator of the health of an immune system—had been steadily falling. "I have so little energy and I'm faced with so much to do," he wrote his agent, Frances Goldin. He did manage to complete his residency at the Getty Center, but his spirits were only "fair." Yet he did remain ambulatory, and even managed, occasionally, to travel and give a reading or talk. The Center for Lesbian and Gay Studies (CLAGS) put on an "An Evening With Essex Hemphill" in 1993, and, before a packed audience, he gave a vigorous, energetic performance and at the dinner for him afterward managed to more than hold his own in a brisk, even forceful conversation.

The effect of AIDS on public opinion had, with the election of Bill Clinton to the presidency in 1992, become something of a double-edged sword; heightened fear of gay men as "carriers" had become increasingly counterbalanced by mounting sympathy for their suffering. In 1993, Hollywood released the big-budget film *Philadelphia* about a sympathetically drawn gay lawyer with AIDS, played by Tom Hanks (for which he won an Oscar). The film went on to earn $125 million at the box office. Soon after, the singer Elton John came out, and a year after that, Greg Louganis, the multiple gold medal winner in Olympic diving, not only came out but revealed that he was HIV-positive.

None of which, needless to add, produced better treatments for AIDS, let alone a cure. By the early nineties, a pronounced demographic shift was taking place: 15 million people in sub-Saharan Africa were becoming infected, the large majority, in contrast with the United States, through heterosexual intercourse. This difference in transmission routes has never been fully examined or explained, though the dominant theory currently suggests that blood products rather than sperm is in Africa the primary culprit. In the United States by the mid-1990s, there were more new cases of AIDS among blacks than whites, with the large majority resulting from male-to-male contact (though a significant number did not self-identify as "gay").

The *New York Times* had greatly increased its coverage of the epidemic over the years, beating out all the other major dailies in the number of published articles on the epidemic. Yet only a shocking 5 percent of AIDS stories published between 1981 and 1993 focused on African Americans, and a mere 1.4 percent on Latinos—and most of those articles were about celebrity blacks like Magic Johnson and Arthur Ashe. (The figures would later go down still further. A Kaiser

Family Foundation study published in 2004 surveyed *all* media coverage on AIDS from 1981 to 2002 and found that only 3 percent focused on minorities.)

Nor was there a steady and reliable uptake in mainstream sympathy. When President Clinton ran into a barrage of opposition to his suggestion that the ban on gays and lesbians serving openly in the military be lifted, he quickly scurried for cover, settling on the "compromise" solution of "Don't Ask, Don't Tell"—which would remain official policy for another twenty years. *Newsweek* would (weirdly) write in 1993 that gay people were "the new power brokers," yet the early nineties saw a 30 percent increase in assaults and hate crimes against them. The dragon of homophobia had hardly been slain, and the seeming increase in respect and attention mostly amounted to a fragile inclusion pretty much confined to those gay people who looked and behaved like "normal" folks—meaning primarily middle-class white men who put their faith in polite lobbying, eschewed the confrontational tactics of a group like ACT UP, and shied away from any left-wing identification.

When I took part in the April 25, 1993, March on Washington, it seemed to me a bland, juiceless event that was more parade than protest—especially when contrasted with the earlier, more overtly political gay marches of 1979 and 1987. And the issue of AIDS no longer seemed in the forefront of concern, as it had been during the 1987 March. It was now one issue among many. If any theme was sounded with frequency, it was the new issue of "gays in the military"—an assimilationist goal that marked a new kind of gay movement, one that included AIDS as one among several issues of concern—along with the right to marry—and, further, replaced the raucous, direct-action demands of ACT UP with a "we're just folks" façade that no longer indicted social inequities but rather *requested* permission to "join up." Left-wing gays, now relegated to the sidelines, deplored the limited new agenda as an affront to the multiple sacrifices made and a dishonest disavowal of the special history and insights of a distinctive subculture. AIDS was being shoved to the margins by a polite new gay movement emphasizing an agenda of traditional values. More and more of its adherents felt it safe to emerge from the closet—even as they pushed the issue of AIDS into it.

Even before the gay movement started its march toward innocuous centrism, Essex had long since rejected it as irrelevant to the needs of black gays and lesbians. He didn't feel the movement had ever understood that for black gays "our sexuality doesn't lessen the chance of us being randomly shot or harassed by the police. Any of the fears black men have, our sexuality doesn't exclude us from them." Even had his health been better, Essex wouldn't have considered joining the vapid 1993 parade. And his health wasn't better. Like Mike, he was by now receiving periodic blood transfusions, which did increase his energy level, but only for a short period. He didn't consider himself depressed, but he did "at times feel mentally debilitated." Never one to zone out on television, he now wasn't much interested in reading, either.

A kind of stasis had set in, during which he listened to an enormous amount of music, "mostly jazz, some classical, and some classic rhythm and blues and pop." Music had always been important to him—Nina Simone a special favorite, a "fine inspiration"—but now it consumed much of his time. It was hard for Essex to accept the "slowdown" in his life "simply because I've always been so driven and so curious about things." Fortunately, he was "in love with" his apartment, and once, when out on an infrequent walk, he came across an old oak school desk in a secondhand store in the neighborhood—and was thrilled. The shop owner suggested that he refinish the surface, covered as it was with pen carvings, ink drawings, "and the names of school kids in love." But Essex chose to clean it with Murphy soap and coat it with polyurethane; he didn't "want to rob the desk of its history."

He did start to write just a little, "but it seems to take so much effort at this time." He slowly got back to revising a long poem that had begun "as a highly internalized poetic narrative," to which he gave the poignant title "Vital Signs." It would appear in 1994 in *Life Sentences*, a collection of memoirs, poems, and interviews relating to AIDS and edited by Thomas Avena, the founder of *Bastard Review*, a literary periodical out of San Francisco (Avena himself later died of AIDS). His connection with Essex went back to 1988, when Avena had published and edited the journal *89 Cents*, in which one of Essex's most powerful poems, "Heavy Breathing," appeared:

> At the end of heavy breathing
> the dream deferred
> is in a museum

under glass and guard.
it costs five dollars
to see it on display.
We spend the day
viewing artifacts,
breathing heavy
on the glass
to see—
the skeletal remains
of black panthers,
pictures of bushes,
canisters of tears.

Essex had found Avena to be a sympathetic, sensitive editor and subsequently gave him two of his other major poems, "Tomb of Sorrow" and "Civil Servant," for the *Bastard Review*. In a letter accompanying the poems Essex urged Avena to "please feel free to be very demanding of this work. I have been quite demanding of it myself, but I can demand more from it. I look forward to your commentaries. And, you don't have to be gentle with the knife." Essex found Avena's subsequent edits incisive and decided to entrust him with "Vital Signs," the longest and among the richest of his poems. The tone throughout is elegiac, a gallant but sorrowful recollection of times past and a future foreshortened:[10]

. . . come stir
the ink blue dusk with me,
come stir it with me
'til it's thick enough
to rub onto our skins,
massage into our thirsty pores and follicles,
so that distant stars
might see themselves
reflected in our shiny
new blackness,
and the planets, too,
and the galaxies
where our new names await us

in full bloom, their succulence,
the taste of victory will dribble
down the sides of our mouths,
sweet juice that will cause us
to be high with liberation
when we announce our new names.

In the internally subtitled "The Faerie Poem," Essex recalls his earlier self:

Once upon a time
I was black and fertile,
I was virile, coltish,
straining leashes,
refusing collars.
Once upon a time
balls of energy
exploded from
my fingertips,
rolled out of me
in brilliant flashes
that blinded
even me.

But that time, he knows, is past. Now, with apparent transparency and acceptance, he quietly laments his changed self:

With twenty-odd T cells
I am nearly defenseless
and counting. I have to learn
multiplication tables, after all,
and put them to wise use.

I am not the wand waver
you may be quick to recall.
I cannot make another thing
disappear. The illusionist tricks
all fail me now,

they draw on my strength
in ways that endanger me.

With deliberate artlessness, Essex gravely considers his remaining options:

In the cluttered afternoons
I rearrange little bits
of my person.
I carefully excavate
those memories
that are most delicate
And for that reason
could still cause
harm and injury.
and I thought
these would be my tasks
when I became an old man,
but I am clearly
not a prophet or a seer.

At the close of "Vital Signs," Essex returns to prose, as if it was the more appropriate form for expressing the factual:

Some of the T cells I am without are not here through my own fault. I didn't lose all of them foolishly, and I didn't lose all of them erotically. Some of the missing T cells were lost to racism, a well-known transmittable disease. Some were lost to poverty because there was no money to do something about the plumbing before the pipes burst and the room flooded. Homophobia killed quite a few, but so did my rage and my pointed furies, so did the wars at home and the wars within, so did the drugs I took to remain calm, cool, collected. . . . Actually, there are T cells scattered all about me at doorways where I was denied entrance because I was a faggot or a nigga or too poor or too black. There are T cells spilling out of my ashtrays from the cigarettes I have anxiously smoked. There are T cells all over the floors of several bathhouses, coast to coast, and halfway around the world, and in numerous parks, and in countless bars, and in places I am forgetting to make room for other memories. My T cells are strewn about like the leaves of a mighty tree, like the fallen hair of an old man, like the stars of a collapsing universe.

In a real sense, Essex had written his own obituary.

He still hoped to revise "Standing in the Gap," the novel that hadn't found any takers on a first go-round, and he hoped, too, to get on with the anthology he'd contracted for of short fiction by black gay writers. At the margins he entertained the notion of a third project as well: "The Evidence of Being," narratives of older black gay men, but there's no indication that he ever started on a series of interviews. There were still a number of days during 1994 when he felt energized and clear-headed enough not only to write, but also to plan on attending and presenting work at this or that event, and he even gave thought to ap-plying for a Guggenheim fellowship. He did manage one trip from Philadelphia to New York City and one to Washington, D.C., to see his mother and his siblings. In the closing section of "Vital Signs" he'd written about "the love and anger my mother and I hold for one another," and the visit to her was "exhausting" for him but made his mother "very happy."[11]

Essex had long felt especially close to his middle sister, Lois Holmes. When growing up he'd helped her with her handwriting and taught her how to play baseball. As an adult he'd always send her some money, when he had any to spare, to help raise her son, and was "always there for her when she needs to talk or get something off her chest." In a poem entitled "Thanksgiving 1993," which he probably wrote after his trip home, he may well have been referring not to his generic "black sisters" but specifically to his own family members:

> I feel sorrow for my heterosexual sisters
> who made the mistake of marrying men
> beyond redemption, men beyond
> the learning of new tricks.
> I feel dread for what hell
> their married lives must be like, sordid
> in how many unimaginable ways?
> their barking, brutish, bullish husbands

are dense to change and insecure
I would wish such misery
upon none that I know,
the curse of having a dullard,
loud-mouthed husband in tow.
I feel sorry for my heterosexual sisters
who have staked their loyalties
in men who fear not the fall of night,
but the start of each new day.[12]

Essex continued to write sporadically, and he even managed a new romance with someone named Roger—though it was soon over ("it is the best decision"). He began, though, to withdraw increasingly "to deal with my stuff"; to Barbara Smith he wrote vaguely of "some interior issue" he had to resolve. As always, he tried hard to stress the positive: "I just remember to say 'thank you' for every day I am able to have. I don't really desire too many things other than the chance to keep creating."

9

Wartime

There were piles of papers everywhere in Mike's tiny apartment—bills to pay, letters to answer, catalogues, books—"*There's so much still to do!*" Mike lamented. He worried about his legacy. "It's begun to dawn on me that some people misinterpret my *message* of hope to mean that everyone with full-blown AIDS won't necessarily die of it. *I have never said any such thing!* Instead, what I've wracked up 180,000 air miles trying to explain is that *no one diagnosed with AIDS needs to die on cue!* That's a very different message. Long-term survival is possible; my own life proves it."[1]

Unexpectedly, he thought for a time that he might even beat KS of the lungs. He put out an all-points bulletin on the PWA grapevine asking if anyone out there had survived pulmonary KS for more than two years. No one replied yes. The sole response he got—both from PWAs and from his doctors—was that chemotherapy was his only option. But he was already doing chemo, and he hated the way it made him feel. After a long internal debate, he decided that quality of life was what he valued most, and he made the decision to stop additional chemo treatments. No sooner had he done so than he worried that the decision was "inconsistent with my AIDS philosophy" to keep fighting. From that, he began to think about exploring some long-shot treatments, though for a decade he'd been advising PWAs *against* trying every touted drug that came along.[2]

As if on cue, he got a phone call from Dr. Joan Priestly, the most famous holistic doctor in L.A. For three months he'd been doing her megavitamin regimen, largely to silence his many New Age friends. She was calling to tell Mike that she'd heard through the grapevine about his pulmonary KS and had managed to get him a free month's supply of aloe vera juice, and had also pulled some strings to get him into the Search Alliance shark-cartilage (the latest "miracle" cure) protocol.[3]

Mike decided that both sounded harmless enough to be worth a try; they met his long-standing condition for experimental treatments—that (unlike AZT) "they couldn't hurt" and *might* help. He gave the aloe vera juice only a halfhearted try, now and then taking a gulp but usually "forgetting" to. The shark cartilage was another matter. The taste and smell were vile—in Mike's words, "dead fish left out in the sun to rot for, oh, say, two weeks, then powdered." He was told to swallow a tablespoon in V8 juice three times a day, but after a week he knew he couldn't continue. He called the doctor running the protocol, who suggested that rather than quit, he should try retention enemas. Mike joked (not to the doctor) that since he "hadn't had sex in eons," he'd give the enemas a try.

Simultaneously, he tried to persuade the radiologist who'd been treating the KS lesions on his leg to irradiate his lungs. After consulting with other radiologists, she gave him a definitive no—a word not in Mike's vocabulary. He kept tenaciously after her and she ultimately consented, against her better judgment, to irradiate *one* of his lungs, and only at a low dosage—and told him frankly that the treatment wouldn't work.

Two weeks later, after completing ten treatments of 100 rads each on his right lung, he went in for an X-ray to see the results. He heard a scream from the control booth, followed by both the technician and the radiologist rushing into the room to tell him, "It's gone! All the KS is gone! Your right lung is whistle clean!" No one, including Mike, could believe it. To check if the results were a fluke, Mike did a repeat X-ray two weeks later. The result was the same: the KS in his right lung had completely regressed. Everyone was nonplussed—except for the doctor running the shark-cartilage protocol. He claimed to have seen the same miraculous results in seven of the ten people in his trial who were taking the cartilage while doing low-dose radiation. His theory was that the combination selectively inhibited the formation of cancerous blood vessels, and he promptly started lobbying the manufacturer of the cartilage to provide funds for additional protocols. Mike's advice to all concerned, and especially to himself, was: "PLEASE remain skeptical!"

Cruelly, his advice proved altogether accurate. Within a short period, KS in his right lung reappeared, and the initial shark-cartilage/radiation sensation could never be replicated. Nor did any plausible explanation for its stunning initial effect ever emerge. Too many people saw Mike's X-rays for the temporary disappearance of KS in his right lung to have been merely the hallucinatory product of wishful thinking. The desperate hope for amelioration from the horrors of AIDS had long produced a series of drugs that had been initially heralded but had failed to live up to the claims in their behalf—from suramin and Peptide T to ddI and ddC. Even Mike, who'd long fought against the promiscuous practice of "drugs into bodies," had briefly succumbed to its siren song—and with the same empty result as from all the preceding "miracles." As it was, he was continuing to take thirty-five to fifty pills a day, mostly preventive medications for MAI (a form of tuberculosis), pneumonia, herpes, antifungal and antiparasitic infections, and the like. He also installed an oxygen tank in his apartment.

Mike, unlike so many, was not easily crushed. Faced yet again with the hard-nosed fact that in all likelihood he had only about a year to live, he started taking imipramine to ward off incapacitating depression and turned all his energy to leaving behind some legacy in music. He was down to 25 percent lung capacity—"I feel like a bicycle tire with a slow leak," he'd say—but remained intent, somehow, on being productively and artistically fulfilled. He was determined—and Mike's determination was no trifle—to leave behind "some semblance of the art I might have made over a normal lifetime." And he wanted to go out "resplendently, redundantly, relentlessly gay-celebratory." He told a group of friends that "before I die I want to see a film that even remotely reflects the sexual reality of my life"—that is, one that would show a man with AIDS continuing to have sex *responsibly*. He also claimed that he'd be leaving $1,000 in his will "for throwing a memorial orgy" and even had what he called the "demented" idea of placing an urn with his ashes in the middle of it.

But then, out of the blue, friends in New York City told him about yet another new drug, DaunoXome, and Mike made any number of failed attempts to secure it. Just as he was about to give up, he got a call from a friend, the philanthropist Judy Peabody—a doyenne of New York society long active on behalf of people with AIDS—imploring him to pursue Doxil (liposomal-coated Adriamycin), another experimental chemo drug. She'd heard that Doxil was working in trials—at least in the sense of gaining additional time—in 65 percent of patients with ovarian or KS cancers.

Mike agreed to try it, and contacted the company that manufactured Doxil. Unlike his previous experience with drug companies, Liposome Technology of Menlo Park reacted with courtesy and kindness. Doxil's principal investigator, Melody Anderson, recognized Mike's name, and when he suggested L.A.—many of his friends, like him, were out of options—as one of the sites for the trial of Doxil, she flew there in person, and within a remarkably short time Mike was one of the first three patients being infused with the drug. He was, as usual, skeptical, since Adriamycin had a bad reputation among PWAs who'd tried various chemical options.

To his surprise, the infusions produced no negative side effects. Better still, he stopped losing hair, his lung capacity slowly began to return, the external KS lesions on his legs seemed to shrink in size, and the swelling in his right leg went down dramatically—though the doctors had told him it never would. "Before I got this drug," Mike wrote a friend, "each day I grew weaker and thinner and something inside my body said quite distinctly: 'Prepare.'" He began to urge others to enlist in Doxil trials, yet always with the caution that long-term toxicities might well develop further down the line. But for the moment at least, he felt "Doxil has given me my life back—in the sense of both length and quality." Yet there was no change in the X-rays of his lungs. Alas, just as Mike had warned, the effectiveness of the drug proved strictly short-term, and in January 1993 he was back in the hospital.

The doctors told him flat out that because he'd already had one remission, when lung cancer returned it would be typically more difficult to treat and he had a 70 percent chance of being dead in two months. Yet when the two months had elapsed, Mike was still alive;

once again, he'd beaten the odds. He decided to go back on chemo every two weeks, and it was soon "kicking the SHIT" out of him. He was released from the hospital, but his apartment took on the look of a ward—three large machines to produce oxygen, pills, needles, and needle disposals stacked high, and an IV pole for IV antinausea medication. He endured a week of incapacitating panic attacks, and having earlier decided to go back into therapy, he now activated the decision. His therapist prescribed a high dose of Xanax and he started sleeping twelve to fourteen hours a day, which wasn't at all like him. In his own estimate, he had only enough energy to accomplish about 10 percent of what he used to be able to do on a given day. His white cell count was also dangerously low, and he had to give himself daily injections.

Despite it all, he refused to give up and wait for death to overtake him. Crucially, he decided to put in a call to Richard and simply said, "Look—I really want to do another album. I don't know if I can do it, but I want to try. Will you help me?" Richard had long been unhappy about their separation and the unresolved anger between them, yet given Patrick's poor health, he told Mike that he'd need a little time to think it over. Patrick cut through Richard's doubts: "Look: Michael loves you; you love Michael; you need to go there and do this. If it involves making music, great. But you guys need to go and hang out. This is a way for you guys to be together at the end of Mike's life. . . . If you don't patch it up with him, you're gonna regret it the rest of your life."[4]

Richard agreed. He flew to L.A. early in 1993 and within a few days he and Mike (who Richard thought looked "deathly") went into a tiny project studio at Trax Recording. They wheeled the oxygen tank into the studio and made a list of songs to work on, starting with the easiest, "Better in the Moonlight," the silliest song Mike ever wrote. Richard sat in the small control room with an engineer he'd never met, and they started. It wasn't a promising beginning, but rather "very fragile, very tenuous." Yet it proved three necessary things: that despite pulmonary KS, Mike could still sing, that it made him "really happy" to be in a studio, and that the two of them "really did love each other and really did want to do this together."

The remaining big question was how to finance the project. It turned out that Patrick, though a nurse by profession, somehow had a knack for fund-raising. He volunteered to write a solicitation letter and sent it out to Mike's huge mailing list; it included most of the people who'd bought *Purple Heart* or *The Flirtations*, supported the PWA Coalition, or simply knew Mike from his years spent on the AIDS front lines. Patrick and Richard also arranged a fund-raiser in New York City at the Perry Street Theatre. In the end hundreds of people contributed— including Mike's good friends womyn's music singers Holly Near, Cris Wiliamson, and Tret Fure. The gay porn star Scott O'Hara gave $1,000. In all, nearly two hundred people gave time or money to the project. And Mike's mother, bucking his father, contributed $4,000 to the effort and enclosed a sweet, short note saying how proud she was to be contributing to the album. It deeply touched Mike.[5]

With the money raised, Richard was able to find three first-rate studios, one each in L.A. and San Francisco, and the famed Sear Sound in Manhattan (Walter Sear's AKG C-12 microphones and the Neve board were fantastic and his clientele included, among others, Paul McCartney, Phish, David Bowie, Steely Dan, Wynton Marsalis, and Norah Jones). Besides raising money, the process of producing a record involved the usual time-consuming tasks of choosing material, finding arrangers, booking musicians and engineers, and scheduling rehearsal sessions. Thanks to technological advances, musicians no longer had to be in the same room on the same day in order to eventually be heard playing together. So Mike, say, might go to Trax in L.A. and record his vocals on one day, and then weeks or months later, musicians at Sear Sound in New York might come in and play along with his recordings, all of it later mixed together into stereo tracks that were then mastered, sequenced, and released.[6]

The process was long. The very first day in a studio, Mike (in his words) "sang the tits off three songs," and Richard said it was some of his best singing ever. With three completed recordings that hadn't made it onto his first album, *Purple Heart*, they already had six songs practically completed "vocally." By the end of March 1993, Mike had recorded no less than thirty-four songs toward what he hoped would be a two-CD album, to which he gave the tentative title *Legacy*. He felt deeply certain that the massiveness of the project was helping to keep him alive.

How could he have possibly made those recordings, given the increasingly desperate state of his health—not to mention the dismal state of his personal finances? The answer surely centers on his astonishing willpower, but at least as essential was the commitment of Richard—along with selfless assistance from Patrick. In the early months of 1993, Mike was still doing chemotherapy every few weeks, and for a week or so after each round of treatment, he'd be knocked out and unavailable, necessitating a rejuggling of schedules all around. Richard, too, had to travel back and forth regularly to New York to keep both his personal and professional lives intact.

With 75 percent of his lung capacity gone, no one could have predicted how well Mike would be able to sing. But it quickly became clear that—somehow—he was singing remarkably well. Had they known that at the top, they would have done all the material on *Legacy* from scratch, avoiding many of the additional hassles that stretched over an eight-month period. As it was, the final two-disc album would run the gamut. It would include three songs recorded in the 1980s: "The Healing Power of Love," "No No" (from a Lowlife recording), and "We've Had Enough," done in the late 1980s for a documentary film produced by the Testing the Limits Collective. Mike's voice had changed two years earlier; he lost three notes off the top and picked up four at the bottom, which meant that the 1993 songs resonated in a distinctly different way from his earlier recordings. Also the technical quality on the three from the 1980s wasn't as good as the music and background vocals—though they were able to redo those in 1993 with far better equipment.

Mike was having such a good time and felt so happy during the sessions that Richard let him give free rein to his perfectionism and do a lot of vocal takes. He describes Mike lying on the floor of the recording booth to rest while Richard worked with the musicians on an arrangement. When that was set he'd signal "okay" to Mike, who'd get himself up from the floor and sing an incredible take. Then he'd have a sip of Coke out of a can and lie down again, until it was once more time to sing. "It was," Richard later said, "one of the most incredibly miraculous things I've ever been involved with. It was transformative . . . and it was certainly perceived that way by the many people who were involved in it." In March Mike reached a different sort of landmark: he became the longest survivor of pulmonary KS in the country.

In April, all hands took a break from working on the album, while Richard fulfilled an earlier commitment to do a monthlong three-band bus tour of the United States. Before leaving, he arranged with Patrick and Carl Valentino (Richard's previous lover) to throw a birthday party for Mike in D.C., where he was scheduled to sing, somehow, at the March on Washington. As it turned out, the leader of the band Richard was touring with came down with appendicitis, which allowed him to show up in person in D.C. to hear Mike sing "Love Don't Need A Reason" at the March—his last big moment in the public eye. Mike told a reporter, "I *had* to be here. The 1987 march was the most amazing day of my life. To see a *million* gay people together . . . We *owned* this town. I need that shot of life again."

That same week in D.C. Mike rejoined the Flirts for three sold-out concerts, his farewell engagements with the group. At the last of the three engagements, with Richard present, Mike took a moment at the end to announce his retirement, telling the audience that "I decided a long time ago that when I could no longer meet my own impossible standards, I would not do the [Judy] Garland thing, where people are thinking, 'Oh my God, will he make it through?'" After the concert, Mike sat out in the lobby of the theater and people came up to him "like it was an audience with the Pope" (as Richard later put it). People knew they were saying good-bye to him. A few of the faces were familiar, but most of them were people he'd never met who wanted to tell him that he'd influenced or touched them in some way. According to Richard, Mike was really able to accept the compliments, unlike earlier in his life when his perfectionism would have had him obsessing about having flubbed this note or said that "wrong" thing. He stayed in the lobby until everyone who wanted to talk to him had managed to.

During his reunion with the Flirts, Mike picked up some negative vibes; as he put it, "things are strangely tense. There's resentment underneath the surface, on my part as well as theirs." It stayed bottled up during the concerts in Washington, but in mid-June 1993, when Mike and Richard were at Sear Sound in midtown Manhattan, for further work on the *Legacy* album, the Flirts made it clear that they resented the limited role assigned them for the recording, and in particular the fact that other singers were doing most of the backups. During his time in L.A. Mike had met some of the best pop backup singers around: David Lasley, Arnold McCuller, and Diane Graselli. Lasley and McCuller had sung on hundreds of records, and toured with James

Taylor for decades, and Lasley, a much-admired songwriter, had written for, among others, Peter Allen, Anita Baker, and Chaka Khan.

It irked Richard that the Flirts chose to air their grievances in a recording studio that was costing $150 an hour. Richard had suggested that they record "Two Men Dance the Tango," but when they refused, he thought they were being willfully uncooperative and got angry; "it's Mike's album," he thought but didn't say. "He's asking you to do this; why would you turn down his last request?" It was finally agreed that the Flirts would do a Henry Mancini song—not a capella, but with a piano—a song they'd had in their repertoire for a while. But when it came time to record, Jon Arterton got busy videotaping the group—while the engineer in the control booth, and Richard, stood by and stewed.

According to Mike, "voices were raised, temper tantrums were thrown"—and a disgusted Richard decided to shut down the session. He told the Flirts, "Look, I'll work on something else. Why don't you guys go in the lounge, and talk about things." And they did, along with Mike. He opened himself up to them completely: "Look, you may not believe it, but I'm dying . . . and I'm trying to make this record. . . . If you guys want to be a part of it, great, let's go in and sing this song. If you don't, fine. But I need to get on with what's remaining of my life." The Flirts finally did go in and do the recording, but Mike "never had the feeling of closure. . . . I barely survived that weekend. I felt like I was a not yet quite-dead carcass whose bones were being picked by the crows." It should be said on the Flirts' behalf that they weren't alone in their skepticism that Mike was actually dying. He'd survived eleven years since his diagnosis back in 1982, and many people thought that either he didn't have AIDS or, if he did and had survived this long, he'd continue to survive. Those who loved him had their own reasons for denying how close to death he actually was.

In New York, Mike suddenly got terribly sick—"I can't recall ever being more weary—cosmically soul weary and physically weary," he'd later write—and he had to fly back to L.A. on an emergency basis. Tests showed that he was anemic and had developed "an out of control, painful candida infection of the esophagus and the LARYNX." He knew that AIDS was "closing in," that he was "running out of gas." In the hospital they gave him daily EPO shots and two units of packed red cells to combat the chemo, his only remaining hope of gaining a little more time.[7]

When he was able to return to his apartment, Mike wrote a very long letter to the Flirts, in which he tried to resolve the tensions between them. He confessed that he'd "felt 'guilty' for some time about not including more of the Flirts, together and/or individually" on *Legacy*. He realized that Cliff Townsend considered the song "Sometimes a Throwaway"—which Mike had asked them to do—to be indeed a "throwaway," but Mike didn't agree. He'd sometimes made fun of the song himself, but he still thought it "an exquisite song" that would be a standout on the album, and he wanted to include it.

Mike thought the difficulties that had arisen between them had deep roots, and in his letter he expressed his willingness to talk them through. He spelled out by mail his own understanding of the assorted grievances on both sides. He confessed, first of all, to having felt hurt that the Flirts hadn't asked him to participate more fully on their recent second album, since he'd been a founding member and at that point hadn't retired. Additionally, he felt that—as with his biological family—he'd learned it was possible to love someone "and at the same time admit that THEY DRIVE YOU NUTS." He'd gradually learned to ignore his "best-little-boy-in-the-world" tendencies to placate and avoid unpleasantness at all cost, and had learned in its place "that healthy fighting is part of healthy loving."[8]

He felt, too, that all along there'd been some tension and jealousy about his separate identity from the Flirts. Unlike the rest of the group, Mike had never felt that the Flirts was his top priority and commitment. He "LOVED being part of the Flirts," he wrote them, "and I have loved each of you in my malformed way." He believed he'd done his best "not to work my divadom—my AIDS notoriety"—and had "RUTHLESSLY fought the tendency," yet he told them frankly that he believed his renown had helped them in getting gigs and interviews (though feathers *would* get ruffled when interviewers singled Mike out for special attention, as they often did). He acknowledged that one source of tension within the group was his "impossible demands for perfection," his cynicism, his "trashing every note and every performance," his inability to relax and enjoy. Richard, he reported, had "always yelled at me to work my individual career more, which I don't think I did."

With *Legacy*, though, Mike had finally put the focus on himself, and he'd had to decide how to use his various friends on the album. He'd already gotten considerable flack from one friend for not including her as a backup singer, even though they'd worked together earlier in Mike's career. In the upshot the Flirts *did* agree to perform "Sometimes Not Often Enough," as well as "Two Men Dance the Tango" and "Redesign the Family." But Mike also insisted on including Cris Williamson, Holly Near, and Tret Fure on the album, all of them dear friends as well as musical partners.

At one point he spent three days with Williamson and Fure at their house in Oregon, recorded backups on several songs for their forthcoming album, and sang with them—along with Holly Near and her accompanist John Bucchino—at the twentieth-anniversary concert for the feminist Olivia Records. Mike had regarded that day as "perhaps the best day of his life," and to celebrate, Patrick hired a stretch limo and the whole group dined in style at Alice Waters' famed restaurant Chez Panisse. The next day they insisted Mike ride on the Olivia float in the San Francisco gay pride parade: "No-one knew," he later wrote, "what to make of this cadaverous man in a FLIRT jacket, but everyone was lovely to me and I nearly swooned with pleasure to be in such august company." On the whole, Mike felt he'd done the best he could and had included on the *Legacy* album as many artist friends as he was able.

By the end of June 1993, nearly all the basic tracks were done, and Mike completed his own lead vocals by August 19. In sum, he'd recorded fifty-two songs—"3 hours, 20 minutes and 7 seconds worth," as he put it. Mike had composed about half of them; the other half he'd been singing for years or were songs "by friends I love." He felt "the only common theme is a celebration of a love of life and a celebration of diversity, especially sexual." He was "immensely satisfied with what's been done so far. I think it's the best singing I've ever done in my life. . . . I'm happier than I've ever been and more artistically fulfilled."[9]

A large amount of additional work was still left to do on *Legacy*—backups, replacing instrumental tracks, artwork, printing, mixing, mastering, pressing, distribution, and so on. And they were almost entirely out of money. The pressure was intense, with Mike having a series of anxiety attacks, one of which landed him in the emergency room. He was lucky, though, with his friends. He and Richard had known the performing artist Tim Miller and his lover Doug Sadownick, the writer (and later therapist), when they all still lived in New York. Tim and Doug had moved to the West Coast before Mike, and when he first arrived in L.A. they'd done a lot to help him get settled. And they stuck with him after his health began to slide. Though Tim sometimes found Mike a little "unforgiving of fools," Doug became one of his closest friends and, as it would turn out, also his chief caregiver in L.A.

As Mike's health began to deteriorate rapidly in early fall 1993, Richard got to L.A. as often as he could manage, but he was also contending with the simultaneous decline of Patrick's health in New York. For lack of a better word, Mike had again taken to referring to Richard as his "lover"; though they essentially lived on separate coasts, he felt that the love between them had deepened, and Richard felt the same, though he also cared deeply for Patrick. Mike had himself come to like Patrick enormously, and the two of them began fantasizing about buying an apartment in L.A. for the three of them. Patrick had cashed in his life insurance policy and suddenly had a considerable sum of money at hand, and he and Mike actually began apartment hunting when Patrick came out to visit in late September. But it was of course a pipe dream. Mike was soon in the hospital more than he was out of it.

By September 1993, he'd lost more than 10 percent of his body weight, was sleeping badly, and was constantly nauseated and cramping, alternating between the runs and severe constipation. He also developed acute anemia; at one point he lay for twenty-four hours on the floor, literally unable to move. He became so sick to his stomach that he—the ultimate chatterbox—was unable to stay on the phone with friends for more than ten minutes at a time before abruptly "having to go." The doctors insisted that he try THC (marijuana) pills to improve his appetite, and when he did, he promptly got the munchies. But though he was on the lowest dosage (2.5 mg.), he got high and paranoid, which he hated; and anyway, no sooner did the THC wear off than he was back to feeling exhausted and crampy. The doctors decided to do a colonoscopy and tried to prepare him for a diagnosis of CMV ulcers or KS of the gut—but to everyone's surprise he turned out to be "whistle clean up there."

While Richard was busy putting together odds and ends for *Legacy*, Patrick kept Mike company in the hospital. At one point, after the nurse had taken Mike's temperature, Patrick casually asked her to take his as well. It was 101.3. Patrick knew he was sick; he'd been developing KS lesions, including some on his penis. But he seemed unfazed and preferred talking about his up-and-coming scuba-diving trip with Diving For Life, an organization he'd put together to raise money for AIDS-related causes. When Richard dropped by the hospital room, Patrick was taking a break in the corridor and Mike used the opportunity to tell Richard about Patrick's temperature reading, to say that he was really worried about him and thought he had TB, or possibly PCP.

Soon after, Mike was released from the hospital, Patrick returned to New York to get ready for his scuba-diving trip, and Richard had to take off for Europe on one of his band tours. Doug Sadownick picked up the slack and organized a small team to care for Mike during the times when he was home. Doug drew up a list of recommendations to coach the group on how they could best be effective: "Mike is one of the most generous and grateful people I know," Doug wrote in a group letter to the team, but "he's not always great at making his needs clear for fear of offending his friends. . . . We all must call before visits and never stop by unannounced. . . . Encourage Mike to rest, rest, rest. He may want to entertain you with his wit when you come over, Diva that he is. . . . I'm getting a cleaning person to come once a week, but no doubt the house will get untidy between then as Mike is not able to vacuum, dust and polish. . . . Never hesitate to call me."[10]

Soon after Richard returned to New York, Patrick had to be hospitalized as well, yet Richard had to fulfill his obligation to perform in Europe. When his band reached Prague, the promoter put up the members in a B and B that lacked phones in the individual rooms. Using the one at the front desk, Richard called Mike and Patrick in their respective sickbeds in L.A. and New York. He thought Patrick sounded despondent, and learned that he'd had to cancel his diving trip. Mike was home, but his building had become filled with druggies, he'd been robbed, and he no longer felt safe. Mike told Doug Sadownick that he wanted "to move into the bowels of West Hollywood," the center of gay life, to die (and live a while) among "my people." He was to an extent being campy; he'd sounded a different note much more often in the past: "I honestly don't believe there is a gay community—as in a monolithic group of people who think alike, work together, and have a common ancestry."[11]

Doug somehow managed to find a two-room apartment in West Hollywood for Mike that was far nicer—it even had a patio—than the dilapidated HUD studio Mike had been living in; the new apartment was mostly paid for by "Section 8" housing—the city of West Hollywood required new developments to have a set-aside (Section 8) for low-income seniors and PWAs. Doug and the O Boys managed the complicated move in late September 1993. True to his role as a "controlling bottom," Mike sent Doug in advance an elaborate list of precautions and reminders that elevated obsessiveness to a charming new level: along with instructions to sprinkle boric acid in the bottom of each carton to avoid transporting roaches and their eggs, he urged Doug "to give free reign to the Jewish mother side and treat all the packers as I would—in other words, feed them well. . . . Please don't be stingy. Use some of the cash to order pizza, beer, whatever people want. Reward yourselves each night with a nice dinner at some place of your choosing. Generosity deserves to be rewarded with generosity."[12]

When Richard next phoned Mike from Prague, Judy Peabody happened to be visiting him and was busy following Mike's directions for making homemade gnocchi. Mike also had a visit from Mary Fisher, the wealthy HIV-positive woman who'd electrified the Republican Convention in 1992; she and Mike immediately hit it off and she told him how much she admired him. By this point, Mike was barely ambulatory, and then only with the help of a cane (Mary Fisher got down on the floor to talk with him). Along with mounting digestive problems, his KS was also continuing to spread; "I'm slowly turning purple," he told a friend, "the color of gay royalty." By November, Mike was in what Doug called "soul-sucking pain."[13]

When alone, Mike read and read, mostly books that were gay related. He also talked a great deal with Doug about the gay-affirmative therapy he'd been in for a year with Richard Levin, one of its leading exponents. Doug himself had entered gay-centered therapy three years earlier and later became a leading figure in the movement. Both men felt (as Doug has put it) "deeply moved by the basic principles of what we were learning therein, namely that a crushed gay child lay in tremulous hiding among the foggy recesses of our uncharted unconscious psyches, a sweet fey youngling badly bashed but not really destroyed by foul heterosexist parenting."[14]

Doug found Mike's "Wildean wit" and his strong androgynous spirit a wondrous combination—"to say nothing of his Martha Stewart panache at orchestrating elaborate, seven-course Marcella Hazan–informed 'Italian Kitchen' meals." Mike could no longer manage the meals, but his wit was intact and the more he read and talked about "gay psychology," the more he entrusted to Doug his wish to die "in the most gay way possible." That meant, among other things, nothing that smacked of standard spiritual or religious ritual. Mike held firmly to his atheism and to his skeptical rejection of any "higher power" other than reason itself. Yet he was powerfully moved by his gay-affirmative readings and his talks with Doug.

What followed was a brief interlude of contentment. Though Mike awoke each day "aware of a decrease in my capacities," his current strategy, as he wrote his friend Holly Near, "is just to float—let the current take me wherever at whatever pace it decides to." While the mood lasted, he focused on what "a good, full life" he'd had, the "wonderful things" he'd experienced, the many "truly amazing people" he'd met. He told one visitor, as if summing up, "The next generation is going to have different problems than we did. Our problem was invisibility—the stigma that kills so many of us. We have shattered that problem for all time. Now you can see us everywhere. . . . But homophobia is firmly, firmly entrenched. I believe [this new generation] has been raised to expect instant success because so much progress was made so quickly. They're going to find a severe backlash that's waiting in the wings."

On December 1, 1993, Mike received the City of Los Angeles Lifetime Achievement Award, and he insisted on being wheeled into the ceremony to accept the honor. He somehow pulled that off, but for the next big event—the premiere of the film *Philadelphia*, in which he and the Flirtations briefly sang "Mr. Sandman" as background to a party scene—he was far too ill to attend. But a friend reported back that at the premiere she'd told Tom Hanks how ill Mike was and Hanks said the news made him very sad; he asked her to tell Mike that he'd prepared in his trailer by listening to the soundtracks from the Flirts and from Mike's *Purple Heart*. She did report all this to Mike, and it did make him happy. Later, when Hanks received the Golden Globe best actor award for his performance in *Philadelphia*, he mentioned Mike in his acceptance speech, saying "the streets of heaven are too crowded with angels."

In the last interview Mike ever gave, he spoke of his deep contentment with having completed all the basic tracks for *Legacy*: "I have never, ever in my life been so fulfilled. . . . I'd love to be around when the album comes out, but it's harder and harder to walk, to stand up." He told the interviewer that he had all the usual fears about "a violent death, and a medicalized death, being a vegetable," but he'd found that "dying can be an amazingly sensual, almost erotic experience because it's very much about the body. I feel that I'm a person who lived in his head all his life and paid very little attention to my body, except during sex, which is why I was addicted to it." But now, though his leg was swollen with KS and throbbingly painful, he'd somehow managed to regard the pain as "a signal that my body is trying to tell me something, it's trying to get my attention and communicate to me. I just sort of feel tactile and sensual." He'd been weepy of late but didn't censor the tears; seeing a beautiful flower or biting into a luscious tomato filled him with unexpected bliss. It had nothing to do with "walking towards the light"—that stuff didn't move him at all: "This life is the light," he said. "If there is a heaven, this is it." A case of denial? That wasn't Mike's temperament. Raw courage would be closer—recognizable to anyone not put off by its association with "sentimentality."

By mid-December, Mike had lost all mobility and instead had to "crawl around on the carpet." Nor could he keep food down, not even Ensure. His lower body had become a mass of purple, leathery KS lesions, with his legs almost entirely covered. Besides longing to be touched again, Mike's ailing body ached with stiffness. He didn't dare ask anyone for a physical massage, but Doug picked up on how desperately he needed it. At first, Doug later confessed, "I was frightened and even disgusted to lay my own hands on the leathery skin," but he somehow managed to put his fear aside and to work regularly and sympathetically on Mike's scarred body.

In New York, meanwhile, Patrick was doing badly. Mike wrote a friend that his "worst fear is that Patrick and I will die around the same time, being a double blow for Richard. . . . he doesn't have a lot of friends, and doesn't make friends easily, and I worry about him being lonely." Patrick was still in Cabrini Hospital in New York City when Richard returned from Europe, and had still not told his family that he had AIDS. Richard felt they had a right to know, regardless of their reaction, and Patrick asked him to make the call. By then, he had so much trouble breathing that he'd been put in a respirator in the intensive care unit. Patrick's mother and two sisters were all nurses, and after getting Richard's call they immediately got on a plane in Portland, Oregon, and rushed to New York. The entire family proved—to use Richard's word—"fantastic," lovingly present for Patrick and expressively grateful to Richard. By now it was early December 1993, and Patrick was clearly losing his grip on life. In L.A., Mike, despite his own suffering, was intent on Patrick's condition and sent him a message, via Richard, to "hang in there . . . I'm coming out there . . . just a few more days"—a clear impossibility, but an accurate gauge of Mike's tendency to worry about others even when himself in extremis.[15]

Richard had the medical power of attorney for Patrick, and after consulting with his family, the decision was made to take him off the ventilator, as he wished. Within a few minutes, while they tightly held his hands, Patrick died. His father made the funeral arrangements at Redden's on Fourteenth Street, and he consulted with Richard about how they should dress Patrick. Together they came up with the idea of putting him in the scuba outfit he'd bought but had never been able to wear. At the cemetery, Patrick's family included and embraced Richard completely, and to this day they've stayed in touch.

Mike, meantime, had reentered the hospital and become wheelchair bound—and he was in agony; he was given a morphine pump, but it proved unable fully to blanket the pain. He and his doctors talked over the advisability of amputating his now-gangrenous foot but finally decided against it. Mike had been hoarding a large batch of the sleeping pill Seconal with the intent of committing suicide at some point. But while in the hospital he couldn't find a doctor who'd help him do the deed. Richard, still in a daze from Patrick's death, decided to leave at once for L.A.

According to Doug, Mike "had made a pact with me about limiting his homophobic parents' involvement" with his dying process. Under Doug's tutelage, Mike had come to fear (in Doug's words) "that their guilt . . . would make them want to coercively overcompensate at his deathbed." Mike's father had indeed held tenaciously to his view of homosexuality as a "disability" and had remained unbendingly rigid about it. Yet even he could sign off a letter to Mike with "love," and he'd once written to him that he'd met very few people in his lifetime who had "what I call 'substance' . . . but you are one of them." His mother had been much more effusive: "You are a great example to many," she'd written Mike, "and you have truly MADE A DIFFER-ENCE!!!" As for his brother, Barry, he and Mike had always been close, and Barry, with his wife, Patty, had come to L.A. the previous month, stayed in Mike's apartment, and made frequent visits to the hospital.[16]

Richard remembers that despite his "pact" with Doug, Mike did toward the end call his parents and tell them that "if you want to see me, you'd better come now." And they did, accompanied by his brother, Barry. Doug was present when they arrived and acknowledges that Mike's mother "did become more warm, present and humane" than her husband, "who remained physically cold, aloof and downcast [though] . . . it appeared like he was fighting back tears a lot." Mike put the question to his parents that he and Doug had planned in advance: could they love him unconditionally for being gay? His mother said yes, but his father (according to Doug) "could only put his head on Michael's sunken-in chest and silently cry." Michael spent some time rubbing his father's head in a soothing way, as if to say, Doug felt, "I understand your limitations." When they left, Mike and Doug had a good cry.[17]

As Christmas approached, Richard got Mike discharged from the hospital, with the intent of taking care of him in his own apartment. But once there Mike, overcome with pain, woke up an exhausted Richard at three a.m. the night of December 23 and told him, "I can't do this. I want to go back to the hospital." Richard tried to persuade him to remain at home, but to no avail. To make matters more difficult still, Mike had been out of the hospital for just enough hours to necessitate going through the entire process of reregistering as a patient—it took from dawn till noon.

On December 24, Christmas Eve, Mike grew very concerned about drawing up a list of some forty-five people who he wanted to leave something to—a book, a record, a cooking pan. At Mike's request a lawyer came to the hospital and they started going over the list "in excruciating detail"—that is, until they reached something like person number twenty, when Mike collapsed from exhaustion and said, "Richard should do what he thinks is right."

On Christmas Day the lawyer returned to finalize the document as Mike's will. An unexpected acquaintance showed up, too, and—much to Richard's annoyance—started talking what he called "some New Age crap about going toward the light." Mike had mocked that sort of thing all his life, but he was now too weak to fight her. At some point around then, Mike's parents called, and with Richard briefly out of the room, the acquaintance took the receiver and told them that "they should tell him they loved him and say goodbye." She held the receiver against Mike's ear as first his brother, then his father, did just that. It was then his mother's turn. She told Mike that she'd bury his ashes under his favorite apple tree in their backyard, and that she'd always love him. "I love you, too, Mom," Mike whispered back, then collapsed in exhaustion.

At that point Doug and Tim arrived in the room. When the acquaintance told Doug about what she characterized as "a miraculous reconciliation" between Mike and his parents, Doug angrily responded that she'd "violated Michael's very being—because Michael didn't want to have anything to do with his family."

Mike began to fade in and out. Since no notary was available on Christmas Day, the lawyer told Richard to get as many witnesses as possible. So he started calling people and explaining that they were needed for Mike's will to be legal. Quite a few showed up, including Richard's brother, Andy. Though he mostly dozed, Mike managed to say hello to everyone who arrived, thanking them for turning out on Christmas. He even started doing his yenta routine on Andy—"Have I got a girl for you!"—extracting a promise from Andy to call her. With the lawyer present, the gathered friends witnessed Mike sign his will. That done, Mike said he wanted to increase the morphine right away.[18]

As the drug took over, Richard rehearsed some last-second details with him—what kind of a memorial service did he want?; should anyone sing, and if so, what?; should the service be in L.A. or New York, or both? Somewhere in there, Mike turned to Richard and said, "No regrets. No regrets." Richard would come to remember "that as the most extraordinary thing to give me to carry forward for the rest of my life." Mike slipped out of consciousness, and Richard had the excruciating task of saying good-bye to each person as they left the hospital room.

Richard spent the night, with Mike off and on aware of his surroundings. Then, on the afternoon of December 27, he became agitated; the nurses took him off the bed, cleaned him up, changed his sheets, and smoothed the covers down. He then became calm again. Richard took a quick break to stretch his legs. When he got back to the room, the nurse told him that Mike had suddenly sat up, looked to the window—and then died. He was thirty-eight years old. It had been seventeen days since Patrick's death. Tim Miller showed up and went off with Richard to the stairwell, let him scream and cry, and gave him big, big hugs.

Thanks to Richard, *Legacy* was released posthumously.

10

Home

Though Essex had earlier publicly revealed that he had AIDS, he
kept the details of the progress of his illness from even his
friends. Yet as one of them has put it, "I don't think Essex or anyone else
was doing a good job of hiding his illness. Everyone knew he had AIDS."
But after his emergency hospitalization and near death while in Chicago in 1994, he talked more openly with close friends like Ron Simmons about his condition. He went into few details about symptoms
or treatments but simply revealed the basic facts. It was typical of how
Essex handled AIDS: he went about his business as long as he was able,
neither clarifying nor lamenting—and certainly never exaggerating—
his condition. And throughout 1993, he did manage to keep to most of
his routine. While still on the West Coast finishing up the Getty fellowship, he continued to put in a number of appearances elsewhere.[1]

At one of them, the University of Oregon, the local branch of the
NAACP called the university and protested his presence, presumably
because he was gay, though the exact reason given isn't known. The
event went on as scheduled, but the audience of mostly straight, black
students proved unusually hostile. Quoting the Afrocentrist Molefi
Asante, they attacked Essex's homosexuality and accused him of "not
doing anything for the race." Essex did his best to be understanding:
"they're trying to protect the little bit of masculinity that's been

constructed . . . an assimilated masculinity—in other words, 'I want to be like what oppresses me.'" It helped to make him realize "that just because one comes from the realm of discrimination and prejudice does not necessarily guarantee that your consciousness is going to open up and you'll understand the connectedness that exists all around. Colin Powell proves that point again for me, just as some members of our own community have proven that point to me, as I've lived and breathed."

Essex extended those thoughts in a prose-poem he called "Loyalty": "We constitute the invisible brothers in our communities, those of us who live 'in the life,' the choir boys harboring secrets, the uncle living in an impeccable flat with a roommate who sleeps down the hall when family visits; men of power and humble peasantry, reduced to silence and invisibility for the safety they procure from these constructions."[2]

Ron Simmons had himself tested HIV-positive in 1989, and in 1991 he had joined a black gay male support group, Us Helping Us. At the time, he'd been teaching for twelve years at Howard University while working on completing his doctoral dissertation. But in 1992 the university had failed to renew his contract. They gave as a reason his insufficient record of publications, though several of his essays were in print, including his seminal "Some Thoughts on the Challenges Facing Black Gay Intellectuals" in *Brother to Brother*, in which he candidly addressed the homophobia that characterized the work of such black leaders and scholars as Amiri Baraka, Nathan Hare, Louis Farrakhan, and Molefi Asante. It seems unlikely that Ron's closing admonition in that essay—"We [black gay people] have been blessed with gifts to share in a society that views love and tenderness between men as a weakness"—did anything to advance his bid for tenure.[3]

When Essex broke the news of his AIDS status, Ron had been seeing an herbalist named Prem Deben for four years in an effort to control his own condition through holistic methods. It was Deben who'd told Ron about Us Helping Us. Ron has stayed with the group down to the present day, and it was only in 2003 that he started taking medication of any kind. Us Helping Us featured internal cleansing, fasting, meditation, the intake of oxygen, and the harnessing of sexual energy (having orgasms without releasing sperm) to aid in the healing process. Ron became executive director of the group, and in 1993 Us

Helping Us got a $20,000 grant—its first—from the Washington AIDS Partnership, a local foundation.

Ron had first met Essex back in 1982, at a benefit for *Blacklight* magazine, but for a number of years they'd known each other only in passing. After Ron became involved in Us Helping Us, he tried to interest Essex in joining but got nowhere. Essex told Ron that he didn't think he could beat "this thing" and had become fatalistic about it. Something the gifted black gay writer Craig Harris, who had died of AIDS in 1991, wrote about his own medical condition is suggestive of Essex's attitude as well: "My quality of life is a control issue. I refuse to be controlled by a daily regimen of oral medications and radiation therapy, controlled by weekly chemotherapy treatments, controlled by the increasing number of side-effects, fatigue or depression, medical bills or reimbursement checks. I refuse to be controlled by limitations imposed upon me by my race/ethnicity, class, sexual orientation, and health. I have made a commitment to relinquish control only as a last resort."

When Ron tried to get Essex to at least give up cigarettes and pot, Essex stopped returning his calls for a while. "That was Hemphill," Ron says philosophically, "sometimes he would get just stuck on . . . [something] that you really couldn't shake." When Ron talked to him about his own Afrocentric views regarding body, mind, and spirit, and the importance of affirming and tending to all three, Essex would vaguely reply "uh-huh," the equivalent of a yawn.

Essex had much more of a falling out with Larry Duckett, with whom he'd performed many times and who'd gone out to the Getty in 1993 to help Essex collect his things for the move back East. What Larry called "our explosion" came while they were still in California—it apparently centered on Essex feeling that Larry had failed to come to his defense when a store clerk had "disrespected" him. But that may have been merely a surface excuse for breaking away from a relationship that had become untenable.

In any case, they had no contact for the last two years of Essex's life. In an unpublished and largely incoherent three-page account of their relationship that Larry later wrote, he wobbles between describing Essex as his lover, his "partner in the arts," and his intimate brother, implying, somewhat bizarrely, that he "allowed" himself "to be distanced from Essex" by certain unnamed brothers who "saw Essex as a sexual boy-toy" and saw Larry "as being in their way." But several of Essex's intimates have described Larry Duckett as being unrequitedly in love with Essex. In any case, Essex was uninterested in repairing the friendship; when he lay ill in the hospital toward the end of his life, Larry asked Chris Prince, a mutual friend, to ask Essex if he could call or visit. Essex said no. Chris tried coaxing him, vaguely suggesting that there might not be another chance to patch things up, but Essex refused to reconsider.[4]

"He was a fierce boy," Chris said by way of explanation. "He was a diva. Humility was not one of his assets . . . [but] he was a warm man . . . and sensitive, not arrogant, not a showoff . . . smoke and mirrors wouldn't fool him." Essex himself referred to his "basic tenaciousness" and as having been, earlier in life, "demanding of attention." He was also, Chris added—as if afraid that his portrait of Essex might come across as stern—"so much fun to be around . . . and that body, child. Ooh, that boy had a fierce body. Before boys were workin' out . . . he was *so* sexy."

Through the latter part of 1993, Essex worked now and then (along with Michelle Wallace, bell hooks, Cornel West, and Angela Davis) with Marlon Riggs on his last film, *Black Is . . . Black Ain't*. But then Marlon's health took a bad turn and he had to be hospitalized. According to Steven Fullwood, a curator at the Schomburg Center for Black Culture, "Much of the final text of *Black Is . . . Black Ain't* was developed by Riggs one night in his hospital room: 'It was as if the film were rolling before me,' Riggs purportedly said, 'and I was just transcribing; I almost couldn't keep up.'" He'd known since December 1988 that he was HIV-positive, but he now became critically ill for months. As he later told an interviewer, "It was all-consuming. The agony of being weak, of vomiting, of nausea, of fever, of blood coming out of all of my orifices, of being disoriented, drugged, having nightmarish dreams because of the drugs. It was a feeling of utter loss of control . . . I wasn't thinking about art: I was driven down too far into the basic consciousness of just staying alive." He was finally able to leave the hospital, but his spirit was diminished, and his once inexhaustible energy reduced to a few hours of early morning work. Riggs never completed *Black Is . . . Black Ain't*, succumbing to AIDS on April 5, 1994. Posthumously, co-producer Nicole Atkinson, co-director/co-editor Christiane Badgley, and Signifyin' Works finished the film.[5]

Eight months later, in December 1994, the writer Don Belton brought Isaac Julien and Essex together for a conversation about Riggs' last film. Essex spoke with particular passion about the ending of *Black Is . . . Black Ain't*, where bell hooks speaks about "communion," which Essex defined as "a willingness to communicate with one another." He and Julien then went on in their discussion to disagree about Louis Farrakhan and black nationalists in general. "I'm as black as anyone," Essex insisted—"but not by the criteria the nationalists construct." Still, he felt that some dialogue with those attracted to black nationalism was essential. Julien felt "the opposite," felt that instead they "should be going back to the communities we are a part of and working on a grassroots level . . . to challenge hetero-normative assumptions."

But the "grassroots level," Essex countered, meant "mostly poor, heterosexual working-class men—the very same men drawn to Farrakhan"—who mocked and denigrated black gay men. And that was precisely the reason, Essex went on, why it was a mistake to ignore them. He believed, adamantly, that they could be reached, that gay men like himself and Isaac Julien should "bear witness," should insist on demonstrating that black gay men had "always been crucial to our communities" and should claim their rightful membership. He believed that if they approached heterosexual black men in a "supportive, caring, trustworthy, and loyal" way that the possibility would open up "of a formidable brotherhood that reaches beyond our sexual desires and connects us to every black male on the planet." It was a view that the Los Angeles–based Black Gay and Lesbian Leadership Forum also shared; after an extended discussion, the group ended up encouraging black gay men to attend Farrakhan's Million Man March.[6]

But Julien remained skeptical. Where Essex argued that opportunities for intervention can unexpectedly appear, Julien discounted the possibility. To him Farrakhan's assumption that black straight men "owned" blackness was impervious to discussion; in Julien's view, moreover, "Black macho discourses of empowerment" inherently denigrated women as well as black gay men—after all, the year before, Ben Chavis had been fired from his position as CEO of the NAACP when it was revealed that, without notifying the board, he'd made a large payoff to keep allegations of sexual harassment from being aired publicly. Picking up on the reference to women, Essex pointed out that "the [negative] things you've heard among gay brothers about women" weren't any different from the disrespectful way straight black men talked about women. In both cases, it disgusted him. He felt passionately that black gay men had the obligation to work actively against sexism—which was exactly what Mike Callen had felt in regard to all gay men.[7]

When Essex's longtime friend Chris Prince asked him early in 1995 how work was going on his novel, Essex quietly told him that he wasn't feeling much like writing anymore. His last spurt seems to have been during the summer of 1994, when he told Wayson, "It feels wonderful to be writing again. I have sorely missed putting pen to paper." Nor was Essex any longer pursuing sex. He'd once thought that he and Chris might take their friendship "to another level" (Chris hadn't been interested), but now, when Chris stayed over at Essex's apartment one night, "he didn't even try anything." Essex had long been "a sexy man," someone who pursued and enjoyed his assorted sexual encounters. He'd never boasted about any of his escapades, though he could be bold about them in his poetry:

> if I am indolent and content
> to lay here on my stomach . . .
> if I choose
> to be liked in this way,
> if I desire to be object,
> to be sexualized
> in this object way,
> by one or two at a time,
> for a night or a thousand days
> for money or power,
> for the awesome orgasms
> to be had, to be coveted,
> or for my own selfish wantonness,
> for the feeling of being
> pleasure, being touched . . .[8]

Or:

> If he is your lover,
> never mind.

> Perhaps, if we ask
> he will join us.

In this, as in all things, Essex held to his own guidelines. He would scold Chris, for example, about going to see gay strip shows—on political, not moral grounds. "You don't know what their, the strippers, stories are," Essex said. "They might have been abused" or "compromised in some way or another. And here you are, objectifying them, and giving them money to take their clothes off."

As Essex's health declined, he was never afflicted with KS lesions but did come down with PCP—though why, given the availability of PCP prophylaxis, is unknown. What we do know is that after being released from the hospital, Essex spent most of his time alone in his apartment. As he put it,

> Some days it seems easier to sort dirty clothes to be laundered than to be sorting my mail and responding, promptly, to what it contains. It seems easier to dust furniture and listen to hours of music from early dawn to late evening. I ignore my telephone. . . . It seems easier to sweep floors and change bed sheets, easier to roast chickens and de-vein shrimp, to weigh potatoes and onions, peppers and broccoli, easier to simply entomb myself in a thousand domestic chores, escape to a land of Joy, Bounty and Cheer. Go there, a fugitive from my present world, a fugitive fleeing terminal illness and death, fleeing to a land of shiny floors, scented soaps and fluffy towels. . . . Never once do I forget that death is so near, but that doesn't cloud my head with fear.[9]

After returning from the hospital, he tried to restore some of his vitality by exercising in his apartment, but then one day he happened to glance into a mirror and saw "the first full-length view of myself":

> I was in the bathroom, at home,
> undressing to take a shower
> I wasn't watching myself undress
> In the wall-to-wall, floor-to-ceiling mirror
> As I finally peeled out of my underwear
> I glanced in to the mirror and was devastated.
> I was as thin as a sheet of paper.

> I could see my ribs, I could see flesh
> sagging from my thighs . . .
> I gathered up my bones
> and showered them,
> while fighting back tears,
> while the mirror fogged over
> what I couldn't bear to see.

What little writing he seems to have done—some poems and a few prose jottings—were privately printed in a nineteen-page limited edition entitled *Domestic Life*. One of the unexpected, dominant themes of that final effort, obliquely but frequently stated, is the return of some semblance of Essex's religious faith. Earlier, in his long poem "Vital Signs," he appears resistant:

> I began looking at the world
> as a leather skullcap of countless
> driven nails meticulously bonneted
> on the head of the Christian God
> many offered me or tried to
> force-feed me. Or more often
> than not this figure was used
> to impose, contain and undermine
> my journey, all in the name
> of salvation, which was
> one more cemetery
> I sadly discovered.
> One more burning flag.

Yet in *Domestic Life* Essex sounds a different note, suggesting a turn toward a kind of faith not explicitly named as Christian: "on the few occasions that I have seriously considered suicide, I have been fortunate enough to return to reason and forge a new peace with my life, reestablish my purpose, affirm my faith. . . . Betrayal and disappointment have been visiting at my door, but so have faith and continuance."

In one of the poems in *Domestic Life*, he moves closer to an ambivalent defining of his "faith" as a possible affirmation of "God":

> . . . there is something
> Nagging to speak, something else
> That has had no voice until now.
> I listen to it calling my name,
> Clearly, gently calling me.
> I answer tentatively
> I have suspicions and doubts,
> But I answer because I think it's God
> Or the distant whistle of my train.[10]

Essex rarely spoke about his failing health, even with Wayson Jones, probably his closest friend. "I don't even really know what his morbidity"—the incidence of disease—"was," Wayson told me years later. Even before Essex learned that he was HIV-positive, he told Wayson that he didn't think he'd live to be very old; perhaps, Wayson thought, because he'd "had a hard life, really." The episodes of abuse and family dysfunction while growing up had left their mark. And in Wayson's opinion, Essex as an adult "had never had a good [lover] relationship. I never met a boyfriend"—there had been only two extended relationships, Mel and Jerry, each lasting about three years— "that I thought was good for him, really." Wayson knew whereof he spoke, since evidence has surfaced that one of the two lovers had assaulted Essex and threatened him with a gun. Chris echoes Wayson's verdict, adding that Essex tended to be attracted to abusive men. Of the two relationships that proved more than casual, neither gave him the sustained comfort he craved. Essex put it this way in "Vital Signs":[11]

> I am searching for whatever
> we relinquished that was
> deemed sacred between us.
> A living memory of this exists
> and I want to find it . . .
> We were not loathsome then,
> We were not dealing in cruelty,
> sabotage, torment, grief . . .
> I am searching
> for the irrefutable clarity
> to all I don't presently comprehend

at any hour
about the hatred in our lives,
the misplaced anger,
the presence of death.

Essex did tell Wayson that he was getting fevers and night sweats and had neuropathy in his legs, and Wayson could see for himself that Essex was becoming perilously thin. Yet as late as May 1995, Essex somehow—his willpower was strong—managed to host a showing of Marlon Riggs' *Black Is . . . Black Ain't* at the University of Toledo Student Union. Only about fifty people showed up, and only a handful attended a community reception the following day. It had hardly been worth what must have been a difficult outing for Essex; the sole consolation was financial—Essex was given a handsome fee.

According to Wayson, Essex not only refused to participate in any of Ron Simmons' Us Helping Us programs, but he "really never took a proactive stance with his own illness." Ron feels that toward the end, Essex may have begun to suffer from dementia. When he reached him by phone one day and asked how he was doing, Essex replied, "I'm busy right now. I'm about to go down to the courthouse." Startled, Ron asked him why. Essex said something about how his last boyfriend kept calling him up and bothering him, even after he'd told him to stop. What did that have to do with a trip to the courthouse? Well, Essex said, "I need to get a restraining order" to keep the man from pestering him. Ron tried to persuade him that maybe the ex-boyfriend was just trying to show his concern and wasn't intent on stalking or harassing him. But Essex wasn't persuaded.[12]

Soon after that exchange, Essex was in and out of the hospital. On one of his better days, a friend gave him a haircut and, finding him "in good spirits," wheeled him around West Philadelphia for an outing. But within days after that, he was reported to be "fading fast," and it became clear that Essex was no longer able to take care of himself. He entered the University of Pennsylvania Hospital in Philadelphia, and very few visitors were allowed to see him. Wayson and Chris saw him for the last time in August 1995. He was having considerable pain from neuropathy, and Wayson sat on his bed and massaged his legs—just as Doug Sadownick had done for Mike Callen. After that visit, one of the few reports that came through said that "Essex was no longer able to speak, he could only point and a horrible rattle came from his throat." Chris called often, trying to reach Essex, but finally gave up. In one of his last poems, Essex had written:

> I am getting ready to depart
> for where, God only knows.
> I have no meaningful guesses,
> I have no hints, no clues
> It is better this way
> that I not be expecting
> more than what may come.

Essex, age thirty-eight—the same age at which Mike Callen had died—passed away on November 5, 1995, with his family around him.[13]

> When I die,
> Honey chil'
> my angels
> will be tall
> Black drag queens.
> I will eat their stockings
> as they fling them
> into the blue
> shadows of dawn.
> I will suck
> their purple lips
> to anoint my mouth
> for the utterance of prayer.
>
> My witnesses
> will have to answer
> to go-go music.
> Dancing and sweat
> will be required
> at my funeral.

> Someone will have to answer
> the mail I leave,
> the messages
> on my phone service;
> someone else
> will have to tend
> to the aching that drove me
> to seek soul . . .

Essex's friends discussed whether or not to attend the funeral service scheduled to be held in his mother's A.M.E. Zion church. They recalled what had happened at the funeral of another black gay writer, Donald Woods; there had been no mention in the service that he'd been gay, which had led an outraged Assotto Saint, who also later succumbed to AIDS, to commandeer the microphone and to say that he was there to honor Woods as an openly proud black gay man. He asked that if anyone else had come to the funeral for that same reason, to please stand up. Half the church stood up, and the Woods family had been horrified.

Barbara Smith, the pioneering black lesbian publisher and writer, told Ron Simmons that in her opinion the funeral belonged to the family and that Essex's gay friends should not attend but should hold a separate event of their own to honor Essex. Wayson agreed with Barbara that it would be inappropriate to "hijack" the family service; indeed, at the request of Essex's mother, Wayson, though uncomfortable, agreed to deliver the eulogy (which was in fact written by the family), and both he and Michelle Parkerson were among the six pallbearers. Ron (and also Phill Wilson of the AIDS Project Los Angeles) also decided to attend. His friends reported back that during the service no mention was made of Essex being a gay man, and that his mother, Mantelene, had spoken of him in his last days as accepting Christ as his Savior. In the program for the services ("Victory Celebration for Essex Charles Hemphill," November 9, 1995, Full Gospel A.M.E. Zion Church), one of the six printed paragraphs of his biography reads: "On September 17, 1995, Essex made the most important decision of his life. He accepted Jesus Christ as his personal Lord and Savior at Full Gospel A.M.E. Zion Church."[14]

Ron's report of the funeral service outraged most of Essex's friends, who refused to accept the family's account of his last days—even though such an outcome was hinted at as at least possible in Essex's final poetry, "Vital Signs" and *Domestic Life* (which in all likelihood only Wayson had seen). His friends held an alternate ceremony at the Hine Junior High School in D.C., which, to their considerable surprise, Essex's mother and one of his three sisters attended. There were choral ensemble readings from Essex's writings, and various people shared anecdotes about their friendships with him, Ron Simmons among them. He spoke frankly about Essex's "perfectionism"—so akin to Mike Callen's—which made working with him sometimes "difficult, sometimes painful. But if you too were willing to accept nothing less than the best in what you brought to that creative process, it would be a joyful thrill unlike any other."[15]

Ron also spoke about the impact of Essex's work on the black gay community:

It was utterly profound. His work gave us a voice we had never heard before. So many of us were living as marginalized souls of internalized guilt and shame, despite our suits and ties, and suddenly there was a writer whose work captured our fears, anger, confusion, frustration, passion and desire as no artist had done before. . . . He encouraged us to celebrate. Imagine that. We who were told that our God despised us . . . And [Essex] dared all of us to envision a new community beyond gay and straight, black and white, male and female.

When the ceremony was over, Essex's mother and sister quietly came up to Ron and thanked him for his remarks. They were apparently as torn between love and unease as Essex himself had been toward them.

Three organizations, Gay Men of African Descent (GMAD), Other Countries, and Black Nations/Queer Nations?, declared December 10, 1995, a National Day of Remembrance for Essex at the Lesbian and Gay Community Services Center in New York City. They urged all those around the country who "knew, loved or were inspired by Essex and his work to join us by staging memorials in your city on that day." We know that at the least, Philadelphia and Detroit, as well as New York City, held such remembrances.[16]

That same month and year, December 1995, the FDA approved the release of saquinavir, the first of a new class of drugs called protease inhibitors, which for many would convert AIDS from a death sentence to a manageable disease.

The FDA announcement came one month after Essex's death.

Acknowledgments

Many people helped to bring this book into being. I'll start my thanks with its publisher, The New Press. This is the fifth book I've published with TNP in the last six years, which is itself a measure of the deep satisfaction I feel about our relationship. Everyone on the staff at The New Press has been consistently kind and helpful, though for this book I want to single out the special contributions of Ellen Adler, Julie Enszer, and Ben Woodward. They've greatly eased my path even as they offered smart, candid suggestions for improving the manuscript. As well, Maury Botton directed all aspects of production for this book and did his usual sterling job.

The two major manuscript depositories for writing this book were the extensive Michael Callen Papers, housed at the Gay History Archives of the Gay Community Center (New York, NY), and a variety of collections (the Joseph F. Beam Papers being central) at the Schomburg Center for Research in Black Culture, a branch of the New York Public Library. At the former, Rich Wandel was a cordial, tireless guide, and at the latter, Steven Fullwood was particularly helpful in locating materials. For a full listing of manuscript collections used, see the list that heads the notes at the back of the book.

I'm heavily indebted to those who sat with me, often for many hours, to share their memories of the two figures whose lives are the centerpiece of this book: Michael Callen and Essex Hemphill. In this regard I owe a great deal to Richard Berkowitz, Richard Dworkin, Wayson Jones, E. Ethelbert Miller, Michelle Parkerson, Chris Prince, Ron Simmons, Sean Strub, Joseph Sonnabend, and Abby Tallmer. Others have sent me documents or correspondence in their private possession; Barbara Smith's letters from Essex were especially significant. Still other people talked with me on the phone or responded to my request for additional information with e-mails, letters, and documents; of special value was the material from Jim Bredesen, Frances Goldin, Jennifer Jackson, Wayson Jones, Jim W. Marks, Tim Miller, Doug Sadownick, and Joseph Sonnabend. Above all, I'm indebted to Richard Dworkin; in multiple interviews, he not only shared with me his intimate memories of Mike Callen, but also provided a significant number of documents and photos from his private storehouse. For photos of Essex Hemphill, I'm comparably indebted to Sharon Farmer. Both she and Richard Dworkin spent countless hours combing arduously through their back files to come up with the unique, vital images that illustrate this book. I'm enormously grateful to them.

Notes

The abbreviations used in the notes are as follows:

For Individuals

MC: Michael Callen
BAC: Barbara Ann Callen
CC: Clifford Callen
EH: Essex Hemphill
RB: Richard Berkowitz
JS: Joseph Sonnabend
JB: Joseph Beam

For Manuscript Collections in Public Depositories

ASSC: Assotto Saint (Yves Lubin) Papers at SC
AVSC: Alexis de Veaux Papers at SC
EH/WJSC: The Essex Hemphill/Wayson Jones Collection, 1981–2008, at SC, plus two boxes of material donated by Wayson Jones in 2010

GCGW: Grace Cavalieri Papers, George Washington University

JBSC: Joseph F. Beam Papers at SC

JSNYPL: Joseph Sonnabend Papers at the New York Public Library at Forty-Second Street, Manuscript and Archives Division

MCP: Michael Callen Papers, Lesbian, Gay, Bisexual & Transgender Community Center, National History Archive, New York City

NYPL: New York Public Library

SC: Schomburg Center for Research in Black Culture, New York Public Library

For Manuscript Collections Privately Held

BSP: Barbara Smith Papers (EH correspondence)

DS: Doug Sadownick (correspondence)

FGAF: Frances Goldin Agency Files (EH unpublished novel, plus fifty unpublished early poems)

MP: Michelle Parkerson (flyers, posters, autographed EH material)

RBP: The Richard Berkowitz Archives (documents, correspondence)

RDP: Richard Dworkin (tapes, photos, documents, correspondence)

SSJS: Sean Strub (transcribed interviews with Sonnabend)

TM: Tim Miller (correspondence)

WJ: Wayson Jones (photos; *Domestic Life*)

For the many individual interviews I conducted, as well as secondary sources, see the notes.

Chapter 1: Before the Storm

Each note cites the material for the paragraph in which it appears and the paragraphs that follow until the subsequent note appears.

1. Multiple interviews with Richard Dworkin; the first two paragraphs are derived from MC to Jon [?], 9 pp., n.d., and the transcript of a microcassette recording between MC and RB, 1982, both MCP. MC was born and spent the first five years of his life in Rising Sun, Indiana, population 550.

2. The family background: MC, "Birth Announcement," 4-p. ms.; MC, "Leave It to Beaver," 26-p. ms.; Barbara Ann Callen to MC, October 4, 1974, October 23, 1977;

MC to "Barbie" [?], August 9, 1977; MC to Jon [?], 10 pp., [1978?]; Dr. David Schmidt, 9-p. typed interview with MC, November 12, 1987; MC to Mary Bemesderfer-McCleary, July 22, 1993, all MCP. MC to Sarah Squires, May 23, 1993 (college), MCP. Three DVDs: "Mike at Home at 29 Jones Street," 1982 (mirrors); "O Boys with Mike on Franklin," October 16, 1993; "Callen on O Boys Video/CDC Part 2" [1993], all RDP; multiple conversations with Abby Tallmer, Jennifer A. Jackson, e-mails to me, March 18, 19, 2013.

3. JS to me, April 1, 2013; JS, interviews with Sean Strub, SSJS; Sean Strub, "The Good Doctor," *POZ*, July 1998; Anne-Christine D'Adesky, "The Man Who Invented Safer Sex Returns," *Out*, Summer 1992; "Callen on OBoys video/CDC Part 2." [1993], courtesy Dworkin. For a survey of the bars, back rooms, and baths from 1969 to 1982, see Arthur Bell, "Where Gays Are Going," *Village Voice*, June 29, 1982. As a result of his reputation as an interferon scientist, JS came to know the cancer researcher Dr. Mathilde Krim, who, as co-chair of the American Foundation for AIDS Research (amfAR—earlier known as AIDS Medical Foundation), would soon become a key figure in AIDS research. James Kinsella, *Covering the Plague: AIDS and the American Media* (Rutgers University Press, 1989); Ronald Bayer and Gerald M. Oppenheimer, *AIDS Doctors: Voices from the Epidemic* (Oxford University Press, 2000); *Morbidity and Mortality Weekly Report*, June 5, 1981; Steven Epstein, *Impure Science: AIDS, Activism, and the Politics of Knowledge* (University of California Press, 1996); Jacques Pepin, *The Origins of AIDS* (Cambridge University Press, 2011).

4. Milton Coleman, "Marion Barry," *Washington Post*, January 2, 1979; David K. Johnson, *The Lavender Scare: The Cold War Persecution of Gays and Lesbians in the Federal Government* (University of Chicago Press, 2004), 193–94, 211–14.

5. Sidney Brinkley, "Making History," in *Smash the Church, Smash the State*, ed. Tommi Avicolli Mecca (City Lights, 2009). The *Blacklight* archive is online at www .blacklightonline.com/archive.html. See, esp., Thomas B. Romney, "Homophobia in the Black Community"; James S. Tinney, "Baldwin Comes Out"; Chasen Gaver, "Interracial Intentions"; the Adrian Stanford poem "Yeah Baby"; and EH's "Homocide: For Ronald Gibson."

6. EH interview in *Network* 1, no. 3 (December 1990), SC. Though I've long taught and written about African American history and culture (see *A Martin Duberman Reader*, The New Press, 2013), in my opinion no one has reflected on the crosscutting identity issues here with more brilliance and persuasiveness than Cathy J. Cohen, in her remarkable *The Boundaries of Blackness: AIDS and the Breakdown of Black Politics* (University of Chicago Press, 1999). I've relied heavily on her insights and perspectives.

I found EH's early poems in the back files of his literary agent, Frances Goldin. I'm grateful to her and to Sam Stoloff of the same agency for making photographic copies of the poems for me, along with correspondence and the manuscript of EH's long-lost novel, "Standing in the Gap." See chapter 7 for my discussion of the novel. A number of EH's close friends have long blamed his family for refusing to turn over his papers to the Schomburg Center for Research in Black Culture at the New York Public Library, as he wished. But as far back as 1998, EH's mother did mail Frances Goldin what she described as all the material he had left behind. Possibly she does still retain some items, but at the least it's clearly an injustice to accuse her of refusing to turn over any material for possible publication. I discuss EH's close relationship with his mother in more detail in this chapter.

7. Thomas B. Romney, "Homophobia in the Black Community," *Blacklight*.

8. EH, "Vital Signs," in *Life Sentences*, ed. Thomas Avena (Mercury House, 1994); EH, "Fixin' Things," in *Ceremonies* (Cleis, 1992); EH interview, *Network*; EH, "Miss Emily's Grandson Won't Hush His Mouth," *Outweek*, August 8, 1990, reprinted in EH, *Ceremonies*; *Vanguard*, August 23, 1991; Albert Williams, "Essex Hemphill and 'Cultural Transformation,'" *Windy City Times*, March 21, 1991; "Where We Live: A Conversation with Essex Hemphill and Isaac Julien," 210, in *([speak my name]): Black Men On Masculinity and the American Dream*, ed. Don Belton (Beacon, 1995).

9. EH, "Ceremonies," in *Ceremonies*.

10. Wayson Jones, interview, May 2009; *Philadelphia Daily News*, December 6, 1990 (Mathis); EH, "The Other Invisible Man," in *Boys Like Us: Gay Writers Tell Their Coming Out Stories*, ed. Patrick Merla (HarperCollins, 1996), 176–85; EH to "David" (at *Gargoyle* magazine), March 28, 1978, GCGW. Many of the details about EH and Jones as roommates derive from Jones' commentary on this book when in manuscript form, and especially from his long e-mail to me of April 15, 2013.

11. EH didn't include "My Funny Valentine/For Southeast" either in *Ceremonies* or in *Brother to Brother* (Alyson, 1991); EH, "Take Care of Your Blessings," *Network* (the manuscript of the poem is in JBSC). Interviews with Chris Prince, Michelle Parkerson, E. Ethelbert Miller, Wayson Jones, and Ron Simmons—all done in May 2009; Wayson Jones commentary on manuscript, April 15, 2013. The Michelle Parkerson poem "Highwire" is courtesy MP. A good deal of material on various aspects of D.C. gay life can be found online at www.rainbowhistory.org/html, including the quotation from a 2001 oral history with Gideon Ferebee Jr. The reference to *Rafiki* is from the guide to the Schomburg Center's February 1 to August 31, 2012, exhibit "Gay Men of African Descent (GMAD) at 25." For early black organizations and their relationship to feminism, see Anne M. Valk, *Radical Sisters: Second-Wave Feminism and Black Liberation in Washington, D.C.* (University of Illinois Press, 2008), esp. chaps. 5–6.

12. EH to Alexis de Veaux, October 19, 1983, September 29, 1985, AVSC; EH to Joe Beam, February 5, 18, 1988, JBSC; Wyatt O'Brian Evans, "Essex Hemphill: The Force Remains With Us," http://wyattobrianevans.com/online/node/49; interviews with E. Ethelbert Miller, Ron Simmons, Chris Prince, Wayson Jones, and Michelle Parkerson, May 2009; phone interview with Jim W. Marks, March 5, 2013; phone conversation with Michelle Parkerson, April 5, 2013; phone conversation with Sharon Farmer, June 7, 2013; Marks e-mail to me, February 28, 2013; Julie Enszer e-mail to me, February 22, 2013 (McCoy); transcript of Brett Beemyn interview with Wayson Jones, June 27, 1998, EH/WJSC; *City Paper*, October 28, 1988. For another example of EH's "ornery" response to authority, see EH to Chris Hayes (The Painted Bride), September 16, 1989, EH/WJSC. In 1986, Essex dedicated his chapbook *Conditions* to "Ray Melrose, Wayson Jones, Joseph Beam and the family." For more on the *Blackheart* collective and the subsequent New York group Other Countries, see Daniel Garrett, "Other Countries: The Importance of Difference" (1987) in *Freedom in This Village: Twenty-Five Years of Black Gay Men's Writing*, ed. E. Lynn Harris, 83–99 (Carroll and Graf, 2005).

Chapter 2: Reading the Signs

1. MC to his parents, November 7, 1979; Clifford Callen to MC, November 13, 1979; MC to Clifford Callen, December 17, 1979; MC to his sister, Linda, March 10, 1981, all MCP.

2. Ronald Bayer and Gerald M. Oppenheimer, *AIDS Doctors* (Oxford University Press, 2000), chap. 1; Sean Strub interviews with Sonnabend, transcripts courtesy Strub; January 27, 2013; discussion between myself, Sonnabend, Sean Strub, Richard Berkowitz, and Walter Armstrong; two DVDS: Gay Cable, *Men and Films* [1984] and *Sandi Freeman Reports* [1984], both courtesy Dworkin.

3. MC, "Leave It to Beaver," 26-p. ms., MCP; Steven Epstein, *Impure Science: AIDS, Activism, and the Politics of Knowledge* (University of California Press, 1996), 46–48.

4. Interviews with RB; RB, *Stayin' Alive: The Invention of Safe Sex* (Westview, 2003).

5. Interviews with RB; JS, Strub, RB, and Armstrong discussion, January 27, 2013; the Rubinstein report is as quoted in Susan M. Chambré, *Fighting for Our Lives: New York's AIDS Community and the Politics of Disease* (Rutgers University Press, 2006), 2.

6. Interview with RB; Deborah B. Gould, *Moving Politics: Emotion and ACT UP's Fight Against AIDS* (University of Chicago Press, 2009), 60, fn. 11.

7. Peter Lewis Allen, *The Wages of Sin: Sex and Disease, Past and Present* (University of Chicago Press, 2000), 120; Randy Shilts, *And the Band Played On* (St. Martin's, 1987). Though Shilts is reliable on the initial lack of federal response, his book is seriously skewed (see Douglas Crimp, "Randy Shilts's Miserable Failure," in *Melancholia and Moralism* [MIT Press, 2004], 117–128).

8. Kate Walter, "High Spirits," *New York Native*, August 26, 1984 (Lowlife); *The Advocate*, October 3, 1984 (Lowlife); interviews with Richard Dworkin; RB, *Stayin' Alive*, 107 (queen), 114 (patriarchy), 117 (sanity); MC, "The Luck Factor," 10-p. ms., MCP; *O Boys with Mike on Franklin, 2 of 2*, DVD, RDP. About as close as JS came to being judgmental was in a letter to Maurice Hilleman, in which he wrote, AIDS "stems from a culture that made possible the sexual excesses of the past ten to fifteen years" (January 8, 1983, JSNYPL). For PCP prophylaxis, JS to me, March 20, April 1, 2013; JS, "Pneumocystis Pneumonia Can Be Prevented," 2006, http://Aidsperspective.net/articles/pcppropylaxis.pdf.

9. MC, "Luck, Classic Coke, and the Love of a Good Man," in *Surviving AIDS* (HarperCollins, 1990); Epstein, *Impure Science*, 56 ff.; Chambré, *Fighting for Our Lives*, 78–79, 114–15; multiple conversations with Abby Tallmer, 2013; Tallmer, e-mail to me, March 21, 2013. The *Voice* finally made AIDS a cover story in its December 21, 1982, issue, but its headline, "Defenseless," angered advocates of self-empowerment like Rich and Mike (RB, *Stayin' Alive*, 166). No better, more poignant description exists of the desperate search for treatment on the part of those diagnosed with AIDS in these years than Paul A. Sergios, *One Boy at War: My Life in the AIDS Underground* (Knopf, 1993), though I've never seen it cited in the AIDS literature.

10. Mirko D. Grmek, *History of AIDS* (Princeton University Press, 1990), 17 (Denmark); MC, 6-p. typescript, no title or date, MCP; Dudley Clendinen and Adam Nagourney, *Out for Good: The Struggle to Build a Gay Rights Movement in America* (Simon and Schuster, 1999), 460–67; Edward Alwood, *Straight News: Gays, Lesbians, and the News Media* (Columbia University Press, 1996), 215–19. The "homophobia . . . junkies" quote is from MC to Ed Kosner, editor of *New York Magazine*, June 15, 1983, JSNYPL. JS made the same argument in a letter to Dr. Marcus Conant, June 22, 1983: "Our view in a nutshell is that repeated exposure to cytomegalovirus on the basis of a mild sperm-induced immunosuppression would be sufficient to explain the

syndrome in gay men . . . a cumulative process as opposed to a single hit by a unique infectious agent," JSNYPL.

11. MC and RB, "We Know Who We Are," *New York Native*, November 8–22, 1982; MD, JS, Strub, RB, and Armstrong discussion, January 27, 2013; Charles Jurrist, "In Defense of Promiscuity: Hard Questions About Real Life," *New York Native*, Dec. 6–19, 1982; "Good Luck, Bad Luck," *New York Native*, November 1982, Dr. Peter Seitzman, "Guilt and AIDS," *New York Native*, January 3–16, 1983; Dr. Nathan Fain, *The Advocate*, February 17, 1983; Dr. Lawrence Mass, *The Advocate*, no. 55; *New York Review of Books*, August 18, 1983; MC and RB, 14-p. transcript and 4-p. reply to Jurrist, both MCA; Clendinen and Nagourney, *Out for Good*, 478–80; Ann Silversides, *AIDS Activist: Michael Lynch and the Politics of Community* (Between the Lines, 2003), 21–23; Gay Cable, *Sandi Freeman Reports*. [1983], courtesy Dworkin. The ms. of MC's 5-p. response ("To the Editors," November 16, 1982) to Dr. Bill Lewis and Michael Lynch, "The Case Against Panic," dated November 16, 1982, is in MCP; Tallmer e-mail to me, March 21, 2013. When the *Native* refused to print their rejoinder, MC and RB took out a two-page ad in the *Native*, "A Warning to Gay Men with AIDS," *New York Native*, November 22–December 5, 1982, emphasizing that chemotherapy, interferon, and ultraviolet light were immunosuppressive, urging gay men to get health insurance, and stating that plasmapherosis *might* prove a helpful treatment, MCP.

12. JS interviewers with Strub; David Roman, *Acts of Intervention: Performance, Gay Culture, and AIDS* (Indiana University Press, 1998), 13; Larry Kramer, *Reports from the Holocaust* (St. Martin's Press, 1989), 39–43; Chambré, *Fighting for Our Lives*, 15–22; MC and RB "A Warning to Gay Men With AIDS." The best account of Mayor Koch's record, and one on which I've relied heavily, is Andy Humm, "Ed Koch: 12 Years as Mayor, A Lifetime in the Closet," *Gay City*, February 3, 2013.

13. For the quote on Apuzzo, see Jeff Escoffier, interview with MC [1987?], MCP; Kramer, *Reports*, xvi.

14. JS interview with Strub; all the quotes about Kramer, Mass, and the GMHC leadership are from a series of mid-1982 to early 1983 transcripts of taped conversations, in various combinations, between MC, RB, JS, and (rarely) Edmund White, MCP.

15. *Mike Talks About War [with GMHC] Again*, DVD, courtesy Jim Bredesen; MC, "Pinned and Wriggling: How Shall I Presume?" 6-p. transcript, MCP. The pre–ACT UP self-empowerment movement has been slighted in the vast literature about AIDS. My account is based largely on a 10-p. transcript, "A History of the PWA Self-Empowerment Movement by Michael Callen (in New York) and Dan Turner (in San Francisco)," MCP; and MC, speech on responsibility, February 3, 1983, 2-p. transcript, MCP.

16. *How to Have Sex in an Epidemic* (Tower Press, May 1983); RB, *Stayin' Alive*, 169–79. In the early eighties Mike held down a daytime job as a legal secretary for the gay lawyer and philanthropist Bill Hibsher, who was so impressed with Mike's intelligence that he urged him to go to law school (Dworkin interviews).

17. *Congressional Record*, May 18, 1983; MC, "Remarks of Michael Callen, AIDS Patient, Before New York State Senate Committee on Investigation and Taxation," June 1, 1983, 10-p. typescript, MCP. JS initially chaired the Scientific Committee of amfAR but resigned that position, while still remaining a member of the committee. In mid-1985 in an angry letter he wrote: "not only is my advice no longer sought . . . [but] executive policy decisions have been directed at disassociating the AMF from

my views." (JS to Terry Beirn, May 21, 1985, JSNYPL.) Yet by the end of the year, amfAR had contributed $126,000 to JS's work (JS to Editor, *New York Native*, October 24, 1985).

18. Gay Cable, *Men and Films* (JS and RB); JS and Harley Hackett interviews with Strub, [2009?], SSJS; JS to J. Grant Halladay, March 11, 1983, JSNYPL (bankruptcy).

Chapter 3: Career Moves

1. JB, ed., Introduction to *In The Life: A Black Gay Anthology* (Alyson, 1986).

2. Martin Duberman, *Left Out: The Politics of Exclusion: Essays 1964–2002* (South End Press, 2002), 285–95.

3. JB to "Steve," June 17, 1984; JB to his parents, May 29, 1976, both JBSC; E. Ethelbert Miller, "Essex Hemphill: Persecution Witness," *Washington Post*, November 12, 1995.

4. JB to "Ken," January 31, 1984; JB to Barbara Smith, August 8, 1984; Smith to JB, November 10, 1984, all JBSC; interview with Michelle Parkerson, May 1, 2009; *Murder on Glass* announcement and program courtesy MP. In most cases, the admiration was mutual. To give one example, in an interview Audre Lorde said, "When I read a poet like Essex Hemphill, my heart just comes up in my mouth and does an African-American folk-dance on the back of my throat. I think, yea that's what the brother is doing—he's making something that has never been made or said before. He gives me hope and strength" (Charles H. Rowell 1990 interview with Lorde in *Conversations with Audre Lorde*, ed. John Wylie Hall, University Press of Mississippi, 2004).

5. EH, *Ceremonies* (Cleis, 1992), 158–59; EH, "Say, Brother," *Essence*, November 1983; Johnson, *The Lavender Scare*, 193–94 (Mattachine); GLBPOC "Tribute," February 16, 2005, and Wayson Jones, commentary on this manuscript, April 15, 2013 (d.c. space). JB's editorial skill in producing the anthology, as well as his difficulties with some of the contributors, can be traced in JB to Isaac Jackson, June 24, 1985; JB to Daniel Garrett, June 8, July 31, 1985; Garrett to JB, July 29, 1985; JB to A. Billy S. Jones, June 7, 1985, all JBSC.

6. Craig G. Harris, "Black, Gay, and Proud," *New York Native*, March 11–24, 1985; "Jacks of Color: An Oral History" (Benjamin Shepard Interviews Liddell Jackson), in *From Act Up to the WTO*, ed. Benjamin Shepard and Ronald Hayduk (Verso, 2002); JB to "Dear Friends," November 18, 1985, JBSC; "Waking Up to AIDS," *Rainbow History Project*, rainbowhistory.org/html/AidsChronology.html; Renee McCoy to Julie Enszer, February 22, 2013, courtesy Enszer; EH's poems "Family Jewels" and "Cordon Negro" are from EH, *Ceremonies*; EH to JB, December 5, 1985; JB to EH, December 14, 1985, both JBSC. The Lost & Found and Whitman-Walker quotes are from EH's unpublished novel, "Standing in the Gap," FGAF.

7. David Roman, *Acts of Intervention: Performance, Gay Culture, and AIDS* (Indiana University Press, 1998), 33–34; Reginald Glenn Blaxton, " 'Jesus Wept': Reflections on HIV Dis-ease and the Churches of Black Folk," in *Dangerous Liaisons: Blacks, Gays, and the Struggle for Equality*, ed. Eric Brandt (The New Press, 1999); Elinor Burkett, *The Gravest Show on Earth: America in the Age of AIDS* (Houghton Mifflin, 1995), 148–52, 184 (quotes from Wilson and Owens); Cathy J. Cohen, *The Boundaries*

of Blackness: AIDS and the Breakdown of Black Politics (University of Chicago Press, 1999), 345, chap. 4. For a thoughtful update on the racial divisions in the gay movement, see Keith O. Boykin, "Where Rhetoric Meets Reality: The Role of Black Lesbians and Gays in 'Queer' Politics," in *The Politics of Gay Rights*, eds. Craig A. Rimmerman, Kenneth D. Wald, and Clyde Wilcox, 79–95 (University of Chicago Press, 2000).

8. James S. Tinney, "Why a Black Gay Church?" in *In The Life: A Black Gay Anthology*, ed. JB, 46–86 (Alyson, 1986). For the reevaluation of black homophobia, see the introduction and the essays by Cheryl Clarke, Keith Boykin, Cathy J. Cohen, and Tamara Jones in Eric Brandt, *Dangerous Liaisons: Blacks, Gays, and the Struggle for Equality*, The New Press, 1999; Gil Gerald, "The Trouble I've Seen (1987), in *Freedom in This Village: Twenty-Five Years of Black Gay Men's Writing*, ed. E. Lynn Harris, 67–82 (Carroll and Graf, 2005).

9. Undated transcripts of MC/RB taped phone conversations, MCP; MC, *Surviving AIDS* (HarperCollins, 1990), 7; John-Manuel Andriote, *Victory Deferred*, rev. ed. (2011); Ann Silversides, *AIDS Activist: Michael Lynch and the Politics of Community* (Between the Lines, 2003), 43–44; Jennifer Brier, *Infectious Ideas: U.S. Political Responses to the AIDS Crisis* (University of North Carolina Press, 2009), chap. 1.

10. Undated transcripts of MC/RB taped phone conversations, MCP; Brier, *Infectious Ideas*, 40–42.

11. MC, "Mike Goes to the Baths," 13-p. transcript, RDP; see also Susan M. Chambré, *Fighting for Our Lives: New York's AIDS Community and the Politics of Disease* (Rutgers University Press, 2006), 54–56; Douglas Crimp, "How to Have Promiscuity in an Epidemic," in *Melancholia and Moralism* (MIT Press, 2004); RB, written comments on this manuscript, April 1, 2013; RB, *Stayin' Alive: The Invention of Safe Sex* (Westview, 2003); JS to me, February 19, April 1, 2013.

That AIDS is primarily a heterosexual disease in Africa has caused a significant debate among specialists that is still in progress, and which I'm unqualified to join. JS is among the experts who dismiss the early theorizing that the lack of circumcision among men and the prevalence of "concurrent partnerships" in Africa are primarily responsible. Circumcision is hardly universal in the United States and Europe, and as for "concurrent partnerships," Africa is a large continent with diverse sexual customs (the assumption that Africa is uniform smacks of more than a little racism). JS, among others, agrees that a growing literature is rightly concentrating on AIDS in Africa as a problem of "blood-borne transmission."

12. Ronald Bayer and Gerald M. Oppenheimer, *AIDS Doctors* (Oxford University Press, 2000), 153–55; Deborah B. Gould, *Moving Politics: Emotion and ACT UP's Fight Against AIDS* (University of Chicago Press, 2009), 77. On the bathhouse issue: MC, "The Case for the Temporary Closure of Commercial Sex Establishments During the AIDS Crisis," 14-p. ms., RDP. Mike had a late (1993) rapprochement with GMHC after the much-admired Jeff Richardson became its executive director.

13. JS, Sean Strub, RB, MD, and Walter Armstrong, discussion January 27, 2013; Gallo and Fauci as quoted in Anne-Christine D'Adesky, "The Man Who Invented Safer Sex Returns," *Out*, Summer 1992; Sean Strub, "The Good Doctor," *POZ*, July 1998; MC, *Surviving AIDS*; MC, "A 'Dangerous' Interview With Dr. Joseph Sonnabend," 18-p. transcript, MCP; MC, "Why I Do Not Believe That HIV Is the Cause of AIDS," PWA *Newsline*, December 1984; MC, "AIDS: The Linguistic Bat-

tlefield," in *The State of the Language*, ed. Christopher Ricks and Leonard Michaels (University of California Press, 1990); MC to Neville Hodgkinson, July 17, 1993; MC to Pam Brandt and Lindsy van Gelder, July 5, 1993; MC to Celia Farber, September 1, 1993, all MCP; Sean Strub to me, October 27, 2012 (constellation of factors).

The controversy over the relationship between HIV and AIDS continues to have a long life. The literature is vast; a good sample exchange is Celia Farber, "Out of Control," *Harper's*, March 2006, vs. Robert Gallo et al., "Errors in Celia Farber's March 2006 article in *Harper's* Magazine," March 2006, http://www.tac.org.za/doc uments/ErrorsInFarberArticle.pdf.

14. JS, Strub, RB, MD, and Armstrong discussion, January 27, 2013; some half dozen DVDs from the 1980s that feature JS, RDP; *Sonnabend Interview with Brent Leung*, December 30, 2011, DVD, RDP. For more on Duesberg and his theories and followers, see Seth Kalichman, *Denying AIDS: Conspiracy Theories, Pseudoscience, and Human Tragedy* (Springer, 2009), esp. chap. 2.

15. The handwritten diary Mike kept off and on during the trip is in MCP.

Chapter 4: The Mideighties

1. JB to Barbara Smith, June 16, 1985; JB to Isaac Jackson, July 19, 1985; JB to Audre Lorde, August 14, 1984, all JBSC.

2. JB to Jackson, July 19, 1985; JB to Smith, June 16, 1985; JB to EH, August 11, November 2, 1985; EH to JB, March 9, 1985, all JBSC; Hizkias Assefa and Paul Wahrhaftig, *The MOVE Crisis* (University of Pittsburgh Press, 1990); Robin Wagner-Pacifici, *Discourse and Destruction: The City of Philadelphia Versus MOVE* (University of California Press, 1994); *Philadelphia Inquirer*, December 4, 1987.

3. JB to Steve [Stephan Lee Dais, an undergraduate at Temple University?], June 8, 1985; EH to JB, December 5, 1985; JB to EH, November 2, 1985, April 29, 1986, all JBSC; EH, "The Tomb of Sorrow," in *Ceremonies* (Cleis, 1992), 94–95; interviews with Ron Simmons and Chris Prince, May 2009.

4. Dorothy Beam to JB, [1985?]; JB to EH, December 14, 1985, both JBSC; JB to Ray [Melrose?], June 24, 1982; JB, "Brother to Brother: Words from the Heart," in *In The Life: A Black Gay Anthology*, ed. JB, 234 (Alyson, 1986).

5. EH, "Untied Inspiration," *Network* 1, no. 3 (December 1990); EH to Alexis De Veaux, September 29, 1985, AVSC; JB to EH, August 11, 1985; EH to JB, December 5, 1985, February 18, [1986?]; JB to "Dear Friends," December 17, 1985; JB to Mosmiller, March 19, 1986; JB to his parents, March 1, 1986, all JBSC. For *Blackheart*, see Charles Michael Smith's blog: http://urbanbookmaven.blogspot.com/2013 /01/hed-tk_9.html. The NCBLG Statement of Purpose is printed in *Black/Out* 1, nos. 3–4 (1987).

6. Abby Tallmer to me, March 26, 2013; Guy Weston, "AIDS in the Black Community," *Black/Out*, Fall 1986 (reprinted from *Au Courant*); PBS Timeline: 30 Years of AIDS in Black America, July 10, 2012, pbs.org; EH, "O Tell Me, Brutus," in *Ceremonies*, 168, originally published in EH, *Conditions* (1986); Charles Henry Fuller, "With Our Heads Held High," JBSC; Larry Duplechan, "Voices of Black Pain," *The Advocate*, November 25, 1986. Wendell Ricketts recalls a symposium he organized in

mid-1993 when Essex appeared on a panel, "AIDS: Images and Analysis in the Arts and Media," along with Bill T. Jones, John Greyson, and Robert Atkins, during which he spoke eloquently about his own condition (WRicketts@aol.com, November 7, 1995), in the Gay, Lesbian, and Bisexual People of Color list GLBPOC "Tribute." Craig G. Harris, who died of AIDS in 1991, wrote movingly of the difficulties black gay men had in gaining access to treatment in "I'm Going Out Like a Fucking Meteor," in *Freedom in This Village: Twenty-Five Years of Black Gay Men's Writing*, ed. E. Lynn Harris, 137–50 (Carroll and Graf, 2005).

7. JB to his parents, March 1, 1986; JB to Isaac Julien, December 29, 1986; JB to Kriss Worthington, December 30, 1986; Barbara Smith to JB, August 14, 1986; JB to Michael Denneny, October 2, 1987, all JBSC; *Thing*, May–June 1991. A flyer for Be Bop Books is in JBSC; Giovanni's Room distributed the books.

8. Wyatt O'Brian Evans, "Essex Hemphill: The Force Remains with Us," wyat tobrianevans.com/online/node49; Brinkley to Harris, March 5, 1986; Colin Robinson to the editor, *New York Native*, March 24, 1986, both JBSC; Kara Swisher, "The Storm over a Stanza," *Washington Post*, September 28, 1987; the Manchester episode and other tributes to EH's growing influence can be found online at GLBPOC "Tribute"; EH to JB, February 18, [1988?]; EH to Assotto Saint, March 2, 1987, ASSC; *Outweek*, August 8, 1990. I haven't come across any evidence that Essex actually marched in the 1987 gay rights demonstration in Washington, but he did participate, along with Michelle, Wayson, and Joe Beam, in "Culturally Yours," an evening of readings and performances held at George Washington University in conjunction with the march; program courtesy MP.

9. "Waking Up to AIDS," *Rainbow History Project*, www.rainbowhistory.org/html/AidsChronology.html; Cathy J. Cohen, *The Boundaries of Blackness: AIDS and the Breakdown of Black Politics* (University of Chicago Press, 1999), 95–99.

10. Aside from MC's own *Surviving AIDS* (HarperCollins, 1990), the best account of PWAC by far—and one on which I've heavily relied—is Susan M. Chambré, *Fighting for Our Lives: New York's AIDS Community and the Politics of Disease* (Rutgers University Press, 2006), esp. chap. 2.

11. Duberman diary, November 10, 1985, in Martin Duberman, *Waiting to Land: A (Mostly) Political Memoir, 1985–2008* (The New Press, 2009), 10; Dudley Clendinen and Adam Nagourney, *Out for Good: The Struggle to Build a Gay Rights Movement in America* (Simon and Schuster, 1999), 514–21. JS himself felt "mortified to see dying people called depraved and dissolute" (JS to Sharon Feinstein, February 3, 1986, JSNYPL). Except for the few excerpts I've published in several of my books, my diary remains in my possession; it will ultimately become part of my papers at the New York Public Library.

12. Clendinen and Nagourney, *Out for Good*, 531–39; MC, "How Should We Presume," 11-p. ms., October 15, 1987, MCP.

13. Duberman diary, May 15, June 6, July 18, August 27, 1985, in Duberman, *Waiting*, 5–9; "Remarks of Michael Callen, American Public Health Association, Annual Meeting, Las Vegas, Nevada, 1986," typescript in MCP; the speech is partly reprinted in Douglas Crimp, ed., *AIDS: Cultural Analysis, Cultural Activism* (MIT Press, 1987).

14. For the original AZT trial, see "AZT: The Clinical Trial That Led to Its Approval," *AIDS Perspective*, January 28, 2011, http://aidsperspective.net/blog/?p=749& preview=true; JS, Sean Strub, MD, RB, and Walter Armstrong, discussion, January

27, 2013; JS, interviews with Sean Strub, [2009?], SSJS; JS to Louis Aledort, April 11, 1983, JSNYPL; Rex Wockner, "Luck, Coke, and the Love of a Good Man," *New York Native*, July 11, 1988; MC, *Surviving AIDS*, 8, 13–14, 51, 193,198, 203–26; Chambré, *Fighting for Our Lives*, 38–39; MC, "Not Everyone Dies of AIDS," *Village Voice*, May 3, 1988 (MC complained that the *Voice* had gutted his article, removing most of his explanation for remaining a "multifactorialist"); MC, "Farewell to Smarm," 17-p. typescript of a speech delivered April 25, 1991, MCP (there is a second MC piece, 13-p. typescript, entitled "A Farewell to Smarm," in MCP, which is *not* a duplicate of the 1991 one); Sean Straub, *Body Counts*, Scribners: 2014.

The "unanswered" questions about HIV are derived from Elinor Burkett, *The Gravest Show on Earth: America in the Age of AIDS* (Houghton Mifflin, 1995), 58–59, 84–85 (AZT). I'm puzzled why Burkett's book—in my view, among the most cogent overviews—is rarely cited in the literature on AIDS. See her astute comments, for example, on Root-Bernstein's *Rethinking AIDS* (pp. 65–68, 74–75) and Dr. Shyh-Ching Lo (pp. 68–72). Root-Bernstein argues that HIV is not present in all AIDS cases, that HIV and antibodies to it can disappear, and that when HIV is injected into monkeys it doesn't produce AIDS (though apparently it does produce what some have called "simian AIDS," which is similar to but not the same as human AIDS). The Nobel Prize winner Walter Gilbert pointed out that at one point cancer was said to be caused by a virus. Even Luc Montanier, the discoverer of HIV, has said that "HIV is not the whole story" (*Day One: Does HIV Cause AIDS*, DVD, and *Q & R 2 Mike TV*, DVD, RDP). JS wrote agilbert@aaas.org, December 19, 1994, JSNYPL, "I continue to believe that the issue of AIDS causation still remains open." MC interviewed twenty-one long-term survivors and felt they shared distinctive personality traits: "very aggressive, able to ask for help, able to say no, able to be clear about what they need; they love themselves and they love life and are able to demand what they need to survive, are incredibly knowledgeable [about AIDS], have a good relationship with their health provider, and believe in the possibility of survival" (DVD, *MC Interview with Tom Brokaw on Widetime*, DVD, 1993, RDP). MC had "studiously avoided feder-ally designed treatment protocols, and insisted that AIDS need not be an automatic death sentence" and was not 100 percent fatal. (MC on *Charlie Rose CBS Nightwatch, March 27, 1989*, DVD, RDP). JS's initial statements on HIV were made on the TV show *Sandi Freeman Reports*, DVD, 1984, and during an interview with John Hochen-berry on *Day One: Does HIV Cause AIDS?* DVD, both RDP.

15. Burkett, *Gravest*, 92; MC, "The Emperor Has No Clothes," 4-p. typescript, MCP; "Statement of Michael Callen, Bethesda, Maryland, June 4, 1992," 6-p. tran-script, MCP; MC to David Groff, June 21, 1993, MCP; JS interviews with Strub; MC, interview with Celia Farber, *Spin*, 1994; Steven Epstein, *Impure Science: AIDS, Activism, and the Politics of Knowledge* (University of California Press, 1996), 194–96, 242–46, 300–309; MC, *Surviving AIDS*, 203–26; MC to Kevin Armington (manag-ing editor, *Treatment Issues*), February 25, 1989 (AZT), MCP.

In the nineties, JS and Elena Klein found that AZT removes interferon from the bloodstream. That gave JS, for the first time, a *rational* use for AZT, since he be-lieved that circulating interferon was "bad for you." As a result, Sonnabend did begin to prescribe a low daily dose of AZT, but for no longer than seven to eight weeks. This didn't contradict his long-standing view that the *chronic* use of AZT was coun-terproductive (MC, "A 'Dangerous' Interview with Dr. Joseph Sonnabend," 18-p. transcript, MCP).

16. Paul A. Sergios, *One Boy at War: My Life in the AIDS Underground* (Knopf, 1993), chap.6.

17. Callen, *Surviving AIDS*, 129.

18. Sergios, *One Boy*, passim; Callen, "Making Sense of Survival," in *Surviving AIDS*, 183–89; Epstein, *Impure Science*, chap. 8; MC, "Remarks of Michael Callen, PWA Health Group," 3-p. ms., April 24, 1987, MCP.

19. Callen, *Surviving AIDS*, 68–69, 186–88; MC, "Are You Now or Have You Ever Been," *PWA Newsline*, January 1989; Jeff Escoffier interview with MC, n.d., MCP.

20. "Remarks of Michael Callen . . . 1986," MCP; Epstein, *Impure Science*, 306; MC, "I Will Survive," *Village Voice*, May 3, 1988.

21. Epstein, *Impure Science*, 258–62; MC to Axelrod, November 10, 1987, MCP; *Buffalo News*, December 24, 1987; the material on GMAD derives from the Schomburg Center's program for its twenty-fifth anniversary exhibit.

22. Cohen, *Boundaries*, 95–102; MC to David Rogers, October 2, 1988, MCP; Wayson Jones commentary on this manuscript, April 15, 2013.

23. Interview with Chris Prince, May 2009; EH, *Domestic Life*, a limited edition for friends of his poetry and prose, courtesy Wayson Jones; *High Performance*, no. 36, August 1986; Michelle Parkerson to me, April 8, 2013.

24. EH, "Letter to the Post: From Essex Hemphill," n.d.; Tod Roulette/EH conversation, printed in *Thing*, n.d., both SC.

25. Lorde to JB [January 1987]; Isaac Julien to JB, March 22, 1987; JB to Julien, March 31, 1987, all JBSC.

26. *Philadelphia Inquirer*, December 31, 1988. A scholarship was set up in Joe Beam's name at Temple University with an endowment, raised from family and friends, of $6,000. A $300 annual award was to be given "to an African-American student on the basis of academic promise, financial need and an essay or literary piece on a topic related to sexual minorities" (*Philadelphia Inquirer*, January 21, 1992).

27. EH, "xix," in *Domestic Life*, private edition, 1994, courtesy Wayson Jones.

Chapter 5: The Toll Mounts

1. JS, Ron Najman, MC, and Mathilde Krim, "Community Treatment Initiative (CTI): A Proposal for the Prevention of AIDS," November 12, 1986, MCP; "Remarks of Michael Callen," PAAC Teleconference, New Orleans, LA, May 17–18, 1989, MCP; Steven Epstein, *Impure Science: AIDS, Activism, and the Politics of Knowledge* (University of California Press, 1996), 216–19; MC, "AIDS Research: Missed Opportunities and Misplaced Priorities," 5-p. transcript, MCP; JS, "Preventing PCP," *AIDS Perspective*, n.d., http://aidsperspective.net/aidsperspective2010_006.htm. "Without Mathilde [Krim]," JS has said, "none of it [amfAR] would have happened." He was a member of CRI's board of directors and Institutional Review Board, and chair of its Scientific Advisory Committee. Due to financial difficulties, CRI dissolved in 1990, but it reconstituted the following year as the Community Research Initiative on AIDS (CRIA). Sonnabend quit amfAR when he felt "that scientific issues were being decided without my knowledge. The most glaring example is the effort in 1985 to put out the message that there would be a heterosexual epidemic for which there was absolutely no evidence at that time" (Sean Strub, "The Good Doctor,"

POZ, July 1998, JSNYPL). The online version of Vanessa Merton's article, "Community-Based AIDS Research," can be found at http://erx.sagepub.com/content /14/5/502.

2. Randy Shilts, *And the Band Played On* (St. Martin's, 1987), 585–89; MC, "AIDS and Passive Genocide," MC testimony given at FDA hearing on aerosol pentamidine, May 1, 1989, printed in *AIDS Forum* 2, no. 1 (May 1989), 13–16. The FDA finally approved aerosol pentamidine in 1989.

3. MC, "AIDS Research: Missed Opportunities," *Los Angeles Times*, December 25, 1988, May 6, 1989; MC, "Turning AIDS into a Chronic Manageable Disease: The Role of Prophylaxis," 6-p. typescript, [1987?], MCP.

4. "Testimony of Michael Callen . . . before Subcommittee on Health and the Environment," September 22, 1987, 4-p. typescript, MCP; MC to Marvin [?], April 15, 1988, MCP.

5. "Remarks of Michael Callen . . . at CRI Press Conference," December 16, 1987, 4-p. typescript, MCP; JS, Najman, MC, and Krim, "A Proposal for the Prevention of AIDS," November 12, 1986, MCP, *New York Times*, March 18, 1988; "Testimony of Michael L. Callen, before the Presidential Commission on the Human Immunodeficiency Virus Epidemic," February 19, 1988, MCP; MC to Governor Mario Cuomo, January 4, 1988, MCP.

6. Dudley Clendinen and Adam Nagourney, *Out for Good: The Struggle to Build a Gay Rights Movement in America* (Simon and Schuster, 1999), 548–49; Epstein, *Impure Science*, 218 ff; Susan M. Chambré, *Fighting for Our Lives: New York's AIDS Community and the Politics of Disease* (Rutgers University Press, 2006), 120–21; John-Manuel Andriote, *Victory Deferred*, rev. ed. (2011), chap. 17; Deborah B. Gould, *Moving Politics: Emotion and Act UP's Fight Against AIDS* (University of Chicago Press, 2009), chap. 2; Steven Chapple and David Talbot, "Burning Desires," reprinted in *While the World Sleeps*, ed. Chris Bull (Thunder's Mouth Press, 2003); "Remarks of Michael Callen," PAAC Teleconference, New Orleans, May 17–18, 1989, MCP.

7. Cathy J. Cohen, *The Boundaries of Blackness: AIDS and the Breakdown of Black Politics* (University of Chicago Press, 1999), 144–48, 162–67; *New York Times*, February 26, 2013 (Koop obituary).

8. Gould, *Moving Politics*, 49–53; EH, "The Occupied Territories," in *Ceremonies* (Cleis 1992), 80–81.

9. MD diary, August 7, 8, October 13, 1987, in my possession but ultimately to be part of my papers at the New York Public Library; Pamela Robin Brandt, liner notes for *Legacy* by MC, recorded 1996; Amin Ghaziani, *The Dividends of Dissent: How Conflict and Culture Work in Lesbian and Gay Marches on Washington* (University of Chicago Press, 2008); MC, "How Should We Presume," 11-p. ms., October 15, 1987, MCP.

10. According to RB (interview of June 9, 2009), JS disapproved of MC taking time out from his AIDS work to devote to making music; MC interview with Dr. David Schmidt, November 12, 1987, 9-p. typescript, MCP (background to "Nobody's Fool" and "Love Don't Need a Reason"). Most of this section on *Purple Heart*, unless otherwise noted—as well as other aspects of Mike and RB's musical history—is primarily based on my multiple interviews with Richard Dworkin. I'm especially grateful to Richard for his help with describing the special qualities of MC's voice. See also Will Grega, "Michael Callen Up Close," in *The Gay Music Guide* (Pop Front Press, 1994), 14–19. Grega's book is dedicated to MC: "Thank you, Michael, for your

generosity of spirit and support for this project. You will always be the spirit of gay music, and the very best of us."

MC had intended to submit "Love Don't Need a Reason" as the love theme for Barbra Streisand's pending film production of Larry Kramer's *The Normal Heart*, but the project never happened. Another song on *Purple Heart*, "Nobody's Fool," derived from the two-year period when MC and his father didn't speak; when MC would call home, his mother would try to persuade him to

> Talk to your Daddy
> He misses you. He does—
> In his own way.
> I know it was rough
> For you and your brother
> But do it for me

11. *Los Angeles Dispatch*, August 3, 1988; *Gay Community News*, August 21–September 3, 1988; *Gaybeat*, June 1988; *New York Native*, July 11, 1988; Grega, *Gay Music Guide*; *San Francisco Sentinel*, July 22, 1988; MC, "Living with AIDS," speech at the American Academy of Dermatologists, December 3, 1989, 7-p. typescript, MCP; MC, "In Defense of Anal Sex," 11-p. typescript, *PWA Newsline*, February 1989; Jim Graham to MC, as printed in the April 1989 *PWA Newsline*; MC to Bruce [?], January 15, 1989, MCP; MC to Kevin Armington, February 25, 1989, MCP.

12. MC, ed., *Surviving and Thriving with AIDS: Collected Wisdom* (People with AIDS Coalition, 1988) in an edition of 12,000. Jim Eigo, "The City as Body Politic/The Body as City unto Itself," in *From ACT UP to the WTO*, ed. Benjamin Shepard and Ronald Hayduk (Verso, 2002). About half the articles in *Surviving* were reprinted from the *PWA Coalition Newsline*, and a few from other publications. Mike was committed to the principle of respecting diversity of opinion, and as a result the book contains a section on "Holistic Approaches," for which in general he held scant regard, and even several arguments in favor of taking AZT. The book was gratefully received; in a typical response, James T. Beal thanked Mike "for taking the time and energy to make such a heroic contribution to our shared condition" (Beal to MC, July 10, 1987, MCP). For the condom study, see Jennifer Brier, *Infectious, Ideas: U.S. Political Responses to the AIDS Crisis* (University of North Carolina Press, 2009), 46.

13. MC, "AIDS 201," in *Surviving and Thriving*; multiple interviews with Richard Dworkin; MC to Holly Near, August 24, 1993 (Gay Men's Chorus), MCP; EH, "The Imperfect Moment," *High Performance*, Summer 1990; Albert Williams, "Essex Hemphill and 'Cultural Transformation,'" *Windy City Times*, March 21, 1991. For a capella, see *New York Times*, June 22, 1997; *Washington Post*, March 12, 1997; *Billboard*, August 23, 1997. At the memorial service for Joe Beam more than a thousand people showed up (*Washington Post*, August 17, 1991).

14. See Black LGBT Archivist Society of Philadelphia (archivistssociety.wordpress .com) for EH and Dorothy Beam's comments on JB; EH to JB, February 18, [1988?]; *Washington Blade*, July 11, 1991 (Dorothy Beam); EH to Barbara Smith, August 1, 1989, BSP; James Baldwin, "If Black English Isn't a Language, Then Tell Me, What Is?" *New York Times*, July 29, 1979; EH, ed., *Brother to Brother: New Writings by Black Gay Men*, conceived by JB, project managed by Dorothy Beam (Alyson, 1991). *Outweek*, August 8, 1990; *Network* 1, no. 3 (December 1990); "Black Talk: A Personal

Interview with Essex Hemphill of *Tongues Untied,*" *Au Courant,* July 29, 1991; Patricia Morrisroe's fine biography, *Mapplethorpe* (Da Capo, 1997), doesn't discuss black anger at his "objectification" but does provide considerable evidence of it. Essex's introduction to *Brother to Brother* is xv–xxxi; the Isaac Julien and Kobena Mercer essay, "True Confessions," 167–73. It's worth pointing out that in his introduction Essex made a point of acknowledging Adrian Stanford's pioneering precursor, *Black and Queer* (Good Gay Poets of Boston, 1977); he also published four of Stanford's poems in *Brother to Brother*; Stanford had been murdered in Philadelphia in 1983. David Frechette, "Renaissance for Black Gay Writers," *City Sun,* April 19–25, 1989; *New Republic,* October 12, 1992. Essex's later collection *Ceremonies* (Cleis, 1992) contains both "Civil Servant" and "To Some Supposed Brothers"; as well, under the essay title "Does Your Mama Know About Me?" Essex reprinted and added to his critique of the white gay world.

The establishment by the OutWrite Conference of an award in JB's name caused considerable controversy. In 1992 Dorothy Beam, at Essex's urging, rescinded her permission to use her son's name. In an extended explanation for the action (the 5-p. transcript is in ASSC, and a 1-p. summary, dated March 1992, in EH/WJSC), Essex cited the fact that "no input was sought from the Black gay and lesbian community" and that the titles nominated failed to include any of the books published in 1991 by black gays and lesbians, but did include two Alyson publications (Sasha Alyson had sponsored the award).

15. To work with Isaac Julien, Essex spent two weeks in London in August 1989; Julien was "a marvelous host" and Essex had "an excellent trip" (EH to Barbara Smith, August 18, 1989, BSP); Frank Broderick interview with EH, n.d., JBSC; Karl Bruce Knapper, "Raw, Fresh, Soothing, Unnerving," *Bay Area Reporter,* May 30, 1991; *Publishers Weekly,* May 10, 1991; Jim Cory review in *Windy City Times,* March 21, 1991; Jim Marks review in *Lambda Book Report,* May–June 1991; interview with Ron Simmons, May 2009; Isaac Julien to JB, May 27, 1987, JBSC; and in *Brother to Brother*: Walter Rico Burrell, "The Scarlett Letter, Revisited," diary entry for February 9, 1989; Assotto Saint, "Hooked for Life"; Craig G. Harris, "The Worst of It"; EH, "Looking for Langston: An Interview with Isaac Julien"; Ron Simmons, "Tongues Untied: An Interview with Marlon Riggs" and "Some Thoughts on the Challenges Facing Black Gay Intellectuals"; and Marlon Riggs, "Black Macho Revisited: Reflections of a Snap! Queen." The typescript of the Riggs essay is in JBSC. EH's essay on Welsing is entitled "If Freud Had Been a Neurotic Colored Woman: Reading Dr. Frances Cress Welsing." It originally appeared in the radical gay Boston publication *Gay Community News* (February 25–March 3, 1991) and was then reprinted in EH, *Ceremonies: Prose and Poetry* (Plume, 1992). For a critique of EH's Welsing essay, see Dwight A. McBride, "Can the Queen Speak?" in *Black Men on Race, Gender, and Sexuality,* ed. Devon W. Carbado (New York University Press, 1999).

16. Phillip Brian Harper, "Eloquence and Epitaph," originally published in Harper, *Writing AIDS* (Columbia University Press, 1993); Elinor Burkett, *The Gravest Show on Earth: America in the Age of AIDS* (Houghton Mifflin, 1995), 186; Harlon L. Dalton, "AIDS in Blackface," originally published in *Daedalus,* summer 1989. Both essays are reprinted in Bull, *While the World Sleeps.*

17. EH to Barbara Smith, December 20, 1990; EH and Dorothy Beam to Barbara Smith, March 14, 1991, both BSP; Don Belton, "Gay Voices, Gay Lives," *Philadelphia Inquirer,* August 25, 1991; see also Phil Harper's review in *Gay Community News,* June

9–15, 1991, in which he finds "the structure of *Brother to Brother* . . . tighter and more cohesive than that of *In The Life*."

Chapter 6: Drugs into Bodies

1. Susan M. Chambré, *Fighting for Our Lives: New York's AIDS Community and the Politics of Disease* (Rutgers University Press, 2006), chap. 5. For a fuller analysis of how the *New York Times* treated AIDS up through 1989, see Douglas Crimp, *Melancholia and Moralism* (MIT Press, 2002), p. 137, fn. 15.

2. Douglas Crimp with Adam Rolston, "Stop the Church," originally in *AIDS Demo Graphics* (1990), reprinted in *While the World Sleeps*, ed. Chris Bull (Thunder's Mouth Press, 2003).

3. Duberman diary, June 1, 1989, in my possession (though I've published this entry in Duberman, *Waiting to Land* (The New Press, 2009), 64–65.

4. Deborah B. Gould, *Moving Politics: Emotion and ACT UP's Fight Against AIDS* (University of Chicago Press, 2009) esp. chap. 4; Jim Eigo, "The City as Body Politic/ The Body as City unto Itself," in *From ACT UP to the WTO*, ed. Benjamin Shepard and Ronald Hayduk (Verso, 2002).

5. Crimp with Rolston, "Stop the Church" and "Seize Control of the FDA," originally in *AIDS Demo Graphics* (1990), republished in Bull, *While the World Sleeps*.

6. Darrell Yates Rist, "The Deadly Costs of an Obsession," *The Nation*, February 13, 1989; follow-up responses, including my own, are in the issues of March 20 and May 1, 1989. For another instance of exasperation over the Rist piece, see Crimp, *Melancholia*, 144–45.

7. John-Manuel Andriote, *Victory Deferred*, rev. ed. (2011), 222–23; Chambré, *Fighting for Our Lives*, 127–29; Gould, *Moving Politics*, 285–86; Crimp with Rolston, "Stop the Church," 171–77.

8. Gould, *Moving Politics*, passim; Maxine Wolfe, "AIDS and Politics: Transformation of Our Movement," originally an October 6, 1989, speech—an edited version is in Bull, *While the World Sleeps*.

9. Jennifer Brier, *Infectious Ideas: U.S. Political Responses to the AIDS Crisis* (University of North Carolina Press, 2009), esp. chap. 5; Elinor Burkett, *The Gravest Show on Earth: America in the Age of AIDS* (Houghton Mifflin, 1995), chap. 6; Wayne Turner e-mail to me, January 28, 2013 (EH had no involvement with ACT UP/DC).

10. EH, "Family Jewels," in *Ceremonies* (Cleis, 1992), 119; Robinson as quoted in Andriote, *Victory Deferred*, 195; Brier, *Infectious Ideas*, 163–71, 184 (Agosto).

11. Celia Farber, interview with MC, *Spin* 10, no. 1 (1994); Gould, *Moving Politics*, 282 (Shilts), 334, 340, 346, 348, 363 (Saunders), 374–83; Harlon L. Dalton, "AIDS in Blackface," *Daedalus*, Summer 1989. JS criticized TAG, as well as Project Inform, on the grounds that it was "collaborationist"—that is, sat "on all these committees with industry and government representatives" (Sean Strub, "The Good Doctor," *POZ*, July 1998). The paragraphs from "As yet . . . to climb" are essentially taken from my *Waiting to Land* (The New Press, 2009).

12. Louis Grant, "Open Letter" of January 4; MC to CRI Board, January 11; Grant to MC, August 10, 17, September 11, 12, 29, November 1, December 26, all 1989, all MCP; Grant to Board, January 4, 1990, MCP; MC, "The Finale," *Genre*,

December 1993; Gregg Gonsalves to MC, July 27, 1993; MC to Gonsalves, August 19, 1993, both MCP. Burkett, *Gravest*, chap. 7 (women); MC's *Speech as Grand Marshal of the Gay Pride Rally, 6/29/91* ("brutal"), DVD, courtesy Dworkin; JS to Paula Treichler, December 27, 1989 ("romantic"), JSNYPL.

13. MC, 3-p. memo to Board of Directors and Staff, May 10, 1989, MCP; MC to Judy and Sam Peabody, February 27, 1989, MCP.

14. MC to Mathilde Krim, April 30, 1989, MCP; *PWA Newsline*, January 1989; MC to Bill Case, July 30, 1989, MCP; MC to Editor, *Time*, June 24, 1989, MCP. Mathilde Krim basically supported amfAR financially for at least the first year and a half of its existence. At some point JS, having been made to feel unwelcome as a result of his opposition to the notion that AIDS would soon spread to heterosexuals, resigned in frustration (JS interviews with Sean Strub, SSJS).

15. Multiple interviews with Richard Dworkin; *Bay Area Reporter*, April 13, 1989; *Bay Times*, May 1989; *The Advocate*, November 21, 1988; Effie Pow, "The Flirtations Tantalize," *The Ubyssey*, February 14, 1991; "Untied Inspirations," *Network* 1, no. 3 (December 1990); *Outweek*, March 6, 1991; Cliff Townsend to me, April 13, 2013.

16. Ron Simmons, "An Interview with Marlon Riggs," 11-p. typescript, [1990?], SC; Thomas Avena, ed., *Life Sentences* (Mercury House, 1994) 265.

17. EH to Gittens and Zalbowitz, May 7, 1990, SC; phone interview with Jim W. Marks, March 5, 2013; *New York Times*, June 25, 1991; *Gay Community News*, February 25–March 3, 1990; *Seattle Post-Intelligencer*, July 16, 1991; Isaac Jackson, "An Open Letter to the Black Gay Community on Loving Black Men and 'Sleeping With the Enemy,'" 5-p. ms., SC; for a more recent critical view of *Tongues Untied*, see John Champagne, *The Ethics of Marginality* (University of Minnesota Press, 1995), chap. 3—but see, too, the persuasive reply, particularly regarding EH, by E. Patrick Johnson, "'Quare' Studies, or (Almost) Everything I Know about Queer Studies I Learned from My Grandmother," in *Black Queer Studies*, ed. E. Patrick Johnson and Mae G. Henderson (Duke University Press, 2005); Chuck Kleinhaus and Julia Lesage, "Listening to the Heartbeat: Interview with Marlon Riggs," UC Berkeley Library, http://www.lib.berkeley.edu/MRC/RiggsInterview.html; Avena, *Life Sentences*, 258–73; Kobena Mercer, "Dark and Lovely Too: Black Gay Men in Independent Film," in *Queer Looks: Perspectives on Lesbian and Gay Film and Video*, ed. Martha Gever, John Greyson, and Pratibha Parmar (Between the Lines, 1993), 238–56.

18. Kleinhaus and Lesage, "Listening to the Heartbeat"; Avena, *Life Sentences*, 267; *Gay Community News*, February 25–March 3, 1990; EH, "Choice," 6-p. typescript, BSP; EH, "Standing in the Gap," FGAF.

19. "Where We Live: A Conversation with Essex Hemphill and Isaac Julien," in *speak my name: Black Men on Masculinity and the American Dream*, ed. Don Belton (Beacon, 1995); Darren Lenard Hutchinson, "'Claiming' and 'Speaking' Who We Are," and Earl Ofari Hutchinson, "My Gay Problem, Your Black Problem," both in *Black Men on Race, Gender, and Sexuality*, ed. Devon W. Carbado (New York University Press, 1999); Keith Boykin, *Beyond the Down Low* (Carroll and Graf, 2005), 216–17, 255–56; Robert F. Reid-Pharr, *Black Gay Man* (New York University Press, 2001), chap. 8.

20. EH's 1990 speech at OutWrite was printed as "Does Your Mama Know About Me? Does She Know Just Who I Am?" in *Gay Community News*, March 25–31, 1990; Chuck Smith, "An Interview with Essex Hemphill," *Vanguard*, August 23, 1991.

21. EH, "Why I Fear Other Black Males," *San Francisco Chronicle*, September 7, 1990; Cathy J. Cohen, *The Boundaries of Blackness: AIDS and the Breakdown of Black*

Politics (University of Chicago Press, 1999), 101–11; EH, "Deliberations," 7-p. transcript, EH/WJSC.

22. Ted Roulette interview with EH, *Thing*, n.d., SC; *Los Angeles Times*, January 14, 1989; *Outweek*, March 6, 1991; *Network* 1, no. 3 (December 1990), SC.

Chapter 7: Stalemate

1. Jennifer Brier, *Infectious Ideas: U.S. Political Responses to the AIDS Crisis* (University of North Carolina Press, 2009), chap. 5; Deborah B. Gould, *Moving Politics: Emotion and ACT UP's Fight Against AIDS* (University of Chicago Press, 2009), chap. 7; Steven Epstein, *Impure Science: AIDS, Activism, and the Politics of Knowledge* (University of California Press, 1996), chap. 8.

2. MC, "Wading into the Deep and Messy Water of Sex in the Age of AIDS," 31-p. typescript, [1990? 1991?], MCP; multiple interviews with Richard Dworkin; *O Boys with Mike on Franklin*, DVD, October 16, 1993; and *MC on the Charlie Rose show Nightwatch*, DVD, March 27, 1989, both RDP. Gayle Rubin's essay is in Carole S. Vance, ed., *Pleasure and Danger: Exploring Female Sexuality* (Routledge and Kegan Paul, 1984). MC also cited the seminal *Powers of Desire: The Politics of Sexuality*, ed. Ann Snitow, Christine Stansell, and Sharon Thompson (New Feminist Library, 1983).

3. The situation would later change somewhat. After the introduction of protease inhibitors in 1995, which for many made AIDS a "manageable disease," there was a notable increase in "bare-backing" (having unprotected anal sex) and a substantial debate about the reasons behind it. For more details, see Gabriel Rotello, *Sexual Ecology: AIDS and the Destiny of Gay Men* (Dutton, 1997); Walt Odets, *In the Shadow of the Epidemic* (Duke University Press, 1995); and my review of the Rotello book in *The Nation*, May 5, 1997, reprinted in Duberman, *Left Out: The Politics of Exclusion* (Basic Books, 1999).

4. Gould, *Moving Politics*, chap. 6; Duberman diary (in my possession). A number of books and anthologies have memorialized artists lost to AIDS; see, for example, Philip Clark and David Groff, *Persistent Voices: Poetry by Writers Lost to AIDS* (Alyson, 2009). Five of Essex's poems are included, along with work by several of his friends—Craig G. Harris, Assotto Saint, and Donald Woods.

5. MC, "Statement of Michael Callen," Bethesda, Maryland, June 4, 1992, 4-p. transcript, MCP; multiple interviews with Richard Dworkin; MC, "A Farewell to Smarm, Swansong," 6-p. transcript, MCP; JS interviews with Sean Strub, SSJS.

6. Martin Duberman, "Masters and Johnson," in Duberman *Left Out: A Political Journey*.

7. EH to Barbara Smith, August 27, 1991, enclosing the exchange of letters (August 20, August 24) in regard to the *Book World* controversy and his letter of August 17, 1991, to Phill Wilson, BSP. In a note to her in 1993, Essex was still employing the brief, vague phrase "my health is good" (EH to Barbara Smith, March 3, 1993, BSP). Since I found no reply from Phill Wilson in EH's papers, I sent him the relevant pages about Essex's charges in order to give him the opportunity to respond. But he's chosen not to.

8. Douglas Crimp, "Accommodating Magic," in *Melancholia and Moralism* (MIT Press, 2002); Randy Boyd, "Just Like Magic," *Frontiers*, December 6, 1991; MC to *Frontiers*, November 26, 1991, MCP.

9. "The Director with Tongue Untied," *Washington Post*, June 5, 1992.

10. EH, *Ceremonies* (Cleis Press, 1992), reissued 2000; "American Wedding" is on pp. 184–85. Thanks to the success of *Ceremonies*, the Apples and Snakes agency sponsored a poetry tour for Essex in England from March 9 to 23, 1992. The flyer announcing the tour also stated that "Essex will be available to work with people around issues of HIV/AIDS awareness." The flyer is in SC.

11. Randy Boyd, "Essex Hemphill's Brutal Honesty," *Washington Blade*, July 31, 1992; EH, interview with Paul Burston "Speaking for Myself," *Capital Gay*, March 20, 1992; Ernest Hardy, "Conversations with the World," *Village View* (L.A.), August 14, 1992; Alden Reimoneng review of *Ceremonies* in *The James White Review*, Fall 1992; conversation with Frances Goldin, February 22, 2013; EH, "Standing in the Gap," passim.

12. Goldin to EH, September 1, 1992; Goldin to Peter Borland (NAL), November 4, 1992, courtesy Goldin. The publicity release for "Bedside Companions," January 25, 1993, is in EH/WJSC. Essex may have misunderstood the Goldin/Borland response to his novel: in a letter to Barbara Smith (August 12, 1992, BSP), he tells her that his editor "phoned back several days after receiving it [the novel] to tell me, with much excitement, that they want it!"—and believed it could be on the stands by fall 1993. To compound the confusion, Essex also wrote Barbara that he was "going to try to negotiate this without an agent" and asked her to read over the pending contract. Yet Borland and Goldin were working hand in hand.

13. EH to Assoto Saint, June 10, 1993, ASSC; Borland to EH, December 15, 1992; EH to Goldin, December 21, 1992, February 16, 1993, July 28, 1993, September 7, 1993; Goldin to EH, January 13, 1993, all courtesy Goldin; Michelle Parkerson to me, April 8, 2013. In EH/WJSC there is also a publicity release for a third book, "The Evidence of Being: Call for Interviews," which Essex intended to co-edit with Ron Simmons. The flyer announces that they "are seeking Black gay men sixty years of age and older to participate in a nation-wide oral history project about Black gay lifestyles in the early twentieth century. . . . This project seeks to uncover a generation of unheard Black gay voices and faces." I've come across no other reference to this project, which leaves me to assume that it never got off the ground.

Chapter 8: Breaking Down

1. Unless otherwise specified, the section that follows largely derives from my multiple interviews with Richard Dworkin and my many conversations with Abby Tallmer. For Tim Miller, see David Roman, *Acts of Intervention: Performance, Gay Culture, and AIDS* (Indiana University Press, 1998), 142–43.

2. The undated letter of apology from Dworkin to Mike is in MCP; MC to Pam Brandt and Lindsy van Gelder, May 28, July 5, 1993, MCP; "Dinosaur's Diary," 8-p. typescript, April 9, 1992, MCP; MC, "An Interview with Harry Hay," February 17, 1992, 7-p. transcript, MCP. For more on the Jacks of Color and other spaces like it, see "Benjamin Shepard Interviews Liddell Jackson" (founder of the Jacks) in *From ACT UP to the WTO*, ed. Benjamin Shepard and Ronald Hayduk (Verso, 2002) 72–77.

3. *New York Native*, July 27, 1992; *Washington Post*, October 4, 1992; MC, "Dinosaur's Diary," February 6, 1992, MCP, is in a few places difficult to decipher. Since

Mike seems to have scribbled the notes in great haste, I've had to make a few changes in tense or spelling for coherence.

4. MC, "Wading the Deep, Messy Waters of Sex: Wear Your Rubbers!" *QW*, June 7, 1992; MC to Tim Miller and Doug Sadownick, January 18, 1992, courtesy Tim Miller.

5. Deborah B. Gould, *Moving Politics: Emotion and ACT UP's Fight Against AIDS* (University of Chicago Press, 2009), chap. 5 (the Sullivan and Shilts quotes are on p. 282); Douglas Crimp, "Right on, Girlfriend!" reprinted in Crimp, *Melancholia and Moralism* (MIT Press, 2004), 130–49; Jeffrey Schmalz, "Whatever Happened to AIDS?" *New York Times Magazine*, November 28, 1993.

6. MC to Karen Ziegler "(and Randa, of course)," June 15, 1992, MCP.

7. *QW*, June 7, August 30, 1992; multiple interviews with Richard Dworkin. Mike even wrote to President Clinton protesting the ban on gay people serving openly in the military; Clinton replied, in what was probably a form letter, "I believe that people should be judged by their conduct, not by their status" (Clinton to MC, February 25, 1993, MCP).

8. Martin Duberman, *Left Out: The Politics of Exclusion* (Basic Book, 1999), 407–12.

9. Cathy J. Cohen, *The Boundaries of Blackness: AIDS and the Breakdown of Black Politics* (University of Chicago Press, 1999), 159–68; Keith Boykin, *Beyond the Down Low* (Carroll and Graf, 2005), 87–88; EH to John Fout, June 22, 1993, JBSC; EH to Goldin, September 7, 1993, March 15, 1994; Goldin to EH, March 29, 1994, courtesy Goldin. The theories about AIDS in Africa include lack of male circumcision, the frequency of "concurrent partners," endemic infections, and blood-borne, non-sexual transmission (e.g., reusing needles, inadequate sterilization of equipment). The circumcision theory has most recently been associated with the much-controverted Craig Timberg and Daniel Halperin book *Tinderbox* (Penguin, 2012). More highly regarded is Jacques Pepin, *The Origins of AIDS* (Cambridge University Press, 2011); also, JS to me, February 3, 2013.

10. Avena to Goldin, December 1, 1995, courtesy Goldin; EH to Alexis De Veaux, September 29, 1985, AVSC; EH, "Vital Signs," in *Life Sentences*, edited and with an introduction by Thomas Avena, 21–57 (Mercury House, 1994).

11. EH to Goldin, July 26, September 9, 1994, courtesy Goldin.

12. EH to Barbara Smith, December 12, 1994, May 16, 1995, BSP. The poem "Thanksgiving 1993," dated November 28, 1993, was enclosed in a letter from EH to Barbara Smith, December 8, 1993, courtesy Smith.

Chapter 9: Wartime

1. MC, "Dinosaur's Diary," *QW*, August 30, 1992.

2. MC, "Reprieve from the AIDS Governor," 9-p. transcript, MCP; MC to Sean Strub, June 22, 1992, courtesy Strub.

3. MC, "Doxil," 4-p. typescript, MCP; MC to Flirts, January 11; MC to Anthony Roberts, February 16; MC to Cris Williamson and Tret Fure, February 19; MC to David Groff, March 19; MC to Wayne [Brasler?], March 19; MC to Nick Mulcahey, March 24; MC to his brother, Barry, March 24; MC to Karen Ziegler, April 20, May 25; MC to Alex Dallas, June 21; MC to Corey Rhodes, September 2,

all 1993, all MCP. Doxil didn't cause MC's KS of the lungs to regress, but it did for a time stop it from advancing. The notion of a memorial orgy is on the DVD *O Boys with Mike on Franklin*, October 16, 1993, courtesy Dworkin. A friend of Mike's, David Roman, the theater historian, describes Mike being "very excited over a breakthrough shark-cartilage treatment" (David Roman, *Acts of Intervention: Performance, Gay Culture, and AIDS* [Indiana University Press, 1998], 217, 221).

4. Unless otherwise noted, my multiple interviews with Richard Dworkin are the source for most of the quotations that follow in this section.

5. MC to Barry and Patty Callen, March 24, 1993; MC to Deborah Tannen, April 1, 1993; MC to Pam Brandt and Lindsy van Gelder, May 28, 1993, all MCP.

6. MC to Alex Dallas, June 21, 1993, MCP; multiple interviews with Richard Dworkin. For more on Sear Sound, see Steve Guttenberg's interview with Walter Sear, "Walter Sear's Analog Rules," March 27, 2005, www.stereophile.com/interviews /305sears/.

7. *Daily News*, April 29, 1993; MC to Karen Ziegler, April 20, 1993; MC to the Flirts, June 23, 1993, both MCP.

8. MC to the Flirts, June 23, July 6, 1993; MC to Tim Rasta, June 23, 1993, both MCP; MC to Pam Brandt and Lindsy van Gelder, July 5, 1993, MCP. Mike's appearance at the April 25, 1993, March on Washington to sing "Love Don't Need A Reason" was described by the journalist Karen Ocamp, who was there: Mike "stood solo, thin as a rail on this massive stage, and sang with such simple joy—he was mesmerizing. . . . I wanted to stand up from my little spot at the corner of the stage and yell, 'Do you guys know what you're witnessing? This is Art defying Death! This is what courage looks like." (Ocamp to me, June 19, 2009.) The Flirtations didn't last very long without Mike; after Cliff Townsend and Aurelio Font both left, Jon Arterton and Jimmy Rutland tried to resurrect the group by adding the lesbian singer Suede; they did put out a record, mostly of songs the Flirtations had earlier recorded, but folded soon after. The moment, culturally and politically, had passed. (Multiple interviews with Richard Dworkin.)

9. MC to Holly Andersen, July 5, 1993; MC to Alix Dobkin, July 5, 1993; MC to Celia Farber, September 1, 1993, all MCP; phone interviews with Tim Miller and Doug Sadownick.

10. Sadownick to Alan [Gassman], Marshall [O'Boy], Shawn Eric [Brooks—Mike's "AIDS Buddy"], Matt [Silverstein], Tim [Miller], and other interested parties, n.d., MCP.

11. MC to Celia Farber, September 1, 1993, MCP; Doug Sadownick, "Gay Psyche Politics," April 24, 2010, and Doug Sadownick, e-mails to me; MC, "The Finale," *Genre*, December 1993.

12. MC to "Doug-alla," September 23, 1993, courtesy Sadownick.

13. Multiple interviews with Richard Dworkin; MC to Holly Near, August 23, 1993, MCP; MC to Dino Sierp, July 5, 1993, MCP; Sadownick, "Agenda," November 10, 1993, courtesy Sadownick.

14. Sadownick, "Gay Psyche Politics," April 24, 2010, 24–25, courtesy Sadownick; MC to David Hofstra and Lynne Tillman, November 12, 1993, MCP.

15. Multiple interviews with Richard Dworkin; Sadownick, "Gay Psyche Politics," April 24, 2010, 29–30, courtesy Sadownick; MC to George Harvey, November 7, 1993; MC to Holly Near, August 24, 1993, both MCP; MC, "The Finale." *Genre*, December 1993.

16. CC to MC, July 3, 1992, MCP; CC and BAC to MC, April 11, 1993, MCP; Sadownick to Barry and Patty, November 24, 1993; Barry to Sadownick, n.d., courtesy Sadownick.

17. Sadownick, "Gay Psyche Politics," April 24, 2010, 31–32, courtesy Sadownick; multiple interviews with Richard Dworkin; MC interview in the *Los Angeles Times*, February 28, 1989 (the light); MC interview with Celia Farber, *Spin* 10, no. 1 (1994). I've deliberately not identified the "acquaintance" by name. A good deal of conflict— accusations and counteraccusations that continue to the present day—developed between her and Doug Sadownick. Though I tend to lean toward Doug's version of Mike's last few days—especially when corroborated by Richard—the "acquaintance" did truly care for Mike and tried to be helpful; I don't wish to cause her needless pain by using her real name. Accordingly, her articles and e-mails to me are not cited, except for one crucial document: "Alice" to me, 9 pp., June 19, 2009, in my possession.

18. Multiple interviews with Richard Dworkin. Barbara Callen later wrote to Doug (March 12, 1994, courtesy Sadownick) that the final exchanges with Mike had been "so very important to all of us, since we were able to clear up some false beliefs that Michael held concerning how we felt about him as our son. *We really did always love him*, and tried to show him our support." And she also wrote to Richard to express her gratitude "for the important part that you played in Michael's life," and to assure him that "you will be welcome and loved" when next they met (n.d., MCP).

Chapter 10: Home

1. Interview with Ron Simmons, May 2, 2009; GLBPOC "Tribute," EH/ WSSC.

2. EH, "Living the Word/Looking for Home," in Martin Duberman, ed., *Queer Representations* (New York University Press, 1997), 305–10; EH, *Ceremonies* (Cleis, 1992), 63–64.

3. Ron Simmons, "Some Thoughts," in *Brother to Brother*, ed. EH, pp. 211–28 (Alyson, 1991); Larry Duckett, "The Unknown Road to Paradise," 3-p. ms., 1999. Larry died the following year in an apartment fire.

4. Interview with Chris Prince, May 2009; EH, *Domestic Life*, 19 pp. of poetry and prose that seem to have been privately published in a limited edition; my copy is courtesy WJ; Craig G. Harris, "I'm Going Out Like a Fucking Meteor," in *Freedom in This Village: Twenty-Five Years of Black Gay Men's Writing*, ed. E. Lynn Harris, 150 (Carroll and Graf, 2005).

5. "Interview: Marlon Riggs," in *Life Sentences*, ed. Thomas Avena, 258–73 (Mercury House, 1994); Steven Fullwood's commentary on the manuscript, April 29, 2013.

6. Don Belton, ed., "Where We Live: A Conversation with Essex Hemphill and Isaac Julien," in *([speak my name]): Black Men on Masculinity and the American Dream*, 209–19 (Beacon, 1995); Robert F. Reid-Pharr, "It's Raining Men: Notes on the Million Man March," in *Traps: African American Men on Gender and Sexuality*, ed. Rudolph P. Byrd and Beverly Guy-Sheftall (Indiana University Press, 2001). The paragraph invoking "racist oppression" is from EH's unpublished novel, "Standing in the Gap," FGAF.

7. EH, *Ceremonies*, 146; Belton, *speak my name*, 217; EH to Wayson Jones, July 23, 1994, EH/WJSC; EH to Barbara Smith, May 16, 1995, courtesy Smith.

8. EH, *Ceremonies*, 77, 79.

9. EH, *Domestic Life*, courtesy Wayson Jones.

10. Interview with Wayson Jones, May 2009; EH, *Domestic Life*, courtesy W.J.

11. Interviews with Wayson Jones and Chris Prince, May 2009; EH, "Vital Signs," in Avena, *Life Sentences*, 36–38.

12. EH, "Vital Signs," in Avena, *Life Sentences*, 50–51; interview with Ron Simmons, May 2009; Regie Cabico, "Poetic Ancestors," *Beltway Poetry Quarterly*, Fall 2012, quoting Chuck Tarver (rattle); Chuck Tarver to GLBPOS, n.d., EH/WJSC.

13. Interviews with Chris Prince and Ron Simmons, May 2009; EH, *Domestic Life*; EH, "The Tomb of Sorrow," *Ceremonies*, 90; Chuck Tarver, "Take Care of Your Blessings," http://www.qrd.org/qrd/www/culture/black/essex/blessings.html; Wayson Jones' commentary on manuscript, April 15, 2013.

14. Interview with Michelle Parkerson, May 1, 2009; program for "Victory Celebration," November 9, 1995, courtesy Barbara Smith.

15. Ron Simmons, "Testimonial for Essex Hemphill Celebration Service," SC. Later, Michelle Parkerson edited a montage of Essex's work in film and video. Lois Holmes, one of Essex's sisters, printed an angry rebuttal to criticisms of the family's behavior: "An Open Letter for Essex, My Brother," *Standards*, January 13, 1996.

16. Soucouyant@aol.com, November 1995, and "James Miles," November 13, 1995, SC; the press release for the Philadelphia celebration, which Sonia Sanchez, Houston Baker, and Dorothy Beam, among others, attended, is from BSP.

Index